ECG in Medical Practice

**Concerned mainly with basic concepts,
abnormalities in cardiac disease and 150 tracings of ECG for practice**

ECG in Medical Practice

Third Edition

ABM Abdullah

MRCP (UK), FRCP (Edin)
Professor of Medicine
Bangabandhu Sheikh Mujib Medical University
Dhaka, Bangladesh

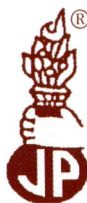

JAYPEE BROTHERS MEDICAL PUBLISHERS (P) LTD

Kolkata • St Louis (USA) • Panama City (Panama) • London (UK) • Ahmedabad • Bengaluru
Chennai • Hyderabad • Kochi • Lucknow • Mumbai • Nagpur • New Delhi

Published by
Jitendar P Vij
Jaypee Brothers Medical Publishers (P) Ltd

Corporate Office
4838/24 Ansari Road, Daryaganj, **New Delhi** - 110002, India, Phone: +91-11-43574357, Fax: +91-11-43574314

Registered Office
B-3 EMCA House, 23/23B Ansari Road, Daryaganj, **New Delhi** - 110 002, India
Phones: +91-11-23272143, +91-11-23272703, +91-11-23282021, +91-11-23245672
Rel: +91-11-32558559, Fax: +91-11-23276490, +91-11-23245683
e-mail: jaypee@jaypeebrothers.com, Website: www.jaypeebrothers.com

Offices in India

• **Ahmedabad**, Phone: Rel: +91-79-32988717, e-mail: ahmedabad@jaypeebrothers.com

• **Bengaluru**, Phone: Rel: +91-80-32714073, e-mail: bangalore@jaypeebrothers.com

• **Chennai**, Phone: Rel: +91-44-32972089, e-mail: chennai@jaypeebrothers.com

• **Hyderabad**, Phone: Rel:+91-40-32940929, e-mail: hyderabad@jaypeebrothers.com

• **Kochi**, Phone: +91-484-2395740, e-mail: kochi@jaypeebrothers.com

• **Kolkata**, Phone: +91-33-22276415, e-mail: kolkata@jaypeebrothers.com

• **Lucknow**, Phone: +91-522-3040554, e-mail: lucknow@jaypeebrothers.com

• **Mumbai**, Phone: Rel: +91-22-32926896, e-mail: mumbai@jaypeebrothers.com

• **Nagpur**, Phone: Rel: +91-712-3245220, e-mail: nagpur@jaypeebrothers.com

Overseas Offices

• **North America Office, USA,** Ph: 001-636-6279734, e-mail: jaypee@jaypeebrothers.com, anjulav@jaypeebrothers.com

• **Central America Office, Panama City, Panama**
Ph: 001-507-317-0160, e-mail: cservice@jphmedical.com, Website: www.jphmedical.com

• **Europe Office, UK,** Ph: +44 (0) 2031708910, e-mail: dholman@jpmedical.biz

ECG in Medical Practice

This book has been published in good faith that the material provided by author is original. Every effort is made to ensure accuracy of material, but the publisher, printer and author will not be held responsible for any inadvertent error (s). In case of any dispute, all legal matters are to be settled under Delhi jurisdiction only.

First Edition: 2004
Second Edition: 2006
Third Edition: **2010**

ISBN 978-81-8448-968-2

Typeset at JPBMP typesetting unit
Printed at Ajanta Offset & Packagings Ltd., New Delhi

*To
my parents
for their never-ending
blessings, love and encouragement*

The value of experience is not in seeing much but in seeing wisely

—William Osler

Preface to the Third Edition

By the good grace of Almighty Allah and blessings of my well-wishers, I have been able to bring out the third edition of this book. Immense popularity and wide acceptability of this book among the students and doctors have encouraged me to prepare this edition.

While I have written this book, my intention was to improve the understanding and interpretation of common ECG in an easy and simple way. Emphasis has been given on the importance of clinical correlation. To what extent this goal has been achieved, only the valued readers and time will tell. However, I can assure that a sincere attempt has been made by me to fulfill this purpose. Many new ECG tracings have been included in this present edition.

In spite of my best efforts, I believe there is still scope of further improvement of this book and make it even better. Any constructive suggestions and criticisms will be highly welcomed and appreciated.

ABM Abdullah

Preface to the First Edition

Despite the advent of many high-tech diagnostic procedures, ECG still remains one of the most basic, useful and easily available tools for the early diagnosis and evaluation of many cardiac problems.

In spite of lot of books on this topic, I have written another new book, which is simple, concise, easy and a practical one that will help any physician, specially the beginners with little knowledge or experience on ECG.

The aim of this book is to guide the students and doctors about the basic concepts in ECG, its interpretation and recognition of cardiac abnormalities. It is also my intention to include common abnormalities in ECG and common cardiac problems that will help the students in any specialty of medicine, specially those who will appear in any examination.

To simplify and also to practice, I have arranged this book in three chapters:

- Chapter I—contains the basic principles of ECG along with normal ECG pattern and the abnormalities.
- Chapters II—contains the ECG abnormalities in different cardiac and extra-cardiac diseases.
- Chapter III—contains 100 ECG tracings of varying difficulty (from simple to more complex) for self practice. Interpretation of these ECG are written in the last few pages (I would advise first to interpret the ECG by yourself, then compare the findings).

Whenever you are going through an ECG, always proceed systematically. Never leave anything to chance and never assume anything. Always describe the basic things and finally look for any abnormality.

Being an internist, I have prepared this book after going through dozens of different ECG books and have tried my best to fill up the gaps, I have noticed in those during my long teaching experience. It is my students and doctor colleagues who have constantly inspired and insisted me to prepare such a book so that they can have a complete and easy grasp over the topic in a short-time. I believe, this book will not only fulfill their demand, but also be of great help for those who are willing to self-learn the basic concepts of ECG.

I was always careful not to overburden the busy clinicians and practitioners with the unnecessary details.

I would like to emphasise that efficiency, skill and fluency in interpreting ECG will only be achieved by going through the ECG tracings repeatedly and reviewing the topics frequently.

I would always appreciate and welcome constructive criticism from the valued readers about this book.

ABM Abdullah

Acknowledgments

My heartiest gratitude and respect to those patients who were kind enough to agree to let me publish their ECG tracings in this book.

I express my sincere gratitude to Prof Pran Gopal Datta, MCPS, ACORL (Odessa), PhD (Kiev), MSc in Audiology (UK), FCPS, FRCS (Glasgow-UK), Vice Chancellor, Bangabandhu Sheikh Mujib Medical University, for his encouragement and valuable suggestions in preparing this book.

I am also highly grateful to Dr Ahmed-Al-Muntasir-Niloy, Medical Officer, BSMMU, Dr Omar Serajul Hasan, MD, internist (USA) and Dr Tanjim Sultana, MD, internist (USA). They have worked almost as co-authors, going through the whole manuscript and making necessary corrections and modifications.

I also acknowledge the contribution of my colleagues, doctors and students who have helped me by providing advice, corrections and encouragement:

- Prof N Islam, IDA, DSc, FRCP, FRCPE, FCGP, FAS, National Professor, Founder and Vice Chancellor, University of Science and Technology, Chittagong.
- Prof Munir Uddin Ahmed, FRCP (London and Glasgow).
- Prof MN Alam, FRCP (Glasgow), FCPS.
- Prof Tofayel Ahmed, FCPS (BD), FCPS (Pak), FCCP, FACP (USA), MRCP, FRCP (Edin, Glasgow, Ireland).
- Prof Md. Fazlul Hoque, FCPS (BD), FRCP (Edin), FRCP (Glasgow), FCPS (Pak), FACP (USA).
- Prof MU Kabir Chowdhury, FRCP (Glasgow).
- Prof Md. Gofranul Hoque, FCPS.
- Prof Taimur AK Mahmud, MCPS, FCPS.
- Prof Md Abdul Wahab, DTCD, MRCP, FRCP.
- Dr Tahmida Hassan, DDV, MD.
- Dr Tazin Afrose Shah, FCPS.
- Dr Shahnoor Sharmin, MCPS, FCPS, MD (Cardiology).
- Dr Md. Razibul Alam, MBBS, MD.
- Dr Samprity Islam, MBBS.
- Dr Monirul Islam Khan, MBBS.
- Dr Sadi Abdullah, MBBS.

I would like to thank Mr Saiful Islam, Kh. Atiqur Rahman (Shamim) and Md. Oliullah for their great help in computer composing and graphic designing of this book.

My special thanks to Shri Jitendar P Vij (Chairman and Managing Director), Mr Tarun Duneja (Director-Publishing), Mr KK Raman (Production Manager), Mr Sunil Dogra, Mrs Yashu Kapoor, Mr Akhilesh Kumar Dubey and Mr Manoj Pahuja of M/s Jaypee Brothers Medical Publishers (P) Ltd., who have worked tirelessly for the timely publication of this book.

Last but not the least, I would like to express my gratitude to my wife and children for their constant support, sacrifice and encouragement. Otherwise, it would have been impossible for me to write this book.

Contents

CHAPTER

I

Basic Concepts of ECG

"Workout the best method for examination and
practice it until it is a second nature to you"

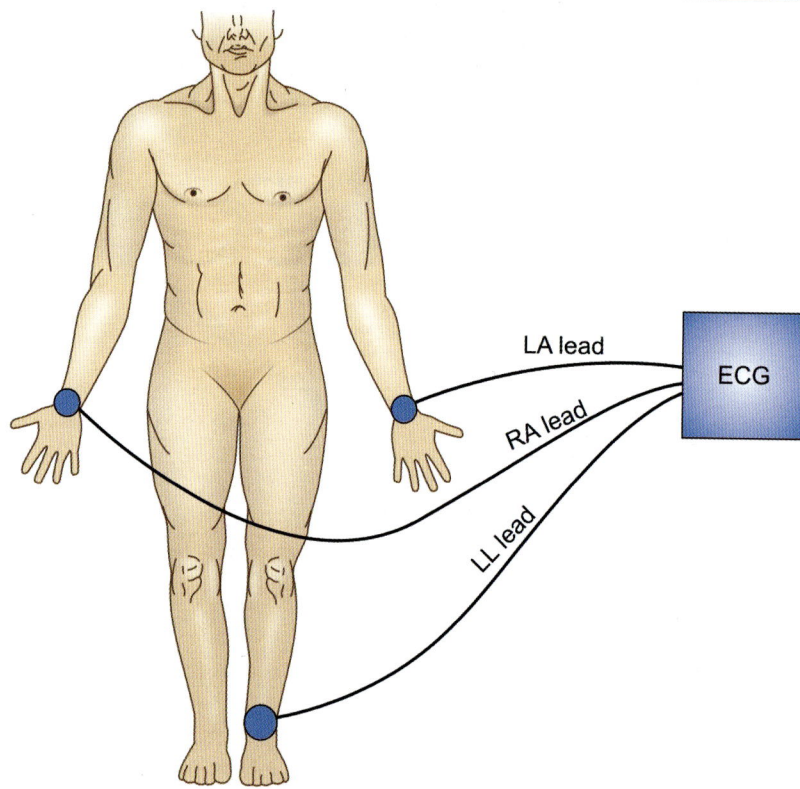

Standard Leads

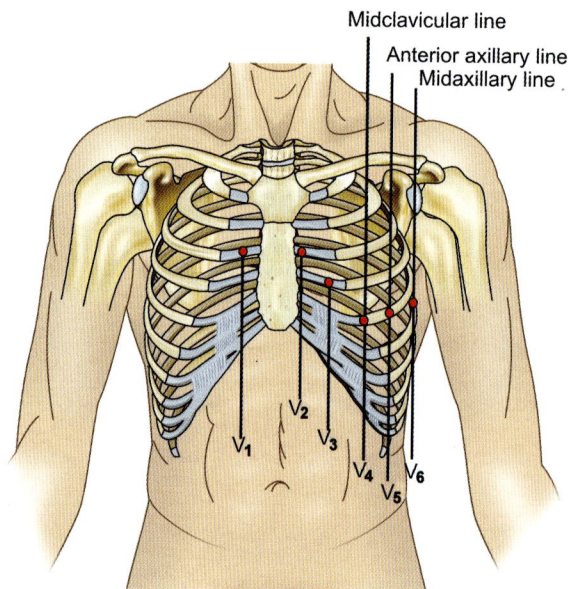

Midclavicular line
Anterior axillary line
Midaxillary line

V₁ V₂ V₃ V₄ V₅ V₆

Chest Leads

SPECIALIZED CONDUCTIVE SYSTEM OF THE HEART

There are 5 specialized tissues called conductive system of the heart. These are:

- SA node.
- AV node.
- Bundle of His.
- Right bundle branch (RBB) and left bundle branch (LBB).
- Purkinje fibers.

These specialized conductive pathways allow the heart to be electrically activated in a predictable manner (see the sequence below).

The impulse arises in SA node (called primary pacemaker), spreads across the atria (by three internodal pathways and Bachmann's bundle), causing depolarization of both atria. From the atria, the impulse reaches the AV node, where there is some delay, which allow atria to contract and pump blood into the ventricles. The impulse then spreads along the bundle of His, then along the left and right bundle branch, finally into the ventricular muscles through Purkinje fibers, causing ventricular depolarization.

First the ventricular septum is activated, followed by the endocardium and finally the epicardium.

Sequence of impulse formation and conduction.

```
                    ┌──────────┐
                    │ SA node  │
                    └──────────┘
                         │────────── By internodal pathway and
                         │            Bachmann's bundle
                         ▼
                    ┌──────────┐
                    │  Atria   │
                    └──────────┘
                         │
                         ▼
                    ┌──────────┐
                    │ AV node  │
                    └──────────┘
                         │
                         ▼
                  ┌──────────────┐
                  │ Bundle of His│
                  └──────────────┘
                     ╱        ╲
                    ▼          ▼
               ┌───────┐   ┌───────┐
               │  RBB  │   │  LBB  │
               └───────┘   └───────┘
                    ╲          ╱
                     ▼        ▼
                 ┌───────────────┐
                 │ Purkinje fibers│
                 └───────────────┘
                         │
                         ▼
                 ┌───────────────┐
                 │   Ventricles  │
                 └───────────────┘
```

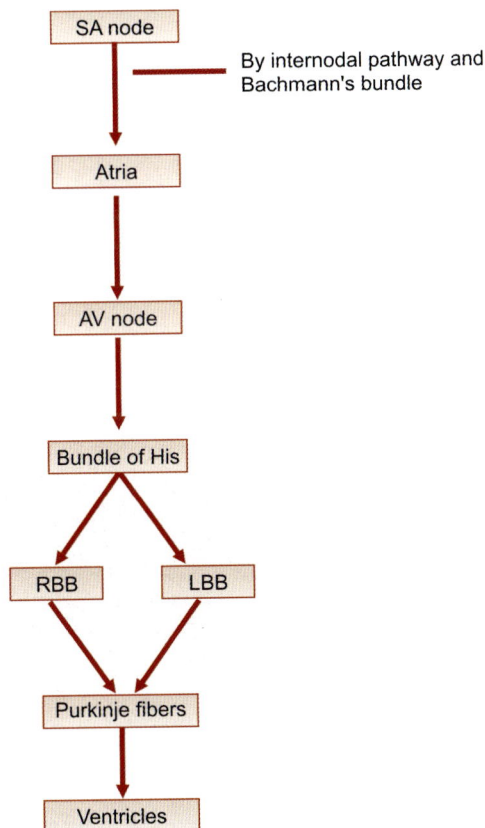

This is the normal sequence of stimulation of the specialized tissue. If any disturbance of this sequence occurs, there is rhythm disturbance, called arrhythmia or abnormality of conduction, called heart block.

SA node is the dominant pacemaker. Other pacemaker sites in the heart are atria, AV node and ventricles. All these are dormant, but can initiate impulse at a slow rate when SA node fails.

ANATOMY OF CONDUCTIVE TISSUE

1. *SA node:* Located in the superior and right side of right atrium, near the root of superior vena cava. Normally, the impulse arises in SA node called sinus rhythm. From SA node, impulse spreads along 3 internodal pathways (anterior, middle and posterior) into both right and left atrium. Finally, these 3 internodal pathways enter into the AV node. An additional internodal pathway called Bachmann's Bundle is present, which transmits impulse to the left atrium. Normal rate in SA node is 60 to 100/minute.

2. *AV node:* AV node smaller than SA node. It is located in the subendocardial surface of right side of right atrium, at the posterior part of interatrial septum, close to the opening of coronary sinus, just above the tricuspid valve.
    If SA node is blocked or fails, AV node can initiate cardiac impulse and perform as a pacemaker. Normal rate of AV node is 40 to 60/ minute. According to the electrical response, AV node is divided into 3 parts:
    *   High nodal (AN region).
    *   Mid nodal (N region).
    *   Low nodal (NH region).
    In ECG, these 3 regions can be detected by looking at the configuration of P wave.

3. *Bundle of His:* It is an extension of the tail of AV node, that extends downward and to the left to enter the interventricular septum, near the junction of muscles and fibrous part of ventricular septum. Then, it is divided into 2 right and left bundle branch.
    When there is AV block, bundle of His can initiate cardiac impulse and perform as a pacemaker. Normal rate of bundle of His is 20 to 40 /minute.

4. *Right bundle branch:* Extends on the right side of interventricular septum and spreads into right ventricle through Purkinje fibers.

5. *Left bundle branch:* It divides into anterior and posterior fascicles. Anterior fascicle spreads into anterosuperior part of left ventricle. Posterior fascicle spreads into posteroinferior part of left ventricle, through Purkinje fibers.

6. *Purkinje fibers:* These are the terminal network of fibers diffusely spread in the ventricular muscles in subendocardial and subepicardial myocardium.
    Normal intrinsic rate of Purkinje fibers is 15 to 40/minute.

NB: Most specialized cardiac fibers contain large number of automatic cells, whereas atrial and ventricular muscle fibers, under normal condition, have no automatic activity.

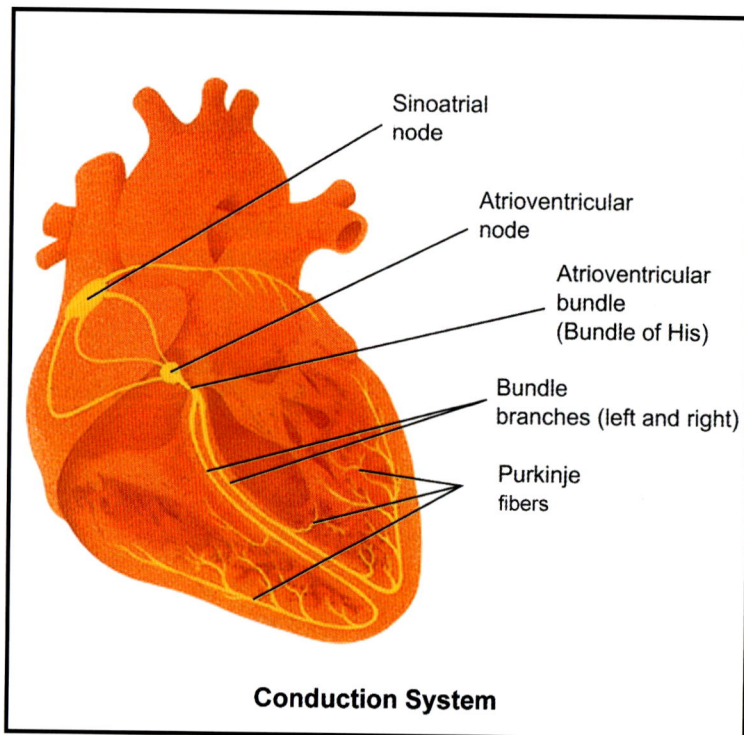

Conduction System

CORONARY CIRCULATION

There are 2 major coronary arteries: (1) Right and (2) Left.

1. Right Coronary Artery

It arises from right coronary sinus of Valsalva, runs along the right atrioventricular groove, gives marginal branch that supplies right atrium and right ventricle. It continues as posterior descending artery, which runs in posterior interventricular groove and supply posterior part of interventricular septum and posterior left ventricular wall.

Right coronary artery supplies the following parts:

- SA node—60% cases.
- AV node—90% cases.
- Right atrium and right ventricle.
- Inferoposterior aspect of left ventricle.

So, the occlusion of right coronary artery results in sinus bradycardia, AV block, infarction of inferior part of left ventricle and occasionally of right ventricle.

2. Left Coronary Artery

It arises from left coronary sinus of Valsalva. Within 2.5 cm of its origin, left main coronary artery divides into 2 branches: (1) Left anterior descending artery and (2) Circumflex artery.

- *Left anterior descending artery:* It runs in anterior interventricular groove and gives branches to supply the anterior part of interventricular septum, anterior wall and apex of left ventricle.
- *Circumflex artery:* It runs posteriorly in left atrioventricular groove and supply by marginal branch to left atrium and lateral and posteroinferior part of left ventricle.

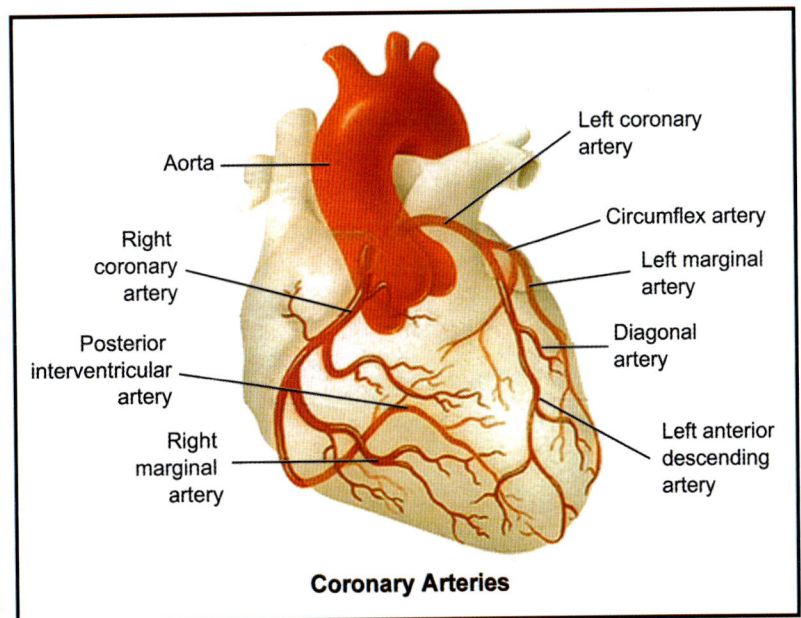

Coronary Arteries

Left coronary artery also supply:

- SA node in 40% cases.
- AV node in 10% cases.
- Bundle of His.
- Right and left bundle branch.

Occlusion of left anterior descending artery and circumflex artery causes infarction of the corresponding territories of left ventricle.

Occlusion of left main coronary artery causes extensive damage and is usually fatal.

Venous system mainly follows coronory arteries, but drains to the coronory sinus in the atrioventricular groove, then to the right atrium.

Coronary vessels receive sympathetic and parasympathetic innervations. Stimulation of α-receptor causes vasoconstriction and β_2 causes vasodilatation. Sympathetic stimulation in coronary artery causes dilatation, parasympathetic stimulation also causes mild dilatation of normal coronary artery. Healthy coronary endothelium releases nitric oxide, which promotes vasodilatation. Systemic hormones, neuropeptides and endothelin also influence arterial tone and coronary flow.

PROPERTIES OF CARDIAC MUSCLES

Cardiac muscles have some special properties:

- *Automaticity:* Without external stimulus, heart muscle can initiate normal cardiac impulse by SA node.
- *Autorhythmicity:* Cardiac muscle can contract after a regular interval, called autorhythmicity.
- *Excitability:* Cardiac muscle can be excited by adequate external stimulus.
- *Conductivity:* Cardiac muscle has the ability to conduct impulse from one muscle cell to another cell.
- *Contractility:* Ability to contract after depolarization.
- *Refractory period:* It is a period during which activated muscle fibers do not respond to further stimulus. It is of 2 types: (1) Absolute refractory period and (2) Relative refractory period.
  — Absolute refractory period—during this period, muscle fibers do not respond to any stimulus.
  — Relative refractory period—with very strong stimulus, muscle fibers may respond.
- *All or none law:* If external stimulus is too little, no cardiac impulse is initiated. But with adequate stimulus, all muscle fibers contract with its best ability.
- *Functional syncitium:* Cardiac muscle fibers are electrically connected with one another by a gap junction. When one muscle fiber is excited, the action potential spreads to whole cardiac muscle fibers, because of presence of intercalated disk. It is called syncytium.

NB: Remember the following points:

- Purkinje fibers transmit impulse faster than any tissue of the heart, at the rate of 4000 mm/sec.
- Atrial muscles transmit impulse at the rate of 800 to 1000 mm/sec.
- Ventricular muscles transmit impulse at the rate of 400 mm/sec.
- AV node transmit impulse at the rate of 200 mm/sec (slowest). This slow conduction in AV node is a protective mechanism. It prevents to transmit rapid atrial contraction or impulse.

NERVE SUPPLY OF THE HEART

The heart is supplied by both sympathetic and parasympathetic (in cardiac plexus).
- Sympathetic (adrenergic) supply both atria and ventricular muscle, also conductive specialized tissue.
- Parasympathetic preganglionic fibers and sensory fibers reach the heart through vagus nerves. Cholinergic nerves supply SA node and AV nodes via muscarinic (M_2) receptors.

Nerve supply is mainly through β_1 and β_2 receptors.
- β_1 receptor is predominant in heart, having both inotrophic and chronotrophic effect.
- β_2 receptor is predominant in vascular muscles and causes vasodilatation.

Under basal condition, predominant effect is parasympathetic through vagus nerve over sympathetic, resulting in slow heart rate. So during sleep, heart rate is slow. Also in athlete, there is predominant vagal effect (so heart rate may show bradycardia).

ELECTROCARDIOGRAM

DEFINITION

It is the graphical representation of electrical potentials produced when the electric current passes through the heart. Electrical activity is the basic characteristic of heart and is the stimulus for cardiac contraction. Disturbance of electrical function is common in heart disease.

Electrocardiogram (ECG) records the electrical impulse on ECG paper by electrodes placed on body surface called waves or deflections.

One beat is recorded as a grouping of waves called P-QRS-T.

- P — Represents atrial depolarization.
- PR interval — Represents the time taken for the cardiac impulse to spread over the atrium and through AV node and His-Purkinje system.
- QRS — Represents ventricular depolarization.
- T wave — Represents ventricular repolarization.

In a normal ECG recording, there are 12 leads:

- 3 bipolar standard leads.
- 3 unipolar limb leads.
- 6 chest leads.

(Leads are different view parts of heart's electrical activity).

1. Bipolar standard leads (also called limb leads) designated as L_I, L_{II} and L_{III}.

> - L_I — Difference of potential between left arm and right arm (LA and RA).
> - L_{II} — Difference of potential between right arm and left leg (RA and LL).
> - L_{III} — Difference of potential between left arm and left leg (LA and LL).

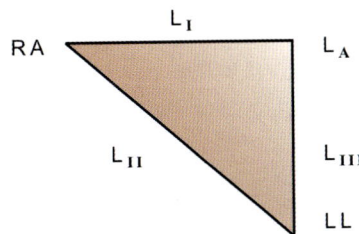

2. Unipolar limb leads (also called augmented limb leads) designated as aVR, aVL and aVF. Three unipolar leads have very low voltage, which cannot be recorded satisfactorily. For this reason, recordings of these leads are increased in amplitude. So, they are called augmented unipolar leads, which are represented as aVR, aVL and aVF.

> - aVR — Augmented unipolar RA lead. Records the changes of potential occurring in the part of heart facing towards right shoulder.
> - aVL — Augmented unipolar LA lead. Records the changes of potential of heart facing towards the left shoulder.
> - aVF — Augmented unipolar LL lead. Records the changes of potential of heart facing towards the left hip.

3. Chest leads (Unipolar) Designated by 'V'.

Electrodes are placed in the following places on the chest wall.

- V_1—4th intercostal space at right sternal border.
- V_2—4th intercostal space at left sternal border.
- V_3—midway between V_2 and V_4 lead on left side.
- V_4—5th intercostal space in left midclavicular line.
- V_5—5th intercostal space in left anterior axillary line.
- V_6—5th intercostal space in left midaxillary line.

VIEW OF THE HEART IN ALL LEADS

By looking the following leads, the site and surface of heart lesion is identified.

- L_I, aVL, V_5 and V_6—Reflects lateral (or anterolateral aspect of heart).
- L_{II}, L_{III} and aVF—Reflects inferior aspect of heart.
- V_1 and V_2—Reflects right ventricle.
- V_3 and V_4—Reflects interventricular septum.
- V_5 and V_6—Reflects left ventricle.
- V_1 to V_6—Reflects anterior aspect of heart.
- L_I, aVL, V_1 to V_6—Reflects extensive anterior aspect of heart or anterolateral.
- L_I and aVL—High lateral.
- L_{II}, L_{III}, aVF, L_I, aVL, V_5 and V_6—Inferolateral.

NB: Remember the following points:

- There is no lead which represents posterior wall of the heart (it is seen in V_1 and V_2).
- Additional leads can be taken from V_3R and V_4R, sites on the right side of chest equivalent to V_3 and V_4. It is helpful for the diagnosis of right ventricular infarction (usually associated with inferior infarction).
- aVR and V_1 are oriented towards the cavity of heart.

INTERPRETATION OF ECG

Before interpreting an ECG, one must know details about the ECG paper, standardization and different waves in ECG, etc. It is a matter of experience and pattern interpretation, which requires a method of systematic ECG analysis.

During interpretation, look at the following points carefully:

1. Standardization (see in the beginning)—like this ⎴ which is 10 mm (1 mV).
2. Paper speed—25 mm/second.
3. Rhythm—by looking at RR interval (L_{II} is usually called rhythm lead), see regular or irregular.
4. Count the heart rate.
5. Different waves:
   - P—whether normal, small or tall, inverted, wide, notched, bifid, variable configuration, etc.
   - PR interval—normal or prolonged or short.
   - Q—normal or pathological.
   - R—normal or tall or short, notched or M pattern.
   - QRS—normal or wide, high or low voltage, variable or change of shape.
   - ST segment—elevated or depressed.
   - T—normal or tall or small or inverted.
   - U wave—normal or small.
   - QT—short or prolonged.
6. Axis—whether normal or right or left axis deviation.
7. Abnormalities—any arrhythmia, infarction, hypertrophy, etc.

One must have some basic idea about the ECG paper, normal ECG tracing, limits of normal value, duration, rhythm, etc.

Q. What are the diseases diagnosed by looking at an ECG?
Ans. As follows:
- Tachycardia or bradycardia.
- Chamber enlargement.
- Myocardial infarction.
- Arrhythmias.
- Block (First degree block, SA block, AV block, bundle branch block).
- Drug effect (such as digoxin).
- Extracardiac abnormalities—electrolyte imbalance (such as hypokalemia or hyperkalemia), hypo- or hypercalcemia, low voltage tracing (in myxedema, hypothermia, emphysema).
- Exercise ECG to see coronary artery disease.

SYSTEMATIC APPROACH IN ECG INTERPRETATION

- Rate—what is the rate ?
- Rhythm—regular or irregular, regularly followed by occasional irregular.
- Characters of individual waves (P, PR, Q, R, QRS, ST, T, U).
- Specific pathological changes.

BRIEF DISCUSSION ABOUT ECG PAPER

ECG paper shows small and large squares. In each small square, thin horizontal and vertical lines are present in 1 mm interval. A heavier thick line is present in every 5 mm (5 small squares) interval. Time is measured horizontally and voltage / height is measured vertically.

1. One small square:
   - Height = 1 mm.
   - Horizontal (in time) = 0.04 second.
2. One big square (5 small squares):
   - Height = 5 mm.
   - Horizontal (in time) = 0.04 × 5 sec = 0.2 second.

   So, 0.2 second = 5 mm.
   1 second = 5/0.2 = 25 mm.

   So, recording speed is 25 mm/sec. (i.e. 1500 mm/min).
   A faster recording speed (50 mm/sec) is occasionally used to visualize wave deflection.
3. *Isoelectric line:* It is the base line in ECG paper. Waves are measured either above (positive deflection) or below (negative deflection).

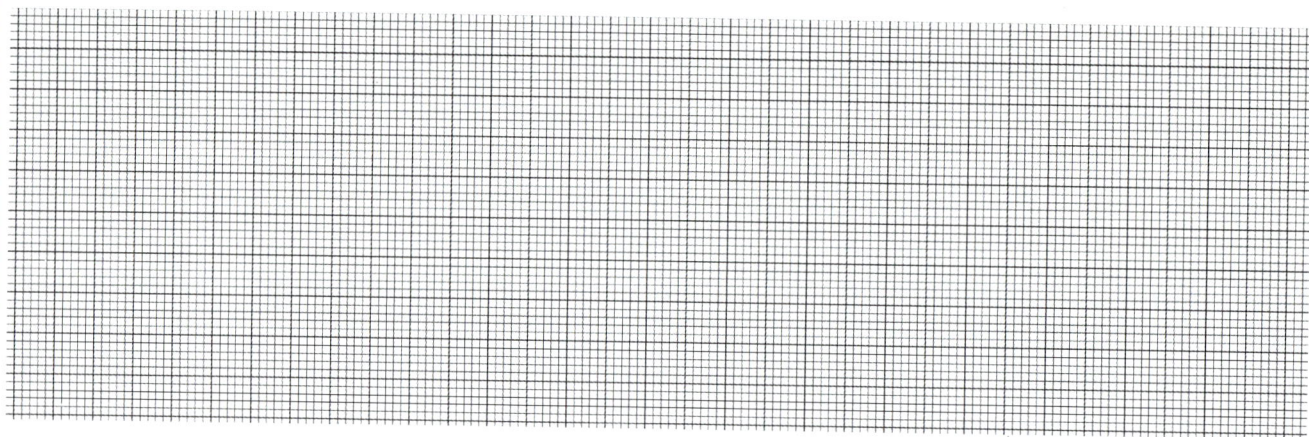

ECG Paper

Standardization of ECG		
• Normally, 1mv current	—	10 mm height (10 small squares)
• Half strength	—	5 mm
• Double strength	—	20 mm
• Recording speed	—	25 mm/second (i.e. 1500 mm/min)

In any ECG, before telling **low voltage or high voltage,** see the normal standardization (i.e. 10 mm in height).

CRITERIA OF LOW VOLTAGE TRACING

- In standard limb leads—QRS < 5 mm (mainly R wave).
- In chest leads—QRS < 10 mm (mainly R wave).

CAUSES OF LOW VOLTAGE ECG TRACING

- Incorrect standardization (i.e. if < 10 mm).
- Obesity.
- Pericardial effusion.
- Chronic constrictive pericarditis.
- Myxedema.
- Emphysema.
- Hypothermia.

ECG CONVENTIONS AND INTERVALS

• Depolarization towards the electrode	— Positive deflection (above the isoelectric line).
• Depolarization away from the electrode	— Negative deflection (below the isoelectric line).
• Sensitivity	— 10 mm = 1 mV.
• Paper speed	— 25 mm/second.
• Each large (5 mm) square	— 0.2 second.
• Each small (1 mm) square	— 0.04 second.
• Normal standardization	— 10 mm.
• Rhythm	— Interval between two successive R R.

Q. What is depolarization and repolarization?

Ans. As follows:

- *Depolarization:* Means initial spread of stimulus through the muscle, causing activation or contraction.
- *Repolarization:* Means return of stimulated muscle to the resting state (recovery from activation or contraction).

NORMAL ECG

CHARACTERS OF NORMAL ECG

- Normal ECG recording consists of P wave (atrial beat), followed by QRS, ST and T wave (ventricular beat).
- Capital letter P, Q, R, S, T—indicates large wave (> 5 mm).
- Small letter p, q, r, s, t—indicates small wave (< 5 mm).

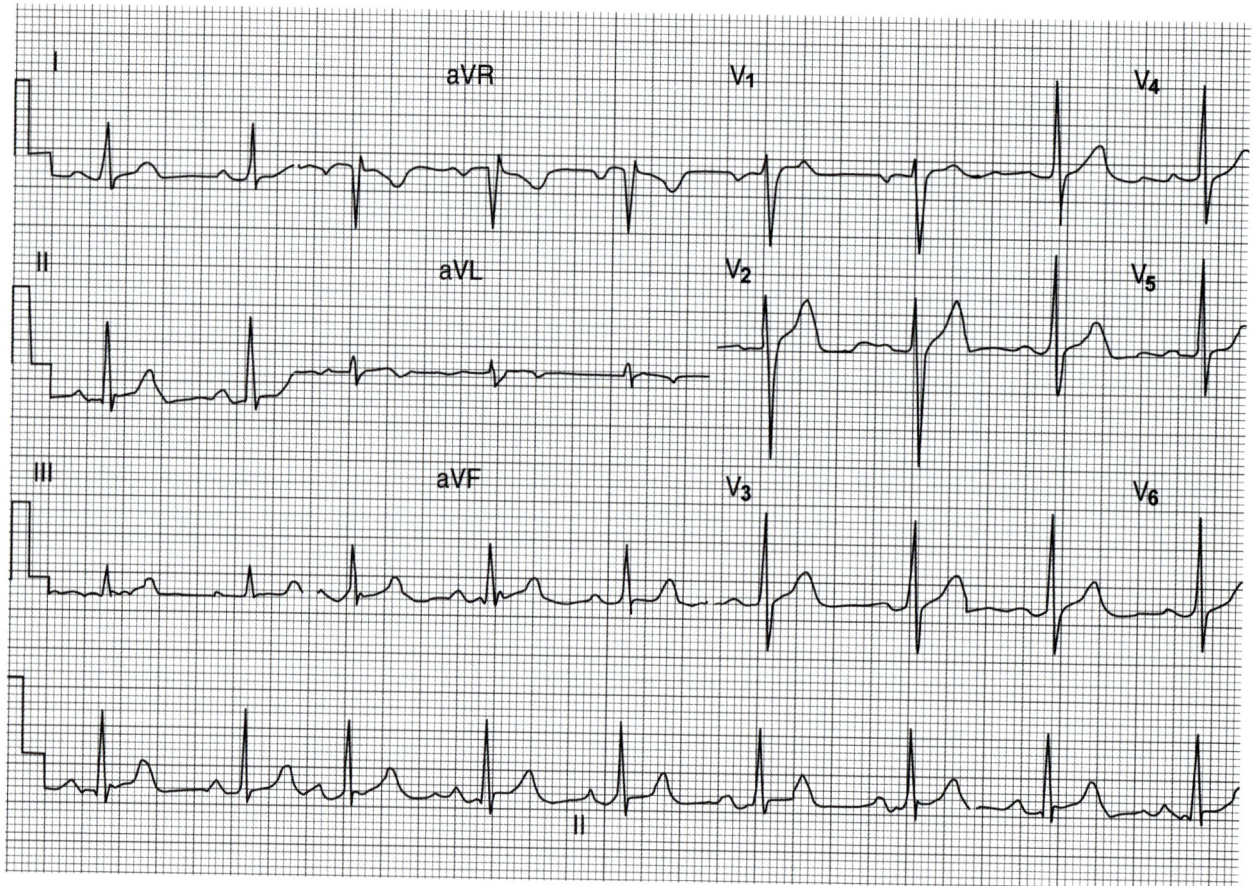

TYPES OF WAVES IN ECG

- P — Deflection produced by atrial depolarization.
- QRS — Deflection produced by ventricular depolarization.
- Q (q) — First negative deflection produced by ventricular depolarization. It precedes R wave.
- R(r) — First positive deflection produced by ventricular depolarization.
- S(s) — Negative deflection after R wave produced by ventricular depolarization.
- T — Indicates ventricular repolarization.

OTHER WAVES

- J — At the beginning of ST segment.
- U — Not always seen. When present, it follows T wave, preceding the next P wave. It indicates repolarization of interventricular septum or slow repolarization of the ventricles.

INTERVALS IN ECG

- PR interval — Distance between the beginning of P to beginning of QRS (Q), ideally called PQ interval.
- PP interval — Distance between two successive P waves. In sinus rhythm, P-P interval is regular.
- RR interval — Distance between two successive R waves. In sinus rhythm, R-R interval is regular.
- QT interval — Distance interval between the beginning of Q wave and the end of T wave.

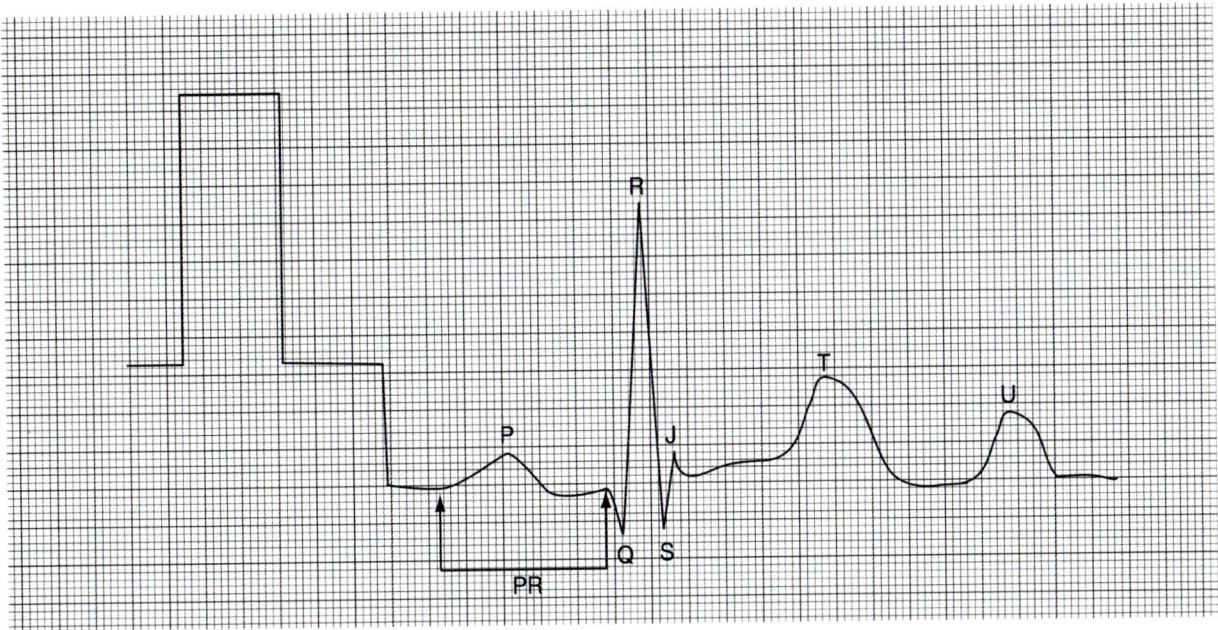

SEGMENT IN ECG

ST—Distance from the end of QRS complex to the beginning of T wave. It indicates the beginning of ventricular repolarization. Normally, it is in isoelectric line, but may vary from – 0.5 to + 2 mm in chest leads.

NB: Remember the following points:

- Ventricles contain majority of the heart muscles (left ventricle contains more than the right). So, QRS is larger than P wave.
- Atrial repolarization is small and is buried in QRS. So, it is not seen in ECG (No wave is seen due to atrial repolarization in ECG).

DETAILS OF WAVES AND INTERVALS

P WAVE

Characters of Normal P Wave

- P wave results from spread of electrical activity through the atria.
- Width or duration (in time, horizontally) - 0.10 sec (2.5 small sq.).
- Height - 2.5 mm (2.5 small sq.).
  (Height × Duration = 2.5 × 2.5 small squares).
- P wave is better seen in L_{II}, as atrial depolarization is towards L_{II} (also seen in V_1), because the impulse spread from right to left atrium.
- P wave is upright in all leads, mainly L_I, L_{II} and aVF (except aVR). (P is inverted in aVR and occasionally in aVL).
- P wave in V_1 may be biphasic (equal upward and downward deflection), notched and wide. (Activation of right atrium produces positive component and activation of left atrium produces negative component).
- Normal P is rounded, neither peaked nor notched.

Abnormalities of P Wave

P wave may be:
- Absent.
- Tall or small.
- Wide, notched, biphasic.
- Inverted.
- Variable and multiple.

Causes of absent P wave
- Atrial fibrillation (P is absent or replaced by fibrillary **f** wave).
- Atrial flutter (P is replaced by flutter wave, which shows **saw-tooth** appearance).
- SA block or sinus arrest.
- Nodal rhythm (usually abnormal, small P wave).
- Ventricular ectopic and ventricular tachycardia.
- Supraventricular tachycardia (P is hidden within QRS, due to tachycardia).
- Hyperkalemia.
- Idioventricular rhythm.

Causes of tall P wave
- Tall P is called P pulmonale (height > 2.5 mm, i.e. > 2.5 small squares).
- It is due to right atrial hypertrophy or enlargement.

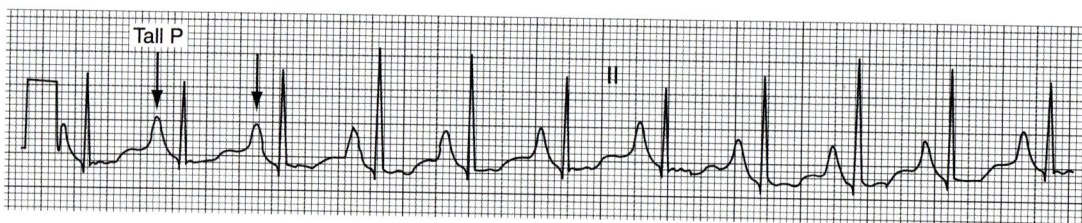

P 4 mm (tall)

Causes of small P wave
- Atrial tachycardia.
- Atrial ectopic.
- Nodal rhythm (high nodal).
- Nodal ectopic (high nodal).

Causes of wide P wave
- Broad and notched P is called P mitrale (duration > 0.11 sec, or > 2.5 small squares).
- It is due to left atrial hypertrophy or enlargement.
- In V_1, P wave may be biphasic with a small positive wave preceding a deep and broad negative wave (indicates left atrial enlargement or hypertrophy).

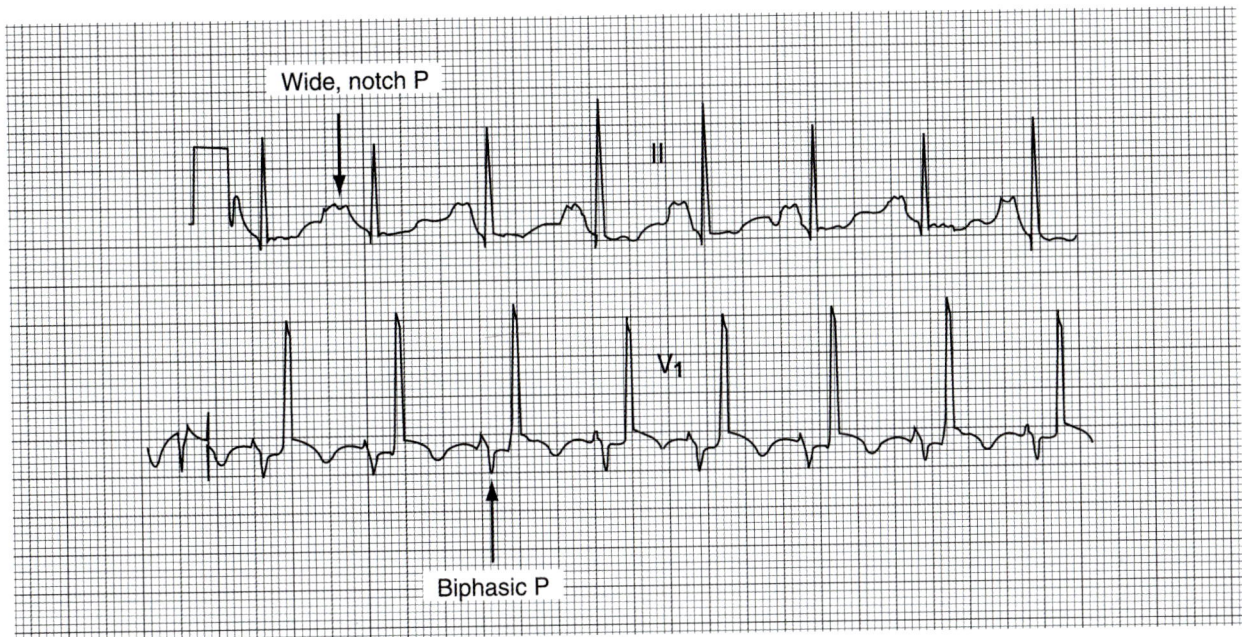

Causes of inverted P wave (negative in L_I, L_{II} and aVF)
- Incorrectly placed leads (reversed arm electrodes).
- Dextrocardia.
- Nodal rhythm with retrograde conduction.
- Low atrial and high nodal ectopic beats.

Causes of variable P waves
Presence of variable P waves indicates wandering pacemaker.

Causes of multiple P waves (consecutive 2 or more)
- A-V block (either partial or complete heart block).
- SVT with AV block.

P-R INTERVAL

Characters of Normal P-R Interval

- It is the distance between the onset of P wave to the beginning of Q wave (if Q wave is absent, then measure up to the onset of R wave).
- It is the time required for the impulse to travel from SA node to the ventricular muscle. (The impulse is transmitted to ventricle via AV node).
- P-R interval varies with age and heart rate. (P-R interval is short, if the heart rate is increased and long, if heart rate is decreased).
- Normal PR interval—0.12 to 0.20 sec (maximum 5 small squares).
  - — In children, upper limit is 0.16 sec.
  - — In adolescent, upper limit is 0.18 sec.
  - — In adult, upper limit is 0.22 sec.
- P-R is short, if it is < 0.10 sec and long, if it is > 0.22 sec.

Abnormalities of P-R Interval

PR interval may be:
- Prolonged.
- Short.
- Variable.

Prolonged P-R interval (> 0.2 second): It is due to first degree heart block. Causes are:
- Ischemic heart disease (occasionally, inferior MI).
- Acute rheumatic carditis.
- Myocarditis (due to any cause).
- Atrial dilatation or hypertrophy.
- Hypokalemia.
- Drugs—digitalis toxicity, quinidine, occasionally β-blocker, calcium channel blocker (verapamil).

Short P-R interval (< 0.12 second): Causes are:
- Wolff-Parkinson-White (WPW) syndrome. In this case, there is delta wave.
- Lown-Ganong-Levine (LGL) syndrome. In this case, there is no delta wave.
- Nodal rhythm.
- Nodal ectopic (high nodal).
- Occasionally, if dissociated beat is present and also in infant, steroid therapy.

Variable P-R interval: Causes are:
- Wenckebach's phenomenon (Mobitz type I): There is progressive lengthening of P-R interval followed by a drop beat.
- Partial heart block (Mobitz type II): PR interval is fixed and normal, but sometimes P is not followed by QRS.
- 2 :1 AV block: Alternate P wave is not followed by QRS.
- Complete AV block: No relation between P and QRS.
- Wandering pacemaker: Variable configuration of P.

Q WAVE

Characters of Normal Q Wave

- Q wave is usually absent in most of the leads. However, small q wave may be present in I, II, aVL, V_5 and V_6. This is due to septal depolarization.
- Small q may be present in L_{III} (which disappears with inspiration).
- Depth—< 2 mm (2 small squares).
- Width—1 small square.
- It is 25% or less in amplitude of the following R wave in the same lead.

Characters of Pathological Q Wave

- Deep > 2 mm (2 small squares).
- Wide > 0.04 sec or more (> 1 mm or 1 small square).
- Should be present in more than one lead.
- Associated with loss of height of R wave.
- Q wave should be > 25% of the following R wave of the same lead.

Causes of Pathological Q Wave

- Myocardial infarction (commonest cause).
- Ventricular hypertrophy (left or right).
- Cardiomyopathy.
- LBBB.
- Emphysema (due to axis change or cardiac rotation).
- Q only in L_{III} is associated with pulmonary embolism (S_I, Q_{III} and T_{III} pattern).

NB: Remember the following points:

- Q wave in V_1, V_2 and V_3 may be seen in LVH and may be mistaken as old myocardial infarction.
- Abnormal Q wave in L_{III} may be found in pulmonary embolism.
- Abnormal Q wave in L_{III} and aVF may be found in WPW syndrome (confuses with old inferior myocardial infarction).

R WAVE

Characters of Normal R Wave

- It is the first positive (upward) deflection, due to ventricular depolarization.
- Duration < 0.01 sec.
- R wave usually small (< 1 mm) in V_1 and V_2. It increases progressively in height in V_3 to V_6 (tall in V_5 and V_6), i.e. R is small in V_1 and V_2, tall in V_5 and V_6.

Normal Height of R Wave

- aVL < 13 mm.
- aVF < 20 mm.
- V_5 and V_6 < 25 mm.

(If R wave is > 25 mm, it is always pathological).

Abnormalities of R Wave

R wave may be:
- Tall.
- Small.
- Poor progression.

Causes of tall R wave

1. Left ventricular hypertrophy (in V_5 or V_6 > 25 mm, aVL >13 mm, aVF > 20 mm).
2. In V_1, tall R may be due to:
   - Normal variant.
   - Right ventricular hypertrophy (RVH).
   - True posterior myocardial infarction.
   - WPW syndrome (type A).
   - Right bundle branch block.
   - Dextrocardia.

Causes of small R wave: Looks like low voltage tracing.
- Incorrect ECG calibration (standardization).
- Obesity.
- Emphysema.
- Pericardial effusion.
- Hypothyroidism.
- Hypothermia.

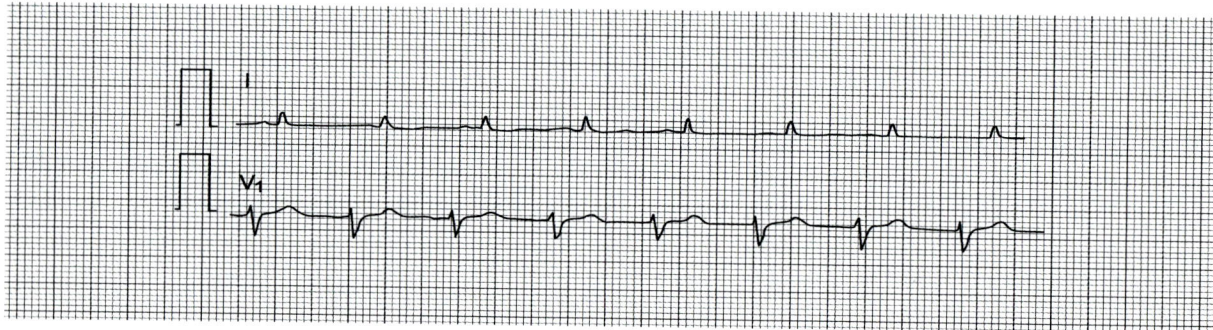

Small R wave

R wave progression: The height of R wave gradually increases from V_1 to V_6. This phenomenom is called R wave progression.

Poor progression of R wave: Normally, amplitude of R wave is tall in V_5 and V_6. In poor R wave progression, amplitude of R wave is progressively reduced in V_5 and V_6.

Causes are:
- Anterior or anteroseptal myocardial infarction.
- Left bundle branch block.
- Left ventricular hypertrophy (though R is tall in most cases).
- Dextrocardia.
- Cardiomyopathy.
- COPD.
- Left sided pneumothorax.
- Left sided pleural effusion (massive).
- Marked clockwise rotation.
- Chest electrodes placed incorrectly.
- Deformity of the chest wall.
- Normal variation.

S WAVE

Characters of Normal S Wave

- It is the negative deflection after R wave (1/3rd of R wave).
- Normally, deep in V_1 and V_2 as impulse is going to the muscles of left ventricle then to the right ventricle.
- Progressively diminished from V_1 to V_6 (small S wave may be present in V_5 and V_6).
- In V_3, R and S waves are almost equal (corresponds with interventricular septum).

QRS COMPLEX

Characters of Normal QRS Complex

- QRS complex represents depolarization of ventricular muscles.
- Depolarization of left ventricle contributes to main QRS (as the left ventricle has 2 to 3 times mass of right ventricle).
- QRS is predominantly positive in leads that look at the heart from left side—L_1, aVL, V_5 and V_6.
- It is negative in leads that look at the heart from the right side—aVR, V_1 and V_2.
- In V_1, S is greater than R.
- In V_5 and V_6, R is tall.
- QRS appears biphasic (part above and part below the base line) in V_3 and V_4.
- Normal duration of QRS is 0.08 to 0.11 second (< 3 small squares) and height < 25 mm.

Various Forms and Components of QRS Complex

- Q wave: Initial downward deflection.
- R wave: Initial upward deflection.
- S wave: Downward deflection after R wave.
- rS complex: Small initial r wave, followed by large S wave.
- RS complex: A complex with R and S wave of equal amplitude.
- Rs complex: A large R wave followed by a small s wave.
- qRS complex: Small initial downward deflection, followed by a tall R which is followed by a large S.
- Qr complex: Large Q, followed by a small r.
- QS complex: Complex with complete negative deflection (no separate Q and S).
- rSr complex: Small r, then deep S, followed by small r.
- RSR complex: Tall R, then deep S, followed by tall R.
- RR complex: When deflection is completely positive and notched (M pattern).

Abnormalities of QRS Complex

QRS may be:
- High voltage.
- Low voltage.
- Wide.
- Change in shape.
- Variable.

Causes of high voltage QRS
- Incorrect calibration.
- Thin chest wall.
- Ventricular hypertrophy (right or left or both).
- WPW syndrome.
- True posterior myocardial infarction (in V_1 and V_2).

Causes of low voltage QRS (< 5 mm in L_I, L_{II}, L_{III} and < 10 mm in chest leads)
- Incorrect calibration.
- Thick chest wall or obesity.
- Hypothyroidism.

- Pericardial effusion.
- Emphysema.
- Chronic constrictive pericarditis.
- Hypothermia.

Causes of wide QRS (> 0.12 second, 3 small squares)
- Bundle branch block (LBBB or RBBB).
- Ventricular ectopics.
- Ventricular tachycardia.
- Idioventricular rhythm.
- Ventricular hypertrophy.
- Hyperkalemia.
- WPW syndrome.
- Pacemaker (looks like LBBB with spike).
- Drugs (quinidine, procainamide, phenothiazine, tricyclic antidepressants).

Causes of changes in shape of QRS
- Right or left bundle branch block (slurred or M pattern).
- Ventricular tachycardia.
- Ventricular fibrillation.
- Hyperkalemia.
- WPW syndrome.

Causes of variable QRS
- Multifocal ventricular ectopics.
- Torsades de pointes.
- Ventricular fibrillation.

ST SEGMENT

Characters of Normal ST Segment

- Measured from the end of S to the beginning of T wave. It represents beginning of ventricular repolarization.
- Normally, it is in isoelectric line (lies at same level of ECG baseline).
- ST elevation is normal up to 1 mm in limb leads and 2 mm in chest leads (mainly V_1 to V_3).
- In Negroes, ST elevation of 4 mm may be normal, which disappears on exercise.
- Normally, ST segment may be depressed, < 1mm.

Abnormalities of ST Segment

ST segment may be:
- Elevated.
- Depressed.

Causes of ST elevation (> 2 mm)
- Recent myocardial infarction (ST elevation with convexity upward).
- Acute pericarditis (ST elevation with concavity upward, chair shaped or saddle shaped).
- Prinzmetal's angina (ST elevation with tall T).
- Ventricular aneurysm (persistent ST elevation).
- Early repolarization (high take off).
- Normal variant in Africans and Asians.
- May be in hyperkalemia.

Causes of ST depression (below the isoelectric line)
- Acute myocardial ischemia (horizontal or down slope ST depression with sharp angle ST-T junction).
- Ventricular hypertrophy with strain (ST depression with convexity upward and asymmetric T inversion).
- Digoxin toxicity (sagging of ST depression—like thumb impression, also called reverse tick).
- Acute true posterior myocardial infarction (in V_1 and V_2), associated with dominant R and tall upright T wave.

Early repolarization (high take-off)
- It is a benign, normal finding in young healthy person, more in black males.
- It is seen in chest leads, commonly V_4 to V_6 (rarely, in other chest lead).
- ST elevation is usually associated with J point elevation.
- It is not associated with inversion of T wave or abnormal Q wave.

NB: Remember the following points:

- Early repolarization syndrome confuses with acute myocardial infarction and acute pericarditis.
- To differentiate from these, detail history, serial ECG tracing (that shows no change) and comparison with old ECG are helpful.

T WAVE

Characters of Normal T Wave

- It indicates ventricular repolarization.
- Follows S wave and ST segment.
- Upright in all leads, except aVR.
- Usually, more than 2 mm in height.
- May be normally inverted in V_1 and V_2.
- Normally, not more than 5 mm in standard leads and 10 mm in chest leads.
- Minimum 1/4th of R wave of the same lead.
- Tip of T is smooth (rounded).

Abnormalities of T Wave

T wave may be:
- Inverted.
- Tall peaked, tented.

Causes of T inversion
- Myocardial ischemia and infarction.
- Subendocardial myocardial infarction (non-Q wave myocardial infarction).
- Ventricular ectopics.
- Ventricular hypertrophy with strain.
- Acute pericarditis.
- Cardiomyopathy.
- Myxoedema.
- Bundle branch block.
- Drugs (digitalis, emetine, phenothiazine).
- Physiological (smoking, anxiety, anorexia, exercise, after meal or glucose).

Causes of tall peaked T wave
- Hyperkalemia (tall, tented or peaked).
- Hyperacute myocardial infarction (tall T wave).
- Acute true posterior myocardial infarction (tall T in V_1 to V_2).
- May be normal in some Africans and Asians.

Causes of small T wave
- Hypokalemia.
- Hypothyroidism.
- Pericardial effusion.

Q. What is juvenile T wave pattern?
Ans. It is a disorder in which T is inverted in V_1 to V_3 (rarely V_4 to V_6). T inversion is neither symmetrical nor deep. It is common in children and young adults, more in female < 40 years. Frequently, it is associated with sinus arrhythmia and high left ventricular voltage.

U WAVE

Characters of Normal U Wave

- It follows T wave.
- It may be present in normal ECG. It is smaller and in the same direction of the preceding T wave.
- It represents slow repolarization of interventricular septum (Purkinje fibers, but actual genesis of U wave is still controversial).
- It is better seen in chest leads (V_2 to V_4).
- Normal amplitude is 1 mm (2 mm in athlete).

Abnormalities of U Wave

U wave may be:
- Inverted.
- Prominent.

Causes of inverted U wave
- Ischemic heart disease.
- Left ventricular hypertrophy with strain (hypertensive heart disease).

Causes of prominent U wave
- May be normally present (usually small).
- Hypokalemia (commonest).
- Bradycardia.
- Ventricular hypertrophy.
- Hyperthyroidism.
- Hypercalcemia.
- Drugs (phenothiazine, quinidine, digitalis).

Q. What is the significance of large U wave?

Ans. The patient is prone to develop torsades de pointes tachycardia.

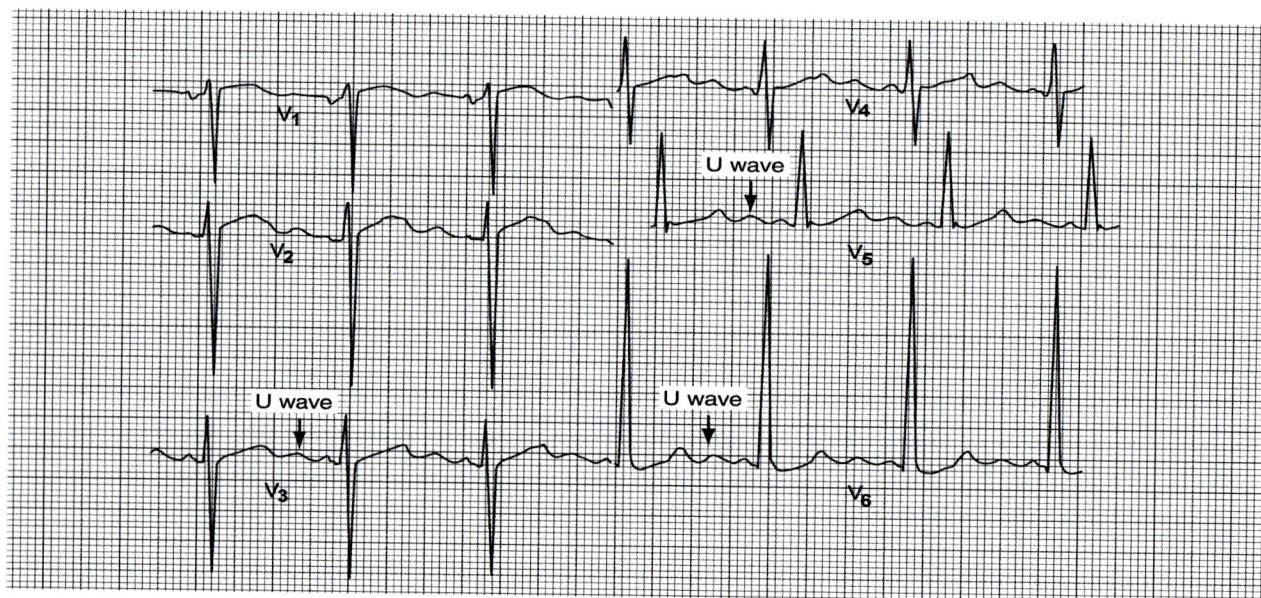

QT INTERVAL

Characters of Normal QT Interval

- It is the distance from the beginning of Q wave (or R wave, if there is no Q wave) to the end of T wave. It represents the total time required for both depolarization and repolarization of the ventricles.
- Normal QT interval is 0.35 to 0.43 seconds.
- Its duration varies with heart rate, becoming shorter as the heart rate increases and longer as the heart rate decreases. In general, QT interval at heart rate between 60 to 90/minute does not exceed in duration half the preceding RR interval.
- It is better seen in aVL (because there is no U wave).
- Corrected formula for real QT is:

$$QTc = \frac{QT}{\sqrt{RR}}$$

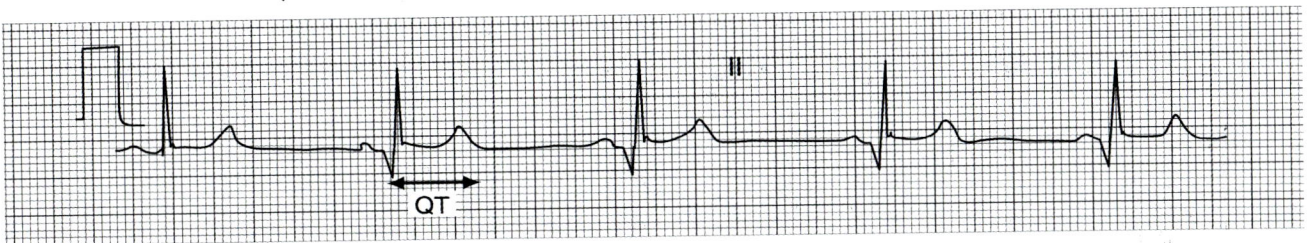

Abnormalities of QT Interval

QT interval may be:
- Short.
- Long.

Causes of short QT interval
- Digoxin effect.
- Hypercalcemia.
- Hyperthermia.
- Tachycardia

Causes of long QT interval
- Hypocalcemia.
- Bradycardia.
- Acute myocarditis.
- Acute myocardial infarction.
- Hypothermia.
- Drug (quinidine, procainamide, flecainide, amiodarone, tricyclic antidepressant, disopyramide, pentamidine).
- Cerebral injury (head injury, intracerebral hemorrhage).
- Hypertrophic cardiomyopathy.
- During sleep.
- Hereditary syndrome:
    (a) Jervell-Lange Nielsen syndrome (congenital deafness, syncope and sudden death).
    (b) Romano-Ward syndrome (same as above except deafness).

NB: Prolonged QT interval may be detected in an asymptomatic individual. It may be associated with ventricular arrhythmia. Rarely, it can cause torsades de pointes tachycardia and sudden death.

RHYTHM OF HEART

To see the rhythm—see the successive RR interval.
- If the RR interval is equal, it is called regular rhythm.
- If the RR interval is irregular, then it is called irregular rhythm.

Causes of Irregular Rhythm

1. Physiological: Sinus arrhythmia.
2. Pathological:
   - Atrial fibrillation.
   - Atrial flutter.
   - Ectopic beat.
   - SA block or sinus arrest.
   - Atrial tachycardia with block.
   - Second degree heart block.
   - Ventricular fibrillation.

CHARACTERS OF SINUS RHYTHM

Sinus rhythm shows the following 5 characters:
- P wave is of sinus origin (means characters of normal P wave).
- P waves and QRS complexes are regular (that means P-P and R-R interval should be constant and identical).
- Constant P wave configuration in a given lead.
- P-R interval and QRS interval should be within normal limit.
- Rate should be between 60 to 100 beats/min (atrial and ventricular rates are identical).

Q. What is arrhythmia?
Ans. It is the abnormality in initiation or propagation of cardiac impulse.

NB: Remember the following points:

- To see any rhythm disturbance, preferably long rhythm strip (L_{II}) should be taken.
- When strong suspicion of arrhythmia, ambulatory ECG (Holter monitor ECG) should be taken.

CALCULATION OF HEART RATE

In any ECG, heart rate should be calculated. Methods vary according to the cardiac rhythm, whether regular or irregular. Standard speed in ECG paper is 25 mm /second. Heart rate is the number of beats /min.

In the ECG paper:

- 0.04 second = 1 small square.
- 0.2 second = 5 small squares or 1 large square.
- So, 1 second = 25 small squares or 5 large squares.
- So, 1 minute = 25 × 60 = 1500 small squares or 5 × 60 = 300 large squares.

Heart rate is determined in the following way:

1. When the cardiac rhythm is regular:

- Calculate the R-R or P-P interval in small squares or large squares (if the rhythm is sinus, R-R or P-P interval is same).
- If small square is calculated:

$$\text{Then the heart rate is} = \frac{1500}{\text{Small squares between R-R or P-P}}$$

- If large square is calculated

$$\text{Then the heart rate is} = \frac{300}{\text{Large squares between R-R or P-P}}$$

Examples

- Suppose, number of small squares between R-R or P-P is 15.

  So the heart rate is $\dfrac{1500}{15}$ = 100/minute.

- Suppose number of large squares between to R-R is 5.

  So the heart rate is $\dfrac{300}{5}$ = 60/minute.

2. When the rhythm is irregular:

- Count the number of R in 30 large squares (it is equivalent to 6 seconds).
- Then simply multiply this by 10 (it becomes rate in 1 minute).

Example

- Suppose, the number of R in 30 large squares is 12.
- So, the heart rate is 12 × 10 = 120 beats / min.

NB: Remember the following points:

- Sinus rhythm means that impulse is arising from SA node.
- PP interval (atrial) and RR interval (ventricular) are equal in sinus rhythm, but varies if the rhythm is irregular.
- To see rhythm, look RR interval.
- Always count atrial and ventricular rate separately (specially important in complete heart block).

CARDIAC AXIS

Definition

It is the sum of all the depolarization waves as they spread through the ventricles as seen from the front.

Axis Determination

- Axis can be derived most easily from the amplitude of QRS complex in L_I, L_{II} and L_{III}.
- The greatest amplitude of R wave in L_I or L_{II} or L_{III} indicates the proximity of cardiac axis to that lead.
- The axis lies at 90° to the isoelectric complex, i.e. positive and negative deflections are equal in any of the lead L_I, L_{II}, L_{III}, aVL, aVR and aVF.

Normal axis is between –30° to +90°.

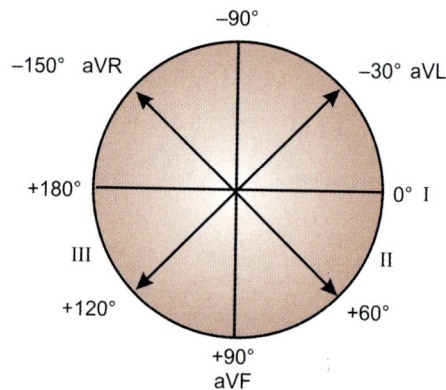

Quick and Simple Way of Determination of Cardiac Axis

- Positive QRS in both L_I and L_{II} means axis is normal.
- Positive QRS in L_I and negative in L_{III} (tall R in L_I and deep S in L_{III})—means left axis deviation.
- Negative QRS in L_I and positive in L_{III} ((tall R in L_{III} and deep S in L_I)—means right axis deviation.

Left Axis Deviation

When the cardiac axis is between –30° to –90°.

Causes are :
- Normal variant (with increased age).
- Left ventricular hypertrophy.
- Left anterior hemiblock.
- Left bundle branch block.
- Inferior myocardial infarction.
- T from apex of left ventricle.
- WPW syndrome (some).
- Pacing from the apex of the right or left ventricle (endocardial pacing).
- Emphysema.

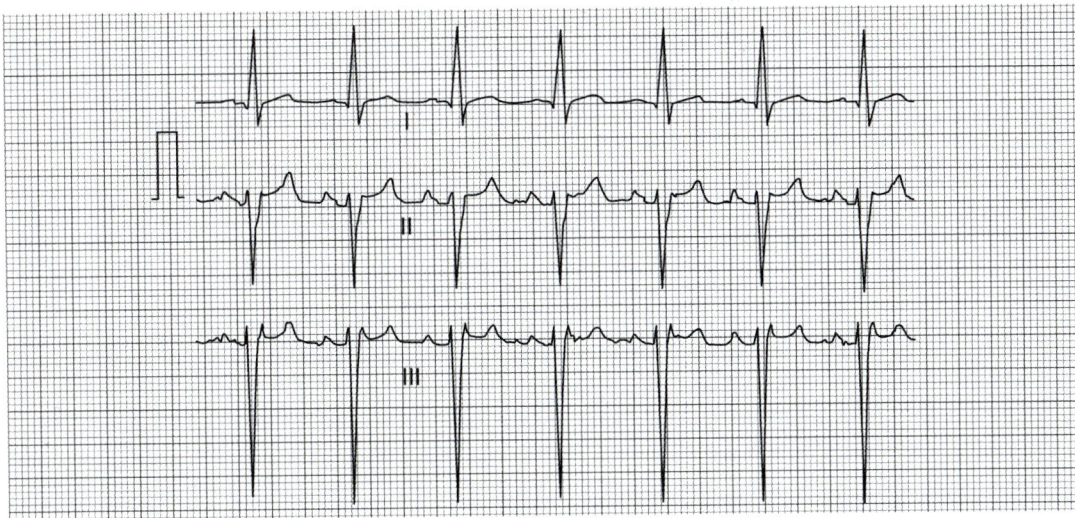

Left axis deviation

Right Axis Deviation

When the cardiac axis is between +90° to +180°.

Causes are:

- Normal variant (common in children and young adult).
- Right ventricular hypertrophy (due to any cause such as—chronic cor pulmonale, pulmonary embolism, congenital heart diseases, i.e. tetralogy of Fallot).
- Anterolateral myocardial infarction (high lateral MI).
- Left posterior hemiblock.
- Dextrocardia.
- WPW syndrome (type A).
- Right bundle branch block.
- Epicardial pacing.

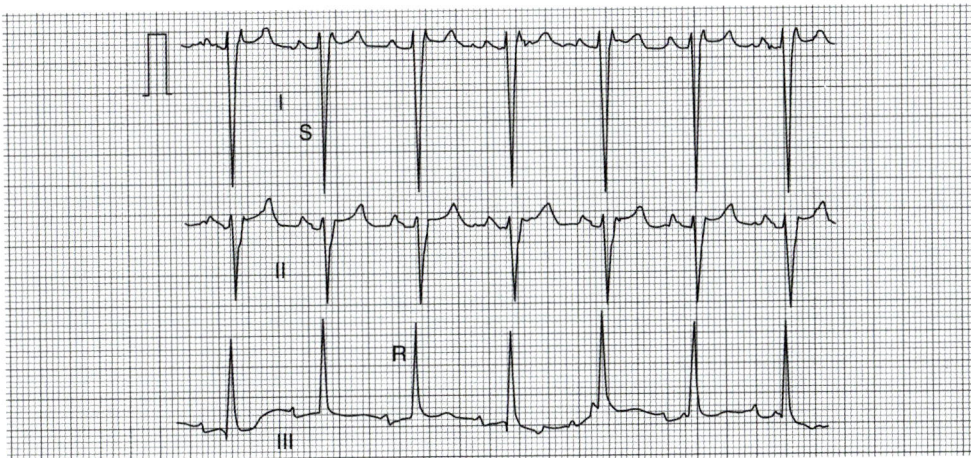

Right axis deviation

Intermediate Axis

Occurs when QRS lies between +180° and –90°. This term is used when the exact axis can not be determined (all 6 limb leads are biphasic).

NORMAL VARIANTS IN ECG

In an ECG, occasionally there are certain findings detected which are the normal variants observed in healthy individuals. These are commonly found in young adults and children:

- Early repolarization syndrome (in young black males).
- Left ventricular hypertrophy (in children and young adults).
- Short P-R interval.
- Right axis deviation (in children and young adults).
- Sinus arrhythmia with or without wandering pacemaker.
- Low voltage in obese people.
- First degree heart block.
- Wenckebach's phenomenon.
- Juvenile T wave pattern in children and young adults.

Careful interpretation is essential for the diagnosis. This should not be confused with underlying pathology. Details history and physical findings should be correlated with the ECG findings.

EXERCISE ECG (ETT)

Exercise ECG is a technique used to assess the cardiac response during exercise. Twelve lead ECG is recorded, while the patient walks or runs on a motorized treadmill. The traditional Bruce protocol is followed. The limb leads are placed on the shoulders and hips, rather than wrists and ankles. Blood pressure is recorded, symptoms are assessed such as anginal pain and ST depression or elevation is noted.

The test is positive, if there is anginal pain, blood pressure falls or fails to rise, ST depression > 1 mm (planar or down sloping depression is more important rather than up sloping ST depression which is non-specific). Sometimes, ST elevation may occur, which indicates transmural ischemia due to coronary spasm or critical stenosis.

The patient who can exercise < 6 min., generally have poor prognosis. Sustained fall of blood pressure indicates severe coronary artery disease.

ETT may be false positive (20%), or false negative. It has a specificity of 80% and sensitivity of 70%.

Indications of Exercise Testing

- To confirm the diagnosis of ischemic heart disease.
- To evaluate stable angina.
- Selecting patient for CABG, PTCA, cardiac catheterization.
- To assess prognosis following myocardial infarction.
- To assess outcome after coronary revascularization (coronary angioplasty).
- To diagnose and evaluate the treatment of exercise induced arrhythmias.

Contraindications of Exercise Testing

- In presence of unstable angina.
- Decompensated heart failure.
- Severe hypertension.

NB: False positive exercise test may occur in—Digitalis toxicity, hypokalemia, ventricular hypertrophy, bundle branch block, pre-excitation syndrome (WPW), mitral valve prolapse and female sex.

CHAPTER

II

ECG Changes in
Different Diseases

"ECG by itself is not to be all and end of the diagnosis.
Correlation of clinical diagnosis is essential and very vital"

LEFT VENTRICULAR HYPERTROPHY

ECG criteria of LVH (voltage criteria):
- S in V_1 + R in V_6 or V_5 > 35 mm (S V_1 + R V_6 > 35 mm).
  (This criteria is applicable only above 25 years of age).

Other criteria of LVH:
- R in V_5 (or V_6) > 26 mm.
- R in aVL > 11 mm (or 13 mm).
- R in aVF > 20 mm (also in L_{II} and L_{III}).
- R in L_I + S in L_{III} > 25 mm.
- R in L_I > 15 mm.
- R in V_6 is equal to or greater than R in V_5 (normally R in V_5 is taller than R in V_6).
- S in V_1 or V_2 > 25 mm.
- Sum of all QRS in all 12 leads > 175 mm.
- Left axis deviation (QRS between –30° and –90°).

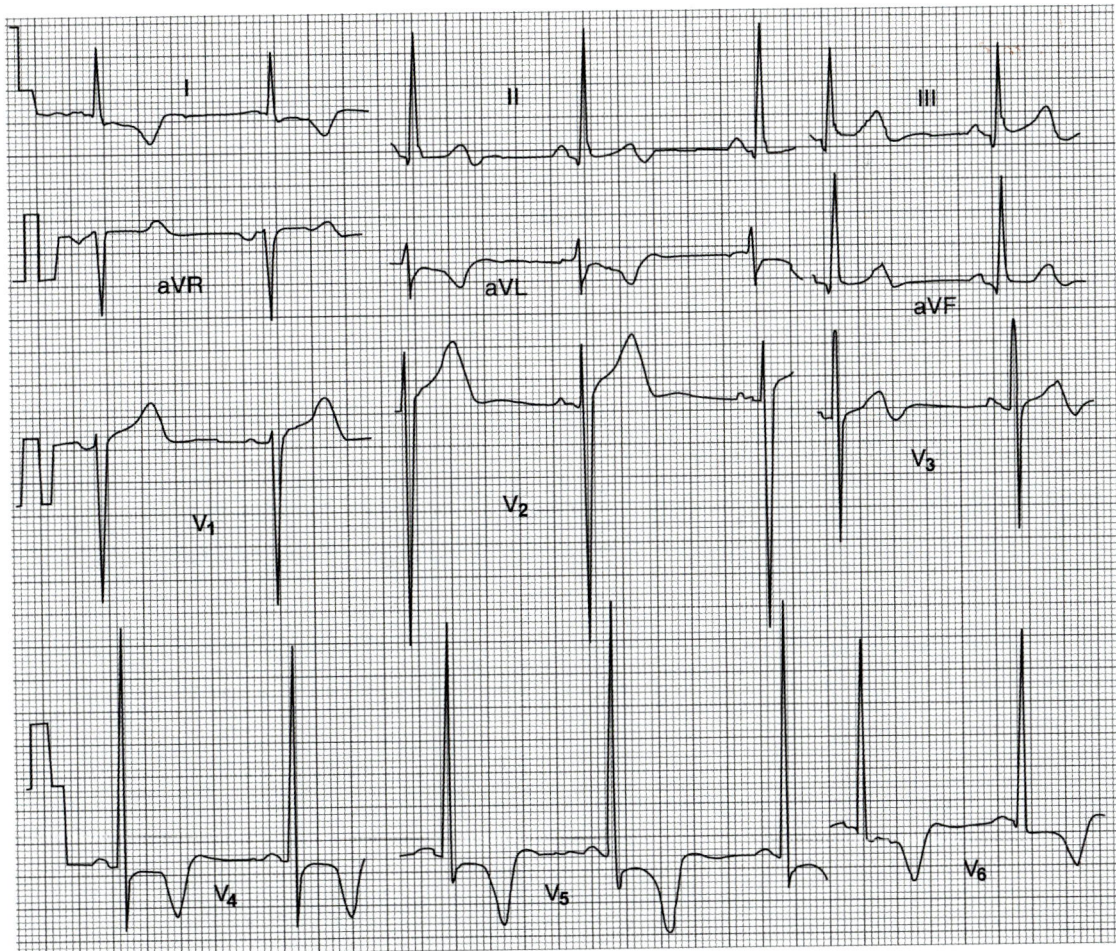

Left ventricular hypertrophy with strain

NB: In young and thin person, this voltage criteria is not diagnostic (in younger person, S in V_1 + R in V_5 or V_6 should be greater than 40 mm).

Q. How to confirm the diagnosis of LVH?
Ans. By echocardiography (M-mode).

Q. What are the causes of LVH?
Ans. As follows:
- Systemic hypertension.
- Aortic stenosis.
- Coarctation of aorta.
- Hypertrophic cardiomyopathy.
- VSD.
- Mitral regurgitation.
- Aortic regurgitation.
- Patent ductus arteriosus.
- Coronary artery disease (long standing).

Q. How to diagnose LVH clinically?
Ans. Apex beat is heaving in nature.
NB: Apex beat is not shifted, as the hypertrophy is concentric type—at the expense of the cavity.

ECG Criteria of LVH with Strain

- Findings of LVH.
- ST depression and T inversion (in L_1, aVL, V_4 to V_6).

Q. What are the differential diagnosis of LVH with strain?
Ans. As follows:
- Hypertrophic cardiomyopathy.
- Subendocardial myocardial infarction (T inversion is the cause of this confusion. However, in this case, T inversion is usually symmetrical, but no signs of LVH).

Q. How to confirm the diagnosis?
Ans. By echocardiography (2D or M mode).

RIGHT VENTRICULAR HYPERTROPHY

ECG Criteria
Tall R wave in V_1 > 7 mm (also deep S in V_5 or V_6).

Other Criteria
- R/S ratio in V_1 > 1 (R is > S in V_1).
- R in V_1 + S in V_5 or V_6 is equal to or > 10.5 mm.
- R in aVR > 5 mm.
- S in V_1 < 2 mm.
- Incomplete RBBB (rSR in V_1).
- QRS-wide.
- Small q in V_1.
- Right axis deviation (between + 90° and + 180°).

Q. What are the causes of tall R in V_1 ?

Ans.   See page no. **18.**

Q. What are the causes of RVH ?

Ans.   As follows:
- Chronic cor pulmonale.
- Mitral stenosis with pulmonary hypertension.
- Pulmonary hypertension (due to any cause).
- Pulmonary stenosis.
- Eisenmenger's syndrome.
- Fallot's tetralogy.
- ASD.
- VSD.
- Tricuspid regurgitation.

Q. How to diagnose RVH clinically ?

Ans.   By palpation of precordium:
- Left parasternal heave.
- Epigastric pulsation.

RVH with Strain
- Features of RVH.
- ST depression and T inversion (in V_1 and V_2).

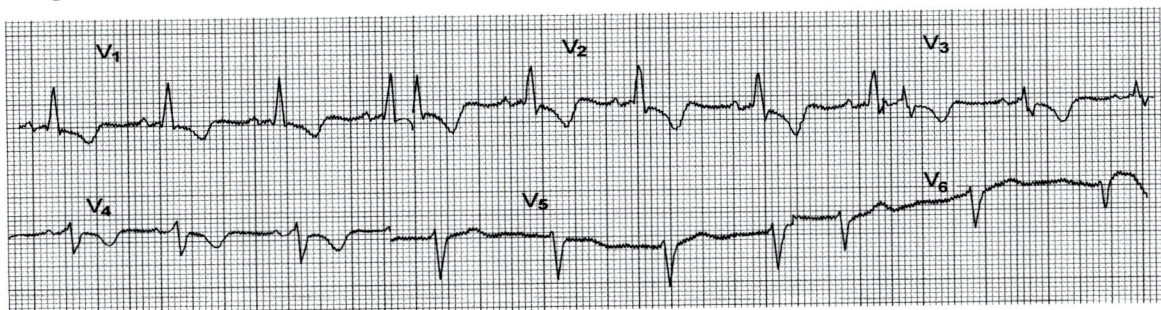

Right ventricular hypertrophy with strain

BIVENTRICULAR HYPERTROPHY
(LVH and RVH)

ECG Criteria

Findings of LVH and RVH as described above.

Other Findings

- LVH + right axis deviation.
- LVH + R > S in V_1.

Q. What are the causes of biventricular hypertrophy ?

Ans. As follows:

- Eisenmenger's syndrome (VSD or ASD or PDA with reversal of shunt).
- Hypertrophic cardiomyopathy.
- Multiple valvular heart diseases (Aortic stenosis + Pulmonary stenosis).

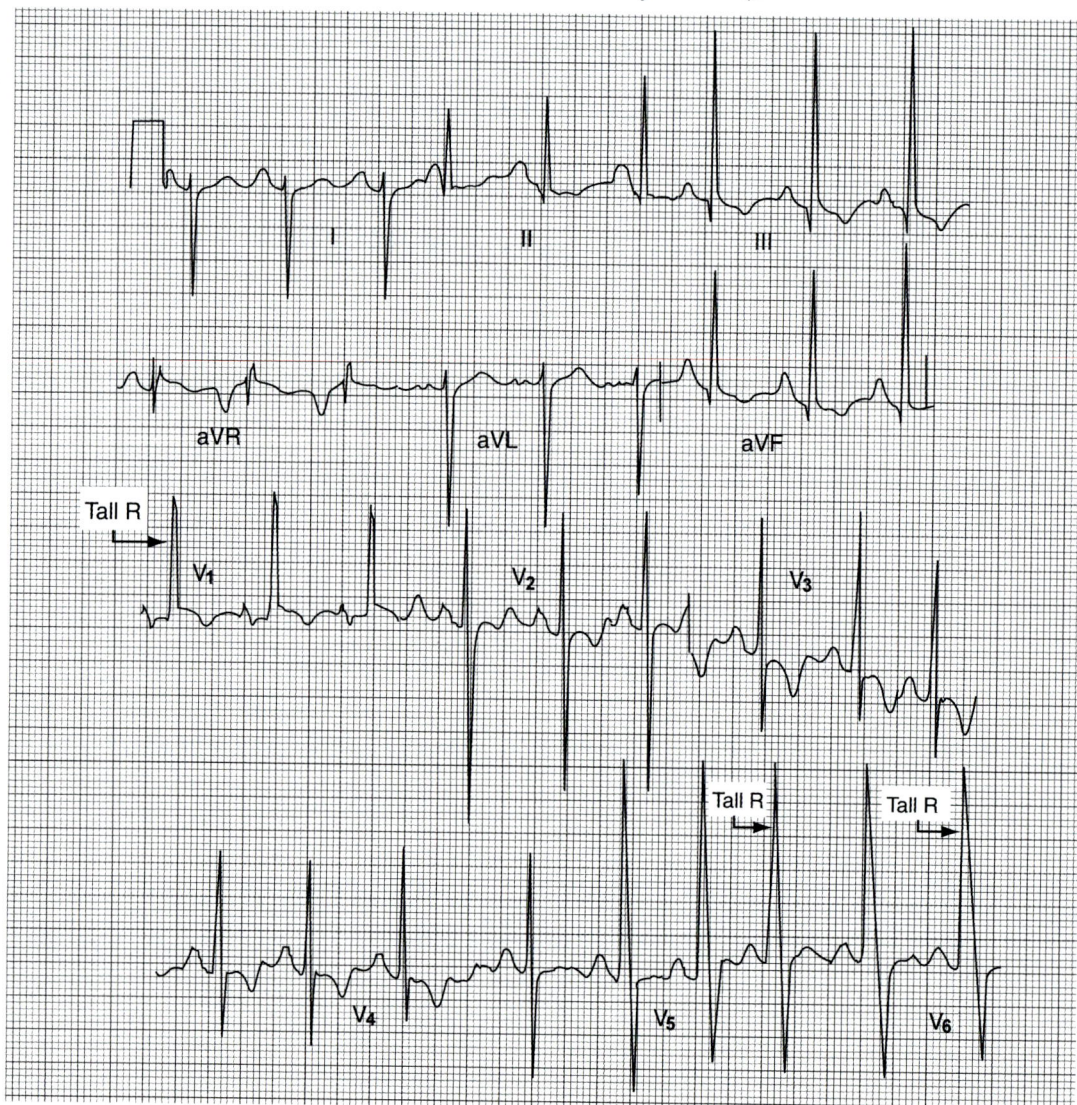

LEFT ATRIAL HYPERTROPHY

ECG Criteria

- P-Wide > 0.12 second (> 2.5 small squares), P may be notched or bifid (like M), called **P mitrale** (It is better seen in L_{II}, also in L_I and aVL).
- P in V_1-Biphasic, with prominent, deep negative deflection (> 1 mm depth) and small initial positive deflection.

Q. What does P mitrale indicate ?

Ans. It indicates left atrial hypertrophy or enlargement.

Q. What are the causes of P mitrale ?

Ans. As follows:
- Mitral stenosis (commonest).
- Mitral regurgitation.

Q. What are the causes of left atrial hypertrophy ?

Ans. As follows:
- Mitral valvular disease (MS or MR).
- Secondary to left ventricular hypertrophy due to any cause.
- ASD.

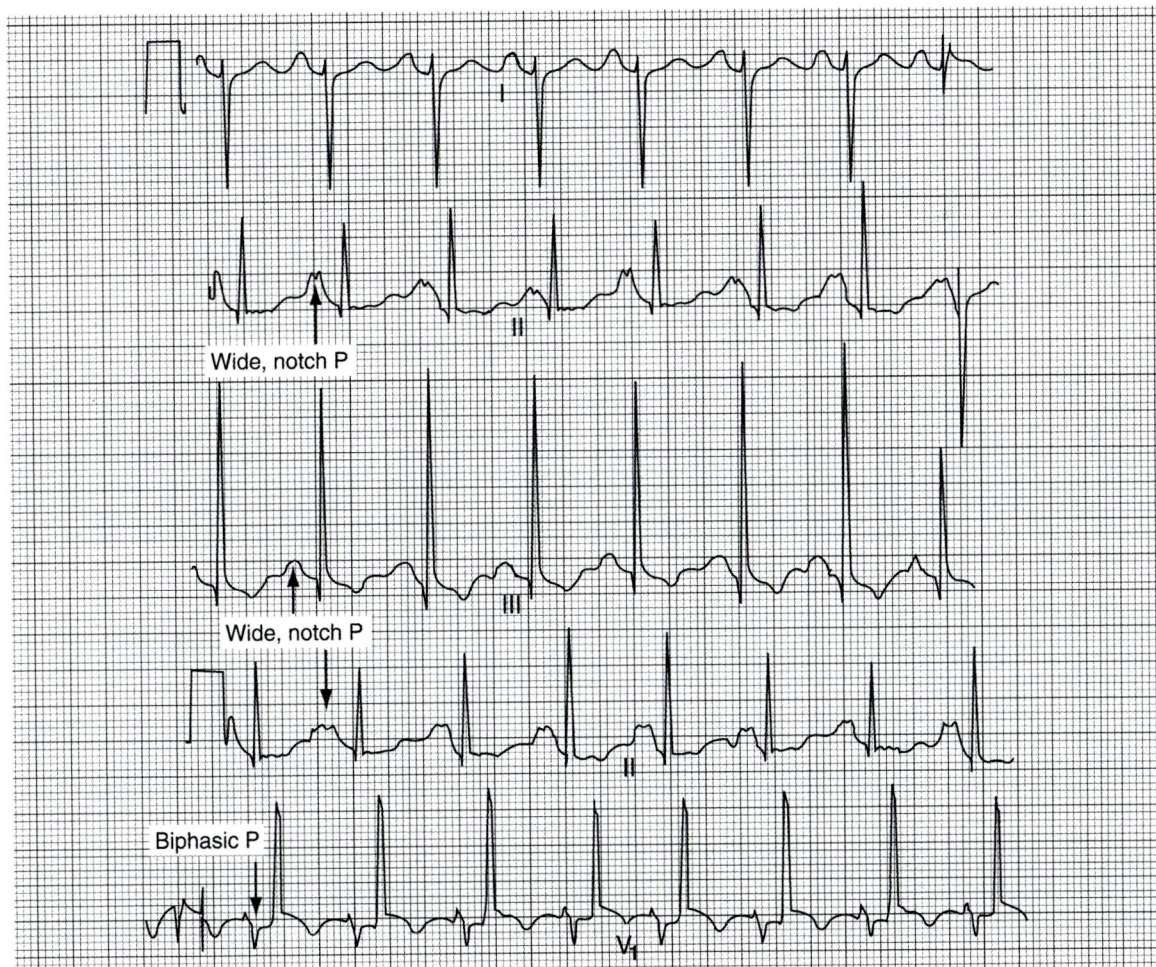

RIGHT ATRIAL HYPERTROPHY

ECG Criteria

- P - Tall, > 2.5 mm (> 2.5 small squares), better seen in L_{II}, L_{III}, aVF and sometimes in V_1 (Tall P is called **P pulmonale**).
- P in V_1 - Biphasic, tall initial positive deflection (> 1.5 mm) with a small negative deflection (only positive deflection may be present).

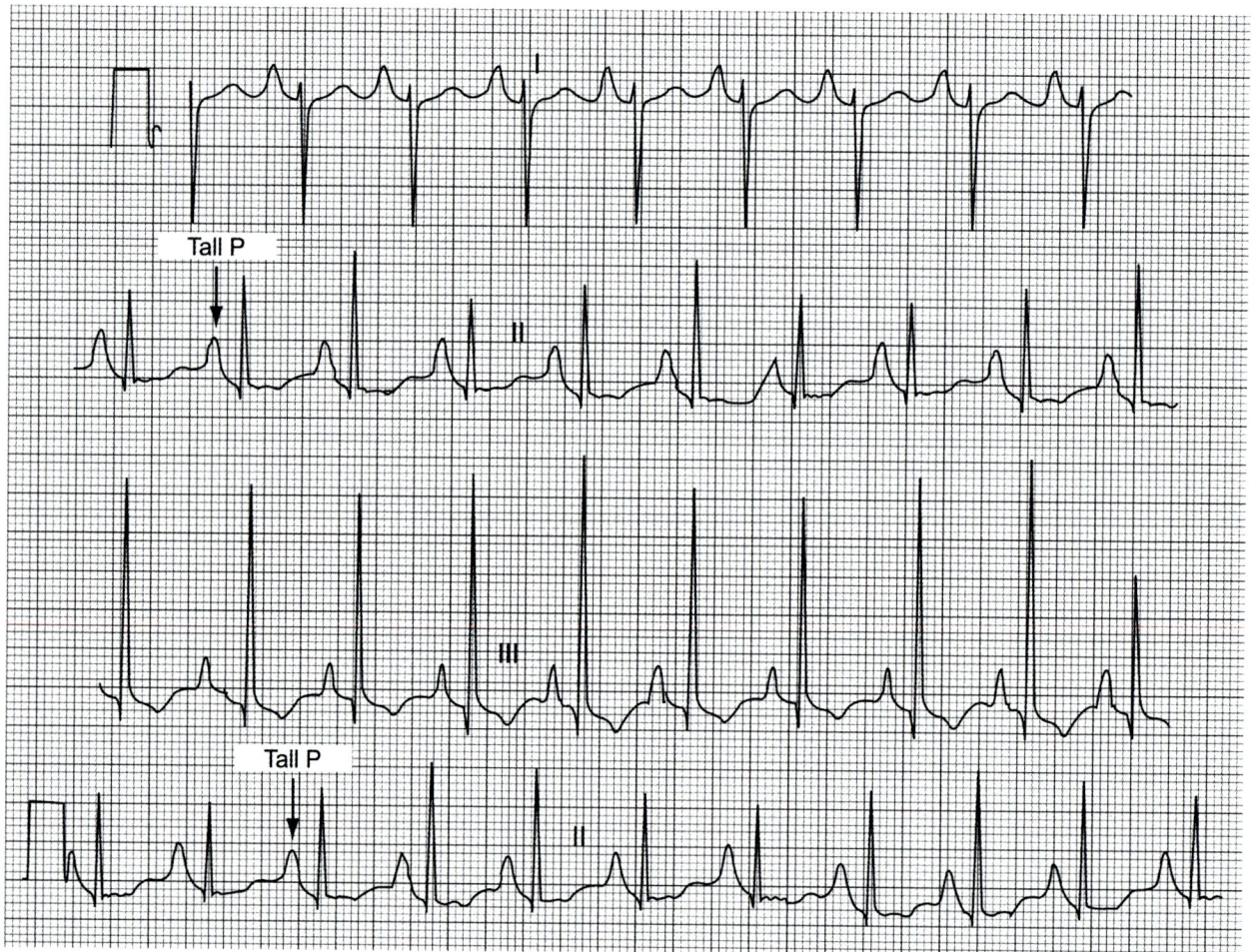

Q. What does P pulmonale indicate?

Ans. It indicates right atrial hypertrophy or enlargement.

(It is called P pulmonale, because it is commonly seen in severe pulmonary disease).

Q. What are the causes of P pulmonale?

Ans. As follows:

- COPD with chronic cor pulmonale (commonest).
- ASD.
- Tricuspid regurgitation or stenosis.
- Pulmonary stenosis.
- Pulmonary hypertension (due to any cause).
- Transient P pulmonale occurs in acute pulmonary embolism and acute severe asthma.

COMBINED LEFT AND RIGHT ATRIAL HYPERTROPHY (BIATRIAL HYPERTROPHY)

ECG Criteria

- Wide and notched P wave in all limb leads, also in V_4 to V_6.
- Tall P in all limb leads, also in V_2 and V_3.

Q. What are the causes of biatrial enlargement ?

Ans. As follows:

- Mitral stenosis with pulmonary hypertension.
- ASD.
- Lutembacher's syndrome (ASD with acquired mitral stenosis).
- Mitral stenosis with tricuspid regurgitation or tricuspid stenosis.

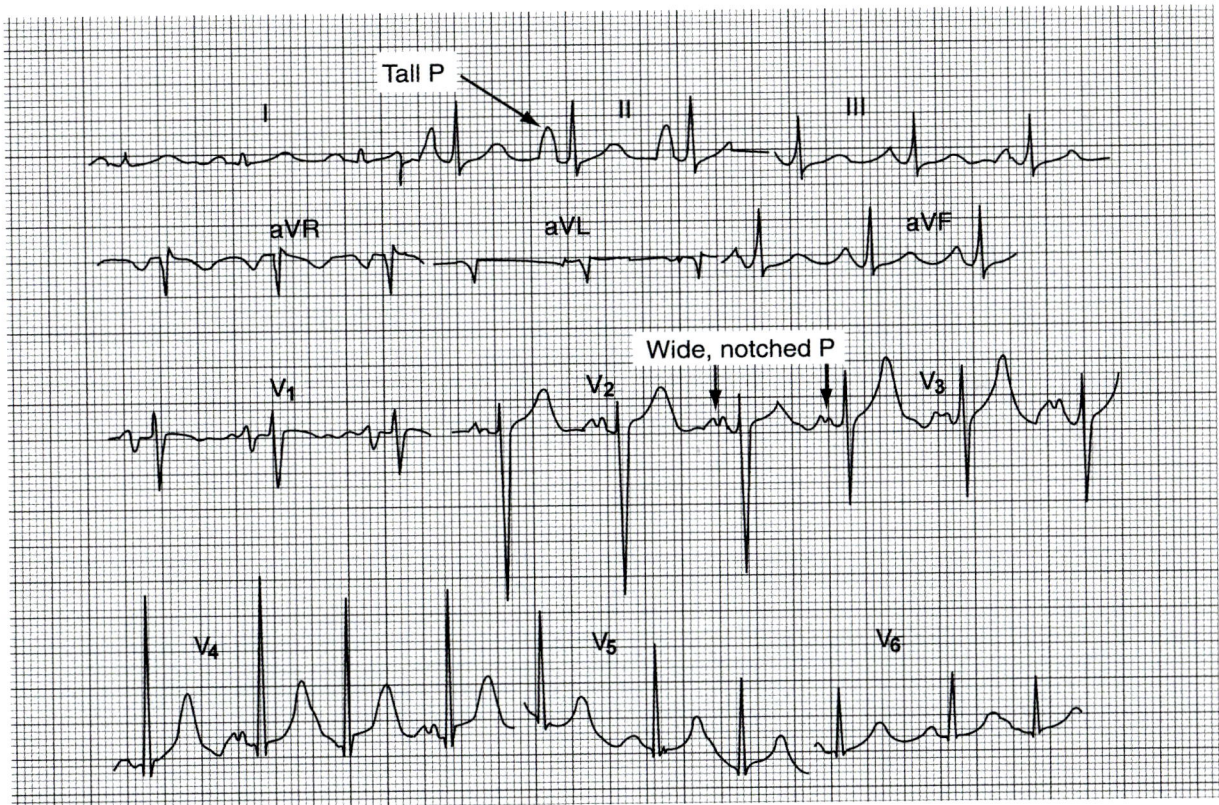

ATRIAL FIBRILLATION

ECG Criteria

- *P wave:* Absent (P may be replaced by fibrillary **f** wave).
- *Rhythm:* Irregularly irregular (R-R interval is irregular).
  (Atrial rate is very high and ventricular rate is less).

According to the rate, atrial fibrillation may be of 2 types:
- *Fast atrial fibrillation:* Heart rate >100 beats/min.
- *Slow atrial fibrillation:* Heart rate <100 beats/min.

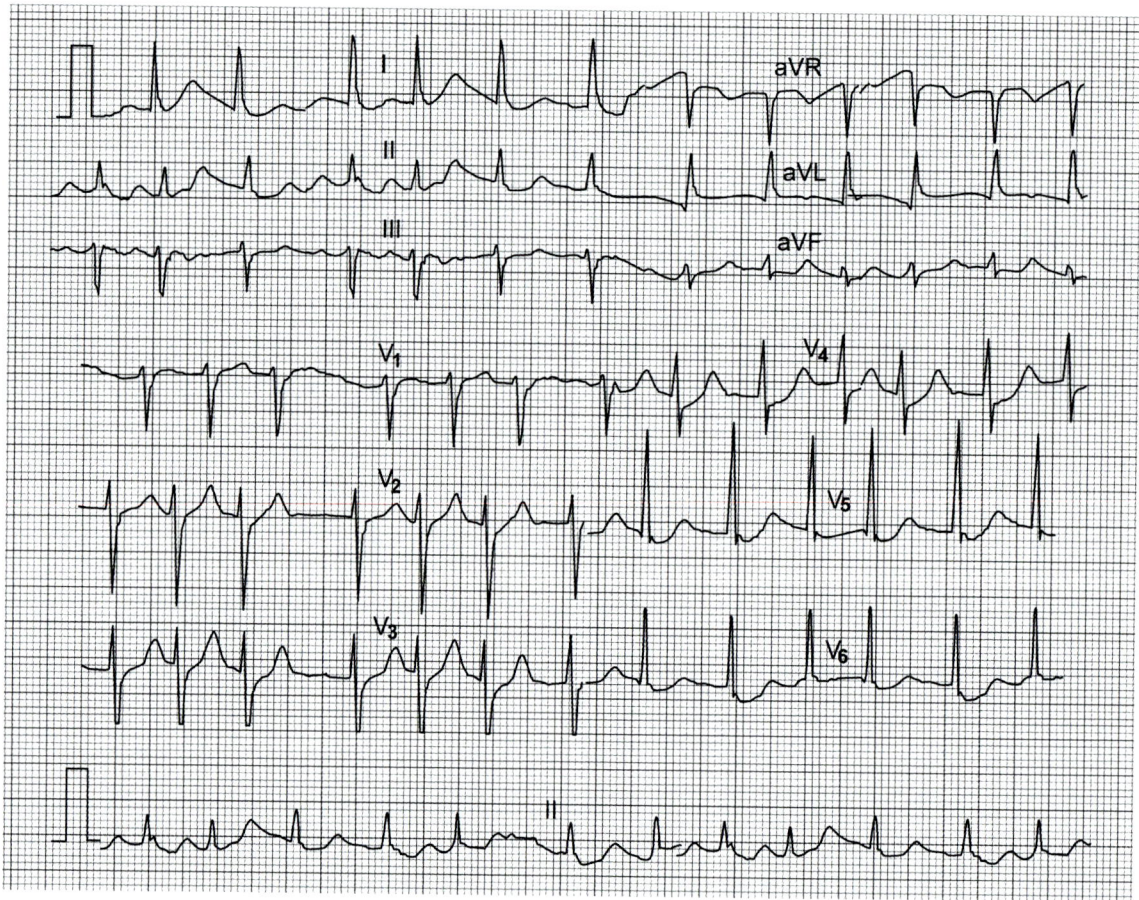

Q. What is atrial fibrillation?

Ans. It is an arrhythmia where atria beat rapidly, chaotically and ineffectively, while the ventricles respond at irregular intervals, producing the characteristic irregularly irregular pulse. Any conditions causing raised atrial pressure, increased atrial muscle mass, atrial fibrosis, inflammation and infiltration of the atrium can cause atrial fibrillation.

Q. What are the types of atrial fibrillation?

Ans. There are 3 types of atrial fibrillation:
- *Paroxysmal*: Discrete self-limiting episodes. May be persistent if underlying disease progresses.
- *Persistent*: Prolonged episode that can be terminated by electrical or chemical cardioversion.
- *Permanent*: Sinus rhythm cannot be restored.

Q. What are the causes of atrial fibrillation?

Ans. As follows:

- Chronic rheumatic heart disease with valvular lesions, commonly mitral stenosis (MS).
- Coronary artery disease (commonly, acute myocardial infarction).
- Thyrotoxicosis.
- Hypertension.
- Lone atrial fibrillation (idiopathic in 10% cases).
- Others—atrial septal defect (ASD), chronic constrictive pericarditis, acute pericarditis, cardiomyopathy, myocarditis, sick sinus syndrome, coronary bypass surgery, valvular surgery, acute chest infection (pneumonia), thoracic surgery, electrolyte imbalance (hypokalemia, hyponatremia), alcohol, pulmonary embolism.

    NB: First 3 causes always top of the list.

Q. If the patient is young, what are the causes of atrial fibrillation?

Ans. As follows:

- Chronic rheumatic heart disease with valvular lesions, commonly mitral stenosis (MS).
- Thyrotoxicosis.
- Others—atrial septal defect (ASD), acute pericarditis, myocarditis, pneumonia.

Q. If the patient is elderly, what are the causes of atrial fibrillation?

Ans. As follows:

- Coronary artery disease (commonly acute myocardial infarction).
- Thyrotoxicosis.
- Hypertension.
- Lone atrial fibrillation (idiopathic in 10% cases).
- Others—see above (unusual or less in chronic rheumatic heart disease).

Q. What are the causes of temporary atrial fibrillation?

Ans. As follows:

- Acute myocardial infarction.
- Myocarditis (due to any cause).
- Pneumonia.
- Electrolyte imbalance.

Q. What are the complications of atrial fibrillation?

Ans. As follows:

- Systemic and pulmonary embolism (systemic from left atrium and pulmonary from right atrium). Annual risk is 5% (1 to 12%).
- Heart failure.

Q. What is lone atrial fibrillation?

Ans. Lone atrial fibrillation means atrial fibrillation without any cause. Genetic predisposition may be responsible.

- Fifty percent patients with paroxysmal atrial fibrillation and 20% with persistent or permanent atrial fibrillation have no cause and heart is normal.
- Lone atrial fibrillation usually occurs below 60 years of age.
- It may be intermittent, later may become permanent.
- Prognosis—low-risk of CVD (0.5% per year). Usually life span is normal.

Q. What history would you like to take in atrial fibrillation ?

Ans. I would take the history of:
- Rheumatic fever.
- Ischemic heart disease.
- History of thyrotoxicosis.
- Other history of any disease (according to cause).

Q. What are the clinical findings of atrial fibrillation?

Ans. As follows:
- Pulse—irregularly irregular (irregular in rhythm and volume).
- BP—may be hypertensive.
- Examination of heart (heart rate to see pulsus deficit, mitral valvular or other cardiac disease).
- Thyroid status (warm sweaty hands, tremor, tachycardia, exophthalmos, thyroid gland size).

Q. If a patient with AF is unconscious, what is the likely cause?

Ans. Cerebral embolism (usually with right sided hemiplegia).

Q. How to treat atrial fibrillation?

Ans. Aim of treatment is as follows:
- Control of heart rate.
- Restoration of sinus rhythm and prevention of recurrence.
- Treatment of primary cause.

Treatment (according to the type):

1. Paroxysmal atrial fibrillation:
   - *If asymptomatic:* Does not require any treatment, follow-up the case.
   - *If troublesome symptoms are present:* β-blocker. Other drugs—flecainide or propafenone may be given. Amiodarone is effective in prevention. Low dose aspirin to prevent thromboembolism.
   - *If bradycardia is present (in sinoatrial disease):* Permanent over drive atrial pacing (60% effective).
   - *In some intractable cases:* Radiofrequency ablation may be required, who does not have structural heart disease (70% effective).

2. Persistent atrial fibrillation:
   - *Control of heart rate:* β-blocker, digoxin or calcium channel blocker (verapamil, diltiazem). Combination of digoxin and atenolol may be used.
   - *To control rhythm:* DC cardioversion may be done safely. It may be repeated, if relapse occurs. Concomitant use of β-blocker or amiodarone may be used to prevent recurrence.

3. Permanent atrial fibrillation:
   - *Control of heart rate:* Digoxin, β-blocker, calcium channel blocker (verapamil or diltiazem).
   - *In some cases:* Transvenous radiofrequency ablation may be done (it induces complete heart block. So, permanent pacemaker should be given).

Q. What is the role of anticoagulant in atrial fibrillation ?

Ans. Usually, warfarin is given who are at risk of stroke. Target INR is 2 to 3. It reduces stroke in 2/3rd cases. Aspirin reduces stroke in 1/5th cases. Anticoagulation is indicated in patient with atrial fibrillation having risk factors for thromboembolism.

Risk factors for thromboembolism in atrial fibrillation:
- Previous ischemic stroke or TIA
- Mitral valve disease.

- Age over 65 years.
- Hypertension.
- Diabetes mellitus.
- Heart failure.
- Echocardiographic evidence of left ventricular dysfunction, left atrial enlargement or mitral anular calcification.

Risk groups with thromboembolism (nonrheumatic)
- *Very high:* Previous stroke or TIA (12%).
- *High:* Age > 65 years and one other risk factor (6.5%).
- *Moderate:* (i) Age > 65 years, no risk factor (4%), (ii) Age < 65 years, other risk factor (4%).
- *Low:* Age < 65 years, no risk factor (1.2%).

NB: Remember the following points:

- In lone atrial fibrillation—aspirin may be given to prevent thromboembolism.
- Age < 65 years and young with no structural heart disease—aspirin may be beneficial. No warfarin.
- Target INR following anticoagulation is 2 to 3.

ASHMAN PHENOMENON

Definition

It is a type of aberrant ventricular conduction that occurs during atrial fibrillation when a long RR interval is followed by short RR interval.

ECG in Ashman phenomenon shows:
- Atrial fibrillation.
- Followed by supraventricular impulse which are aberrantly conducted in ventricles, resulting wide QRS (confuses with ventricular ectopics), i.e. wide QRS in between atrial fibrillation.

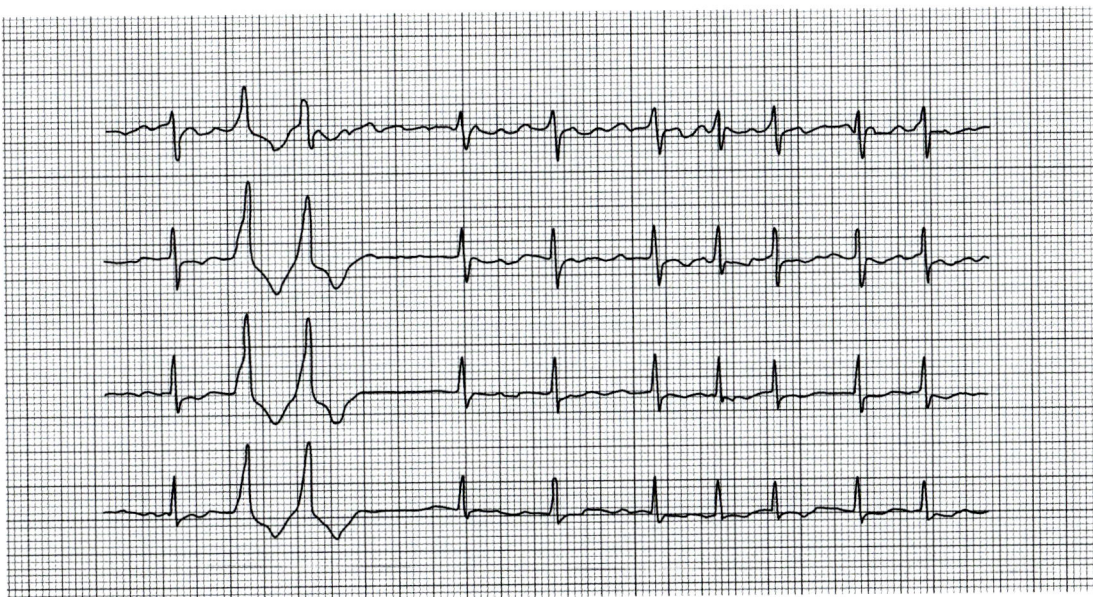

ATRIAL FLUTTER

ECG Criteria

- P—saw toothed appearance (normal P is replaced by flutter or F wave. Better seen in lead II, III, aVF, and V_1).
- RR—regular (may be irregular, when there is variable block).

  (Atrial rate—250 to 350 beats /minute, ventricular rate—variable, may be 2:1, 3:1, 4:1, it is then called flutter with variable block).

NB: Occasionaly, atrial fibrillation and flutter may be present together, it is called flutter fibrillation.

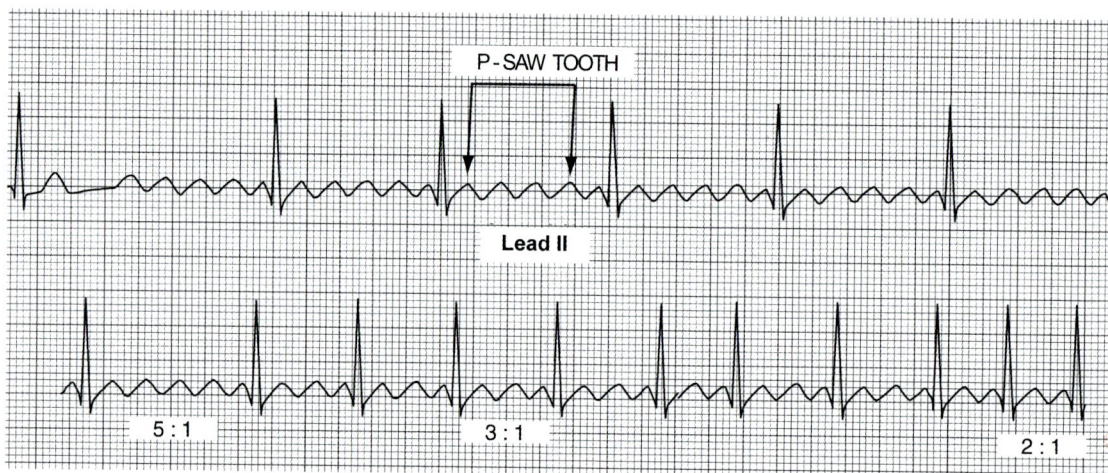

Q. What is atrial flutter ? What are the causes of atrial flutter?

Ans.   Atrial flutter is characterized by large re-entry circuit within the right atrium, usually encircling the tricuspid annulus. For causes, see in atrial fibrillation (same causes).

Q. What is the treatment of atrial flutter?

Ans.   As follows:

- To control heart rate—digoxin, β-blocker or verapamil may be used. Amiodarone, propafenone or flecainide may be used and these can be used to prevent recurrence.
- If no response and patient has troublesome symptoms—DC cardioversion or atrial overdrive pacing may be done.
- In persistent or troublesome symptoms—radiofrequency catheter ablation.

NB: Digoxin sometimes converts flutter to atrial fibrillation, due to shortening of atrial refractory period. This may be followed by conversion to normal rhythm, when digoxin is stopped.

Q. What is the differential diagnosis of atrial flutter?

Ans.   When atrial flutter is associated with regular 2:1 AV block, it is difficult to differentiate from supraventricular or sinus tachycardia, because flutter waves are buried in QRS complex.

In such case, diagnosis can be done by carotid sinus massage or intravenous adenosine which temporarily increases the degree of AV block and reveals the flutter waves (F wave).

NB: Remember the following points:

- Atrial flutter is always associated with organic heart disease.
- Drugs which can restore and maintain sinus rhythm are—sotalol, flecainide, disopyramide, propafenone.
- DC cardioversion is the easiest way to convert sinus rhythm.

VENTRICULAR ECTOPIC

ECG Criteria

- P—absent.
- QRS—wide > 0.12 second (3 small squares).
- T—opposite to major deflection.

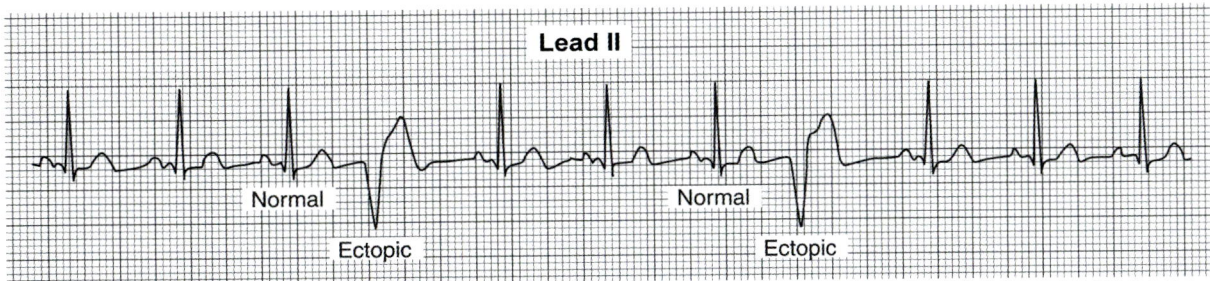

Q. What are the types of ventricular ectopics?

Ans. Ventricular ectopics may be of different types:

- *Unifocal:* Similar configuration of ectopics in all leads and originates from a single ectopic ventricular focus (QRS-similar).
- *Multifocal:* Variable configuration of ectopics in same lead, because ectopics originate from different focus of ventricle (QRS-variable).
- *Interpolated ventricular ectopics:* It means when ventricular ectopics occur between two normal sinus beat without compensatory pause (it is usually associated with sinus bradycardia).

Other Types

- *Couplet:* Two ventricular ectopics in a row, multifocal.
- *Triplet:* Three ventricular ectopics in a row (runs of ectopic, three or more ventricular ectopics in a row, may be taken as ventricular tachycardia).
- *Ventricular bigeminy*: Every one normal beat followed by ventricular ectopic.
- *Ventricular trigeminy:* Every two normal beats followed by ventricular ectopic.
- *Ventricular quadrigeminy:* Every three normal beats followed by ventricular ectopic.
- *Grouped ventricular ectopics*: 2 to 5 consecutive ventricular ectopics.

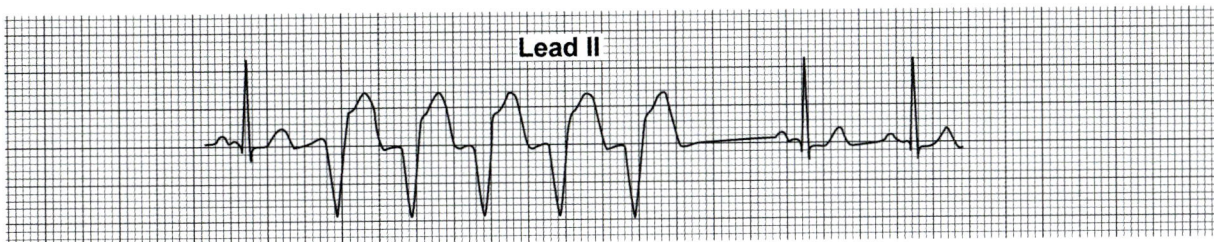

Runs of ventricular ectopics

NB: Remember the following points:

- Ventricular ectopics originating in left ventricle resembles RBBB pattern.
- Ventricular ectopics originating in right ventricle resembles LBBB pattern.

Q. What is R on T phenomenon?

Ans. It means R wave of ventricular ectopic occur on or near the peak of previous T wave. It is common in acute myocardial infarction (rare in other case). This is also called malignant ectopic, as it may induce ventricular fibrillation or ventricular tachycardia.

Q. How grading is done for ventricular ectopic ?

Ans. Grading is done according to the severity of ectopic.

In acute myocardial infarction, Lown's classification is as follows:
- Grade 1—no ventricular ectopic.
- Grade 2—ventricular ectopics < 30/hour (not > 1/minute).
- Grade 3—frequent ventricular ectopics > 30 /hour.
- Grade 4 A—couplet (2 consecutive ventricular ectopics).
- Grade 4 B—repetitive (3 or more consecutive ventricular ectopics).
- Grade 5—multiple ventricular ectopics (R on T).

Q. How to treat ventricular ectopics?

Ans. As follows:
- In the absence of any heart disease and in asymptomatic case—no treatment is necessary. β-blocker may be used.
- With organic heart disease—treatment of primary cause.
- Antiarrhythmic drug does not improve, and may even worsen the prognosis.

NB: Remember the following points:

- Ventricular ectopics may be found in normal people, incidence increases with age.
- Ventricular ectopic in normal heart is prominent at rest and disappear with exercise. No treatment is necessary, occasionally β-blocker may be given for palpitation. Prognosis is good.
- Multifocal ventricular ectopics and also in pairs are always abnormal. Usually, indicates serious myocardial disease.

Q. What are the causes of ventricular ectopic?

Ans. As follows:
- Normally in young adults, also in anxiety, excess caffeine, alcohol.
- Acute myocardial infarction.
- Myocarditis.
- Cardiomyopathy.
- Valvular heart disease.
- Mitral valve prolapse.
- Hypertensive heart disease.
- Electrolyte imbalance (specially hypokalemia).
- Digoxin toxicity.
- Hypoxemia.

VENTRICULAR TACHYCARDIA

ECG Criteria

- P wave—absent (Dissociated P wave may be seen).
- QRS—broad > 0.14 second, abnormal or bizarre pattern.
- Rate > 100 beats /minute (usually, 140 to 220 beats/min).

Other Criteria

- Occasional capture beat is present (normal sinus P, QRS and T in between ventricular tachycardia).
- Fusion beat (conducted sinus impulse fuses with impulse from tachycardia).
- QRS—in chest leads (V_1 to V_6) either all positive or all negative (called ventricular concordance).

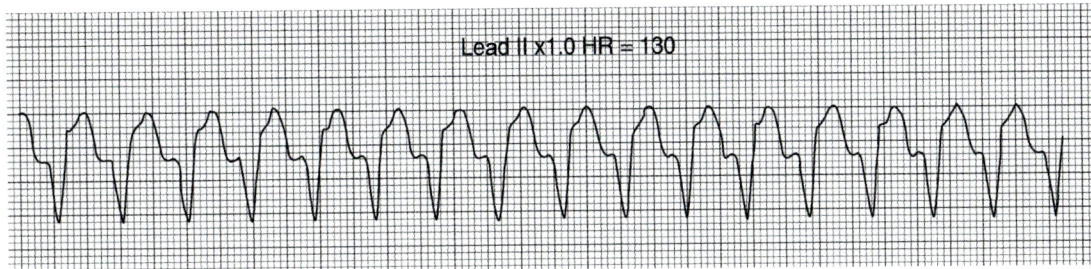

Lead II x 1.0 HR = 130

Q. What are the causes of ventricular tachycardia?

Ans.   As follows:
- Acute myocardial infarction.
- Myocarditis.
- Cardiomyopathy.
- Chronic ischemic heart disease (specially with poor left ventricular function).
- Ventricular aneurysm.
- Mitral valve prolapse.
- Electrolyte imbalance (mainly hypokalemia and hypomagnesemia).
- Idiopathic.

Q. What is the differential diagnosis of ventricular tachycardia (VT)?

Ans.   Ventricular tachycardia is confused with supraventricular tachycardia with bundle branch block or WPW syndrome (aberrant conduction). Ventricular tachycardia is more common.

Q. How to differentiate between VT and SVT with bundle branch block?

Ans.   In ECG, points suggesting VT are as follows:
- History of myocardial infarction.
- QRS > 0.14 sec.
- Extreme left axis deviation.
- AV dissociation (Dissociated P wave may be seen).
- Narrow QRS capture complex beat (normal sinus beat in the middle of VT).
- Fusion beat (conducted sinus impulse fuses with impulse from ventricular tachycardia).
- Ventricular concordance (either all positive or all negative in chest leads).
- Bifid R in V_1 with a tall first peak in V_1 and deep S in V_6.
- RR interval is regular.
- No response to carotid sinus massage or IV adenosine (but it terminates SVT).

Q. What are the types of ventricular tachycardia?

Ans. Two types:

- Sustained ventricular tachycardia (lasts > 30 sec.). Heart rate is 150 to 250/minute.
- Nonsustained ventricular tachycardia (lasts < 30 sec.), consists of short salvos (> 3 or more).

VT may be present in normal healthy heart (called normal heart VT), because of abnormal automaticity in right ventricular outflow tract or one of the fascicles of left bundle branch. In these cases, prognosis is good and catheter ablation can be curative.

Q. What is nonsustained ventricular tahchycardia (NSVT)?

Ans. It is defined as VT > 3 or more consecutive beats, but last < 30 seconds, at a rate > 100/min.

- NSVT that occurs in normal heart (6%)—no treatment is necessary.
- NSVT with heart disease—treated with β-blocker. In some cases, specially with myocardial infarction and ejection fraction 30% or less, Implantable Cardioverter Defibrillator (ICD) may be helpful.

Q. How to treat sustained ventricular tachycardia?

Ans. As follows:

- If the patient is hemodynamically unstable (such as hypotension, systolic < 90 or heart failure)—cardioversion (DC shock).
- If the patient is hemodynamically stable—IV amiodarone bolus followed by IV infusion. IV lignocaine 100 mg bolus (1 to 2 mg/kg). It is followed by lignocaine infusion–2 to 4 mg/minute for 24 to 36 hours. It depresses left ventricular function causing hypotension or acute heart failure.
- If fails—cardioversion should be done.
- To prevent recurrence—β-blocker, oral amiodarone may be used.
- Correction of hypokalemia, hypomagnesemia, hypoxemia and acidosis should be done.
- If all fail—automatic implantable cardioverter defibrillator device (ICD) or radiofrequency ablation of focus of ventricular tachycardia should be done.

Q. What is accelerated idioventricular rhythm? (also called slow VT).

Ans. It means slow ventricular tachycardia (rate slightly higher than the sinus rate). There is enhanced ectopic ventricular rhythm at the rate of 100 to 110 / minute (faster than intrinsic ventricular pacemaker rate of 15 to 40 beat /minute).

- Accelerated idioventricular rhythm is most commonly seen within the first 48 to 72 hours of acute myocardial infarction and frequently after successful reperfusion during acute myocardial infarction (following thrombolysis or angioplasty). Also, after cardiac surgery.
- It is more likely a benign arrhythmia.
- It is asymptomatic, transient, self-limiting and does not require treatment.

Q. What are the causes of wide-complex tachycardia?

Ans. As follows:

- Ventricular tachycardia.
- Supraventricular tachycardia with aberrant conduction.
- WPW syndrome.

Q. What is bidirectional ventricular tachycardia?

Ans. When ventricular tachycardia is associated with two different QRS complex alternating with every other beat, it is called bidirectional ventricular tachycardia. It may occur in severe digoxin toxicity, prognosis is grave in that case.

TORSADES DE POINTES

ECG Criteria

- QRS—wide, bizarre, irregular of different or changing amplitude from upright to inverted position (different configuration of QRS).
- QT—prolonged.
  (ECG looks like ventricular tachycardia with different configuration of QRS).

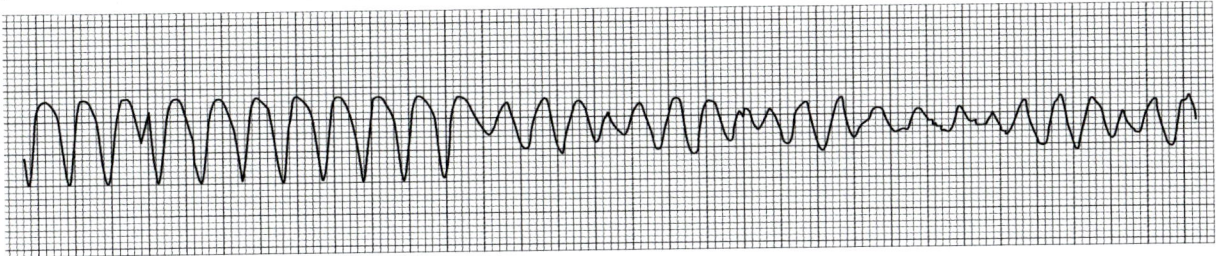

Q. What is torsades de pointes?

Ans. It is a type of polymorphic ventricular tachycardia characterized by "twisting of the points" of QRS in ECG, which shows rapid irregular complex from upright to inverted position. During the period of sinus rhythm, ECG shows prolonged Q-T interval.

It is usually nonsustained, occurs in repetitive burst, lasting for few seconds.

- It may progress to ventricular fibrillation and sudden death.
- Torsades de pointes is usually initiated by a ventricular ectopic with prolonged QT interval and broad T wave (may be R on T phenomenon).
- It is more common in women, triggered by multiple drugs and hypokalemia.

Q. What are the causes torsades de pointes?

Ans. As follows:

- Electrolyte imbalance—hypokalemia, hypomagnesemia, hypocalcemia.
- Drugs—quinidine, procainamide, amiodarone, disopyramide, sotalol, tricyclic antidepressant, erythromycin, cisapride, chlorpromazine and other phenothiazines.
- Acute myocardial infarction.
- Acute myocarditis.
- Bradycardia (as in sinus node disease, complete heart block).
- Congenital syndrome such as Jervell-Lange-Nielson syndrome (autosomal recessive), Romano-Ward syndrome (autosomal dominant).

Q. What is the treatment of torsades de pointes ?

Ans. As follows:

- Electrolyte imbalance should be corrected.
- Causative drugs should be stopped.
- IV magnesium—8 mmol for 15 minutes, then 72 mmol over 24 hours should be given in all cases.
- The problem is best treated by cardiac pacing (atrial, or in AV block—ventricular or dual chamber).
- If no pacing is available—isoprenaline infusion is a suitable alternative (it is avoided in congenital long QT syndrome).
- If all fail and there is history of sudden death in family—implantable defibrillator.
- In congenital long QT syndrome—β-blocker is helpful. Other treatment—left stellate ganglion block, or implantable cardioverter defibrillator may help.

VENTRICULAR FIBRILLATION

ECG Criteria

QRS—Chaotic, wide, bizarre, irregular.

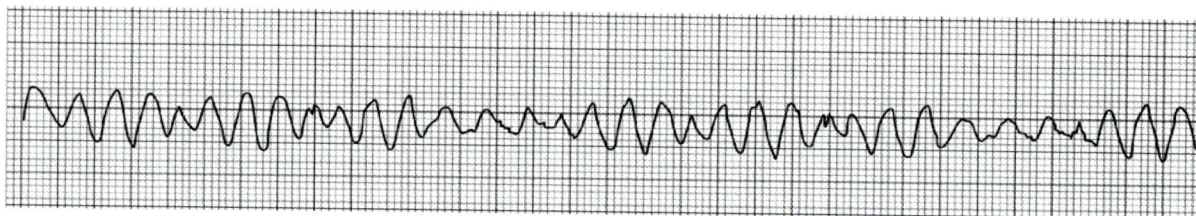

Q. What is ventricular fibrillation?

Ans. This is a type of ventricular arrhythmia characterized by rapid, irregular, ineffective and uncoordinated ventricular activation with no mechanical effect. There is chaotic electrical disturbance of ventricles, with impulse occuring irregularly at rate of 300 to 500/min. Ventricular contraction is uncoordinated and ventricular filling and emptying ceases. Cardiac output falls to zero. Ventricular fibrillation is the more common cause of sudden death. It may occur as a primary arrhythmia or as a complication in acute myocardial infarction.

Q. What are the findings, if you examine the patient clinically?

Ans. As follows:
- Pulse—absent.
- BP—not recordable.
- Respiration—ceases or absent.
- Patient—unconscious.
- Pupil—dilated, less or no reaction to light.
- Heart sounds—absent.

Q. What are the causes of ventricular fibrillation?

Ans. As follows:
- Acute myocardial infarction.
- Electrolyte imbalance (hypokalemia, hypomagnesemia).
- Electrocution.
- Others—drowning, drug overdose (digitalis, adrenaline, isoprenaline).

Q. What is the treatment of ventricular fibrillation?

Ans. As follows:
- Immediate defibrillation—200 Joules. If no response, another shock with 200 Joules is given. If still no response, another shock with 360 Joules is given.
- If three shocks unsuccessful—adrenaline is given IV, followed by cardiopulmonary resuscitation.
- If defibrillator is not available—cardiopulmonary resuscitation should be given.
- The patient who survives from VF in the absence of identifiable cause is at high-risk of sudden death. This case is treated with implantable cardioverter defibrillator.

NB: Remember the following points:

- VF is invariably fatal, immediate treatment is necessary if death is to be prevented.
- Effective circulation and ventilation must be obtained within 4 minutes to prevent, if irreversible brain damage.
- Sinus rhythm can usually be restored by defibrillation.

HEART BLOCK

Heart block or conduction block may occur at any level in the conductive system of the heart. Block in AV node or His bundle result in atrioventricular (AV) block and block lower in conducting system produces bundle branch block.

Q. What is heart block ?

Ans. Heart block is defined as defect in either initiation or conduction of cardiac impulse.

Q. What are the sites of heart block ?

Ans. Sites may be:
- SA node.
- AV node.
- Bundle of His.
- Branches of bundle of His.

Q. What are the types of heart block ?

Ans. Heart block are of different types. Such as:
1. SA block.
2. Atrioventricular block
   It is of 3 types:
   - 1st degree AV block.
   - 2nd degree AV block. It is of 2 types:
     — Mobitz type 1 (Wenckebach's phenomenon).
     — Mobitz type 2.
   - Complete heart block or 3rd degree heart block.
3. Bundle branch block:
   - Right bundle branch block (RBBB).
   - Left bundle branch block (LBBB).

Q. What is hemiblock?

Ans. It means when there is block involving one of the fascicles of left bundle branch.

It is diagnosed by seeing the axis deviation in ECG.
- When there is left axis deviation—it is called left anterior hemiblock.
- When there is right axis deviation—it is called left posterior hemiblock.

NB: There may be more block either two or three. In that case it is called bifascicular or trifascicular block.

SA BLOCK

ECG Criteria

- Absence of one P-QRS-T complex.
- P-P (or R-R) is double than the next P-P (or R-R).

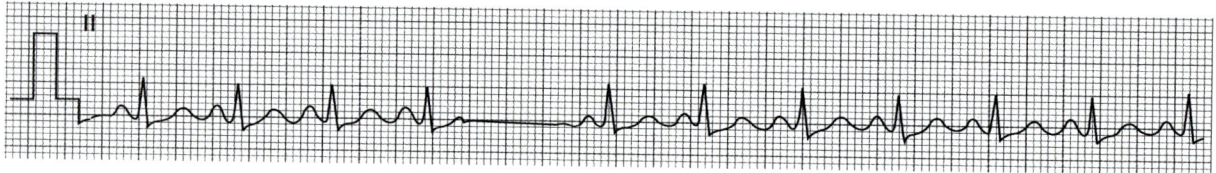

Q. What are the differential diagnosis?

Ans. As follows:

- Sinus arrest.
- Sinus standstill.

Q. How to differentiate between these two ?

Ans. In sinus arrest, P-P (R-R) is not exactly the double of next normal beat.

Q. What are the causes of SA block?

Ans. As follows:

- Degenerative changes in elderly.
- Ischemic heart disease (involving SA node).
- Drugs (digoxin).
- Increased vagal tone.

(May present like sick sinus syndrome).

Q. How to diagnose SA block?

Ans. As follows:

- Clinically—drop beat and no heart sound at the time of drop beat.
- ECG—complete absence of one complex (P-QRS-T).
- Holter monitoring—may show the block.

Q. What is the treatment of SA block?

Ans. As follows:

- No treatment, if asymptomatic.
- Withdraw the offensive drug, if any.
- If any syncopal attack or sick sinus syndrome—permanent pacemaker should be given.

Q. What is sick sinus syndrome?

Ans. It is the dysfunction of SA node characterized by attacks of sinus bradycardia, sinus arrest, or junctional rhythm which may lead to dizziness or syncope, followed by episodes of paroxysmal tachycardia, so called tachy-brady syndrome.

Q. What are the causes of sick sinus syndrome?

Ans. It is due to fibrosis, degenerative changes or ischemia of sinoatrial node. Probable causes are:

- Elderly (due to degeneration).
- Ischemic heart disease.
- Drug (digoxin).
- Cardiomyopathy.
- Rheumatic heart disease.
- Idiopathic in many cases.

Q. What are the presentations of sick sinus syndrome?

Ans. Dizziness, syncope, palpitation.

Q. Why bradycardia or tachycardia occurs in sick sinus syndrome?

Ans. As follows:
- Bradycardia due to—sinus bradycardia, SA block or arrest, junctional bradycardia.
- Tachycardia due to—atrial fibrillation, or atrial flutter or paroxysmal atrial tachycardia.

Q. How would you diagnose sick sinus syndrome?

Ans. By Holter monitoring (single ECG may sometimes be normal).

Q. What is the treatment of sick sinus syndrome?

Ans. As follows:
- If asymptomatic—no specific therapy. Follow-up the case.
- If symptomatic—permanent pacemaker (it does not improve prognosis).
- Antiarrhythmic drug—may be required.

FIRST DEGREE AV BLOCK

ECG Criteria

*   PR interval—prolonged > 0.22 second (normal 0.12 to 0.20 second).
*   QRS—normal.
*   Rhythm—normal.

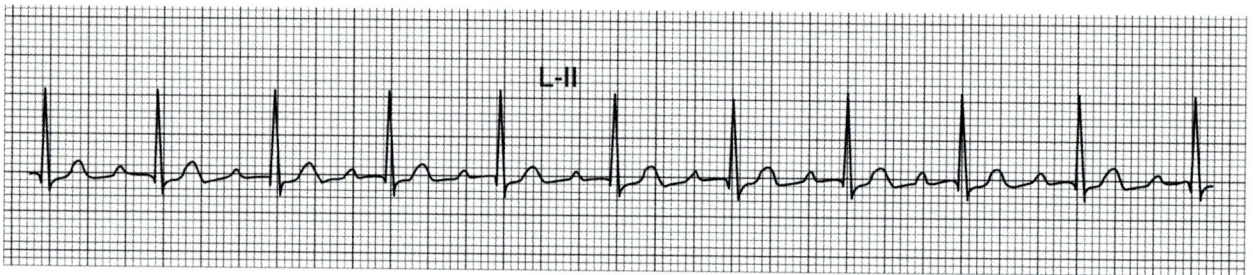

First degree heart block

Q. What are the causes of first degree AV block ?

Ans.   As follows:

*   Normally in athlete (due to increased vagal tone).
*   Drugs (digitalis toxicity).
*   Acute myocardial infarction (common in inferior MI).
*   Acute rheumatic carditis.
*   In elderly (atherosclerosis).
*   Hyperkalemia.

Q. What is first degree heart block ?

Ans.   It is the simple prolongation of PR > 0.22 sec. Every atrial depolarization is followed by conduction to the ventricles, but with delay.

Q. What are the clinical features of first degree AV block ?

Ans.   Usually asymptomatic.

Q. What is the treatment of first degree AV block ?

Ans.   As follows:

*   No specific treatment is necessary.
*   Treatment of the primary cause should be done.

NB: Markedly prolonged PR interval may progress to Wenckebach's atrioventricular heart block.

SECOND DEGREE AV BLOCK

Second degree AV block may be of 3 types:
- Mobitz type I (Wenckebach's phenomenon).
- Mobitz type II.
- 2 : 1 or 3 : 1 heart block.

MOBITZ TYPE I (WENCKEBACH'S PHENOMENON)

ECG Criteria

- Progressive lengthening of PR interval followed by absent QRS complex (one P is not followed by a QRS complex).
- PP—constant.
- RR—irregular.

  (Progressive shortening of R-R interval until block occurs).

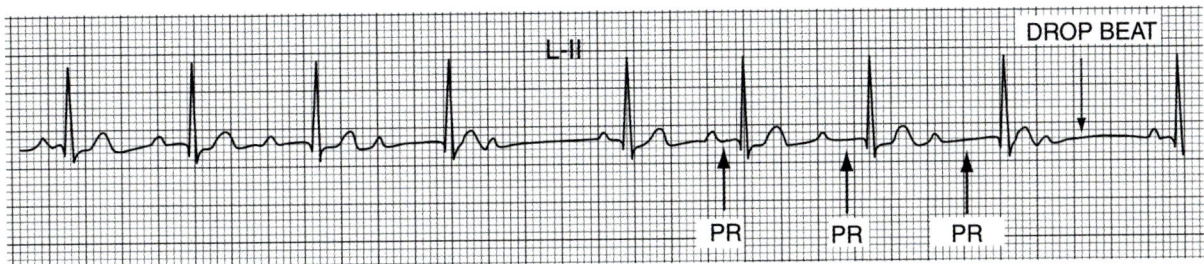

Q. What is Mobitz I block ?

Ans. Progressive prolongation of PR interval until a P wave fails to conduct. PR interval before the blocked P wave is much longer than the PR interval after the blocked P wave.

Q. What is the site of block in Mobitz type I AV block ?

Ans. The block is in the higher area of AV node (proximal to bundle of His).

Q. What are the causes of Wenckebach's phenomenon ?

Ans. As follows:
- Physiological—in athlete, during rest, sleep (due to increased vagal tone).
- Drugs—digoxin toxicity.
- Acute myocardial infarction (commonly inferior MI).

Q. What are the features of Mobitz type I AV block ?

Ans. As follows:
- Usually asymptomatic.
- Features of primary disease.
- Pulse is irregular (drop beat occurs).

Q. How to treat Mobitz type I AV block ?

Ans. As follows:
- No treatment is necessary.
- Primary cause should be treated.

Q. What is the prognosis of Wenckebach's phenomenon ?

Ans. It is a benign condition. Prognosis is good.

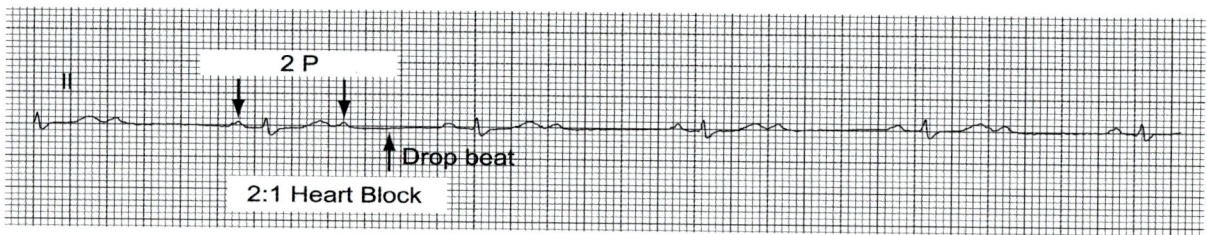

MOBITZ TYPE II AV BLOCK

ECG Criteria

- Some P waves are not followed by QRS complexes.
- PR interval is constant (also PP interval constant).
- QRS—wide.

  (In 2 :1 AV block, alternate P wave is conducted. It may be 3:1, 4:1).

  This type of AV block is rare and more severe. It is generally a sign of severe conduction system disease.

Q. What is the prognosis?

Ans. It is more serious than Mobitz type I. There may be:
- Complete heart block.
- Stokes Adam's syndrome.
- Heart failure.

Q. What is the site of lesion in Mobitz type II AV block ?

Ans. Disease of His-Purkinje system.

Q. What are the causes of Mobitz type II AV block ?

Ans. It is commonly seen in acute anterior myocardial infarction (not in digoxin toxicity).

Q. What is the treatment of Mobitz type II AV block ?

Ans. As follows:
1. If associated with inferior myocardial infarction:
   - If asymptomatic—close monitoring and follow-up.
   - If symptomatic—Inj. atropine 0.6 mg IV. If fails, temporary pacemaker. Majority will resolve in 7 to 10 days.
2. If associated with anterior myocardial infarction—temporary pacing followed by permanent pacemaker is required (because complete heart block may develop).

Q. What is 2:1 or 3:1 block ?

Ans. This type of block occurs when every second or third P wave conducts to the ventricles. This form of second-degree block is neither Mobitz I nor II. Permanent pacemaker is usually indicated in 2:1 block.

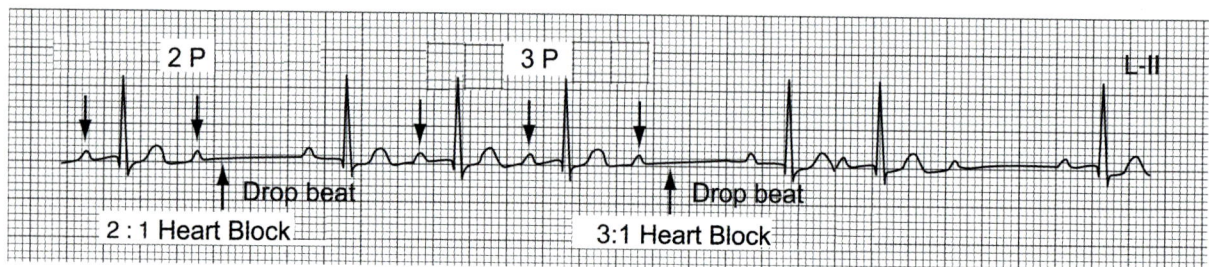

FASCICULAR BLOCK (HEMIBLOCK)

Left bundle divides into anterior and posterior fascicles.

* Anterior fascicle spreads in anterior and superior part of left ventricle.
* Posterior fascicle spreads in posterior and inferior part of left ventricle.

Fascicular block is diagnosed by looking at the axis deviation.

Fascicular block are of 2 types:

* RBBB with left anterior hemiblock (block in anterior fascicle).
* RBBB with left posterior hemiblock (block in posterior fascicle).

ECG in RBBB with Left Anterior Hemiblock

* RBBB with left axis deviation.

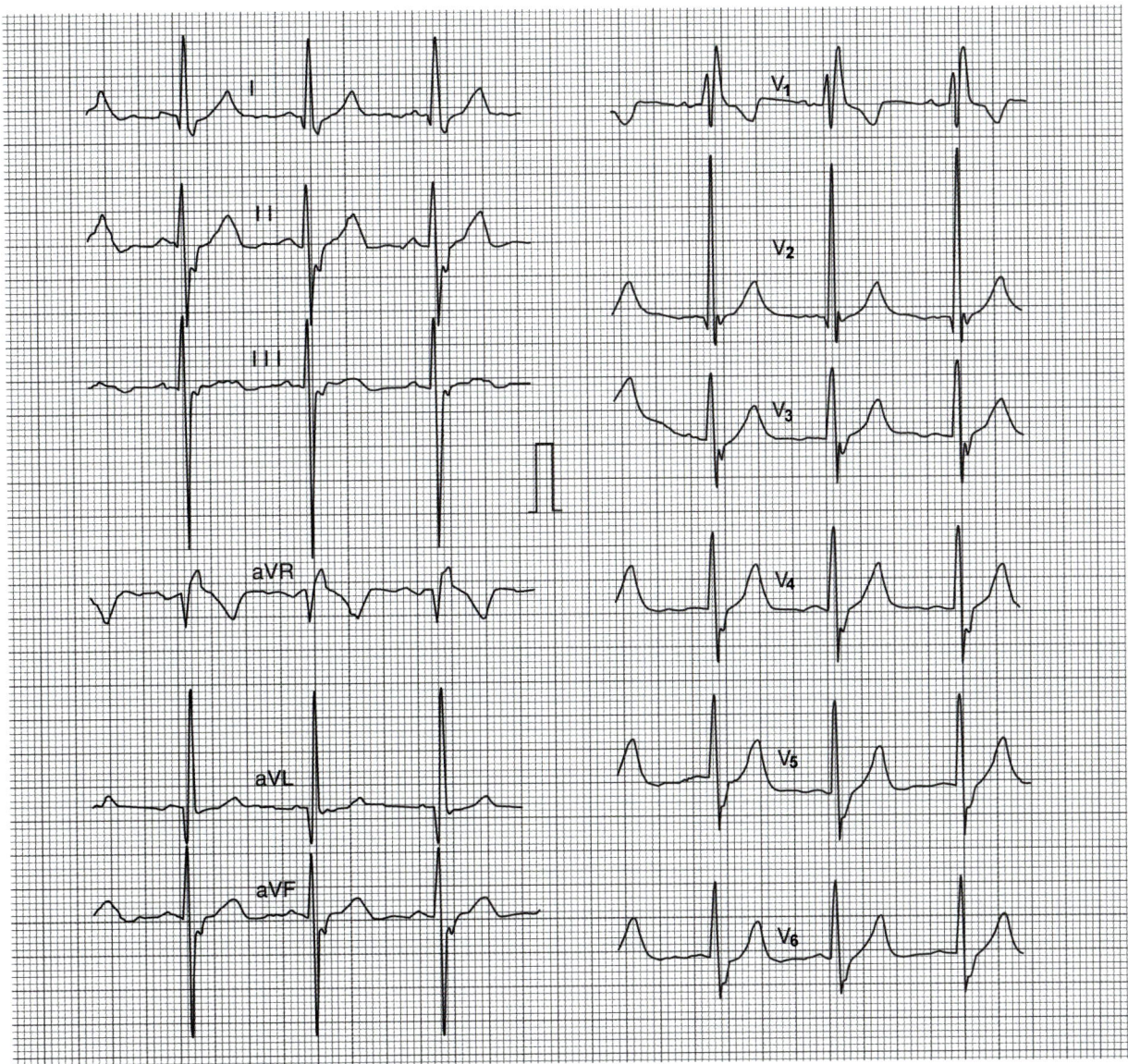

RBBB with left axis deviation

ECG in RBBB with Left Posterior Hemiblock

RBBB with right axis deviation.

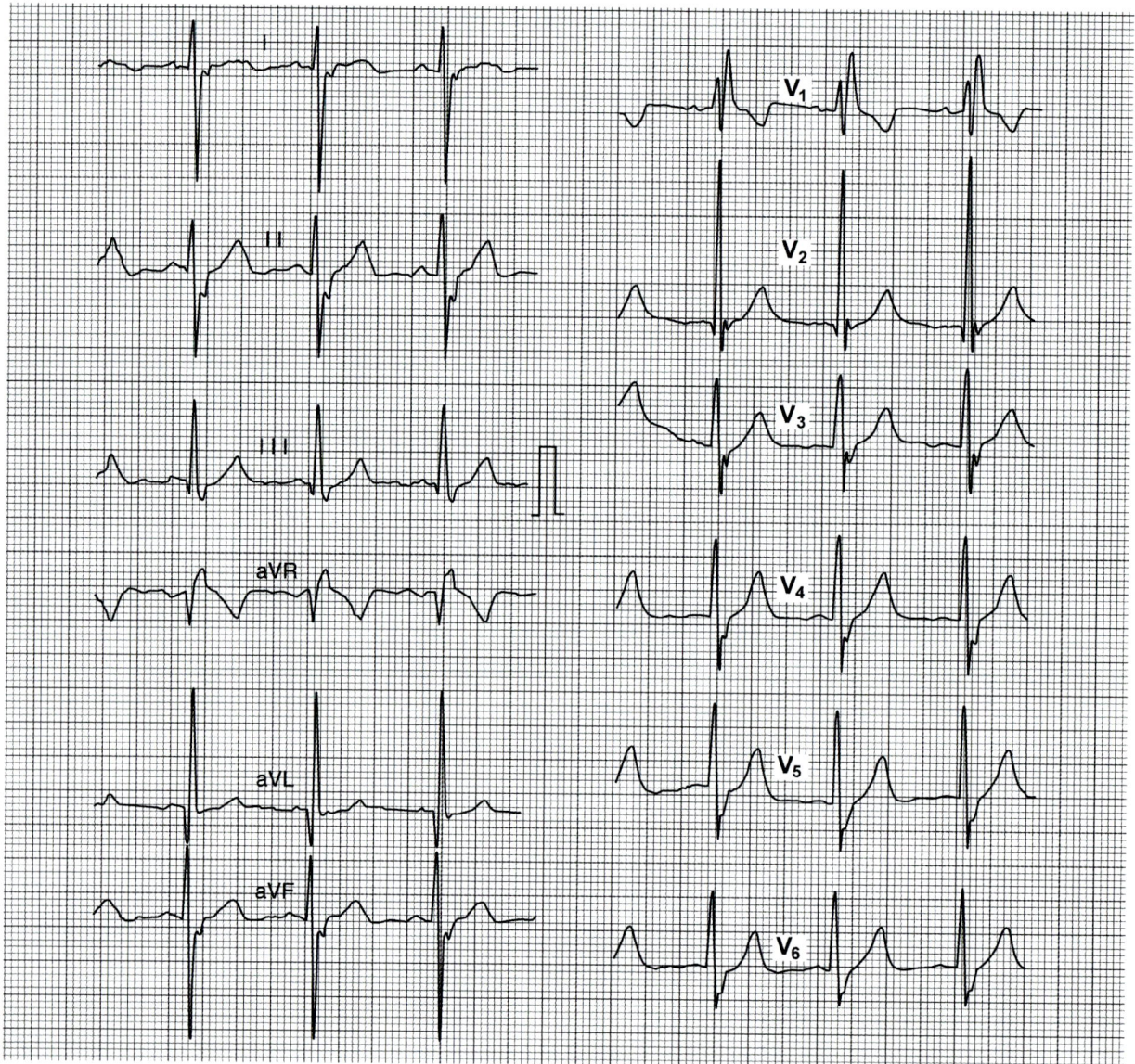

RBBB with right axis deviation

NB: Remember the following points:

- The combination of RBBB with left anterior or posterior hemiblock is called bifascicular block.
- Left anterior hemiblock is common, left posterior hemiblock is rare.
- Isolated finding of left anterior or left posterior hemiblock does not have any clinical significance.

Q. How to treat bifascicular block?

Ans. In asymptomatic case—no treatment is necessary.

NB: Complete heart block with acute anterior infarction is sometimes preceded by sudden appearance of bifascicular block. In that case, temporary pacemaker may be needed.

LEFT BUNDLE BRANCH BLOCK

ECG Criteria

- RSR′—in V_5 and V_6, also in L_I and aVL (M pattern).
- QRS—wide, > 0.12 second (3 small squares).

(ECG - QRS looks wide from L_1 to all leads—**A clue** for diagnosis).

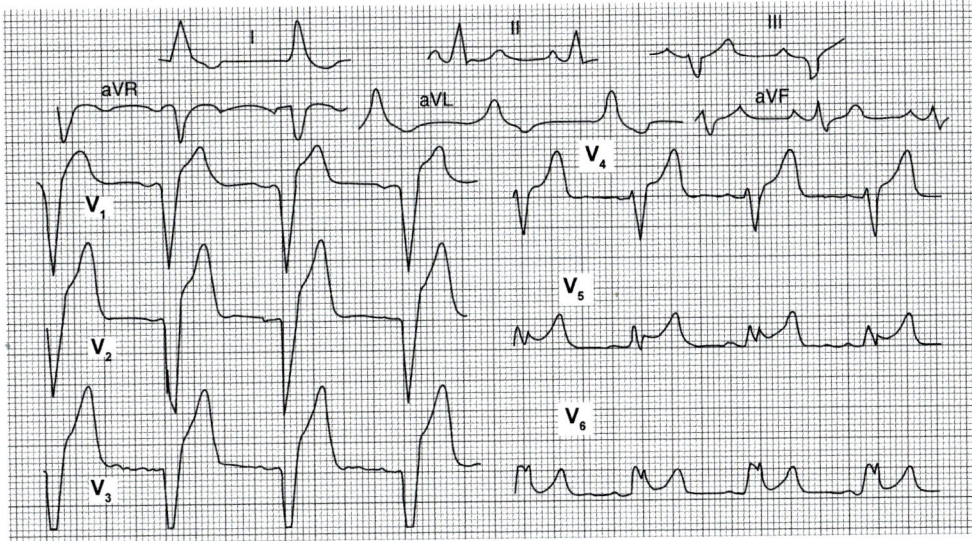

Q. What are the causes of left bundle branch block?

Ans. As follows:

- Severe coronary artery disease (Two or three vessels disease).
- Acute myocardial infarction.
- Cardiomyopathy.
- Aortic valve disease (stenosis or regurgitation).
- Left ventricular hypertrophy.
- Hypertension.
- Myocarditis.

Q. How to diagnose LBBB clinically?

Ans. On auscultation, there is reverse splitting of second heart sound.

Q. How to treat LBBB?

Ans. As follows:

- Treatment of primary cause.
- In acute myocardial infarction—if there is new LBBB, temporary pacemaker is indicated.

NB: Remember the following points:

- RBBB may be a normal variant.
- LBBB is always pathological (it indicates underlying heart disease).
- In presence of LBBB, acute MI is difficult to diagnose.
- When LBBB occurs in acute myocardial infarction, complete heart block may develop.
- Old anterior MI may also be difficult to diagnose in presence of LBBB.
- Small q in V_1 to V_2 may be present normally in LBBB.

MYOCARDIAL INFARCTION

Before diagnosing myocardial infarction, remember to mention the following points:
* Criteria of infarction (by looking for ST elevation, Q wave, T inversion).
* Site of infarction (whether anterior, inferior, septal, lateral).
* Recent or old.

Sites of Myocardial Infarction is Detected in Different Leads

* Inferior MI — L_{III} and aVF (may be in L_{II}).
* Extensive anterior MI — V_1 to V_6.
* Anteroseptal MI — V_1 to V_3 or V_4 (mainly V_2 to V_4).
* Lateral MI — L_I, aVL, V_5 and V_6.
* Posterior (true) MI — V_1 and V_2 (may be V_1 to V_4).
* Subendocardial MI — Symmetrical T inversion in all chest leads (non Q wave MI).
* High lateral — L_1 and aVL.
* Anterolateral — L_1, aVL, V_1 to V_6.
* Right ventricular infarction — V_3R and V_4R.

ECG Criteria of Acute MI (Fully Evolved Case)

* ST elevation (with upward convexity).
* Pathological Q wave.
* T inversion.

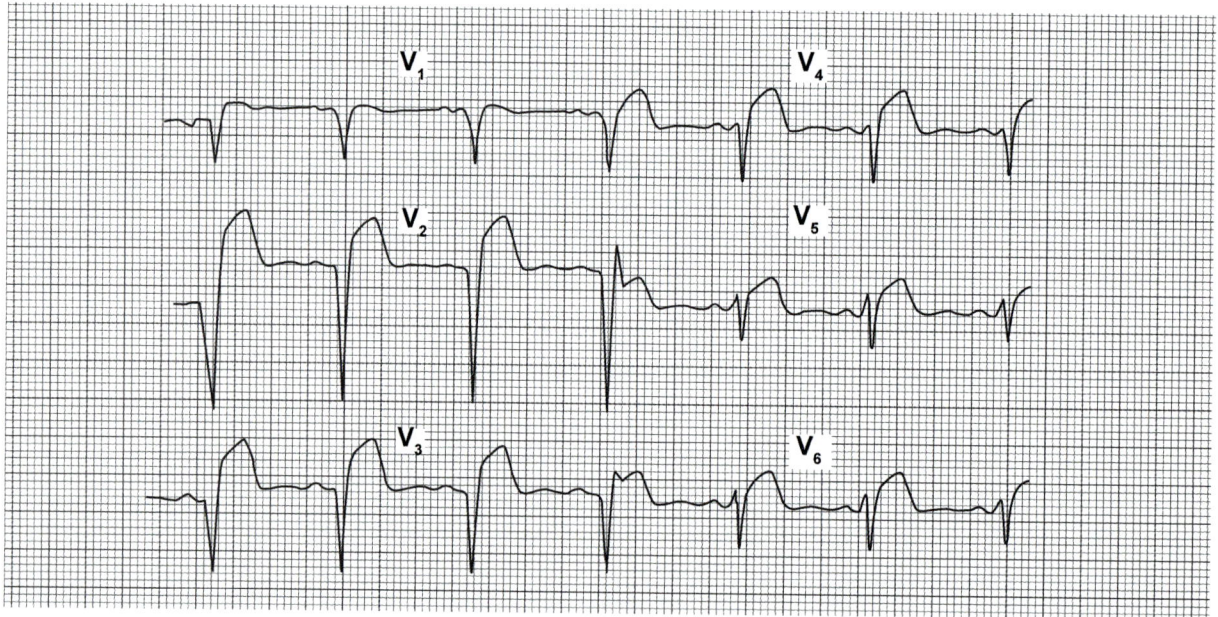

Acute anterior myocardial infarction

ECG Criteria in Old MI

* Pathological Q wave.
* ST—in baseline.
* T—normal or inverted.

Q. What does the pathological Q, ST elevation and T inversion signify in MI?

Ans. As follows:
- Q wave is due to myocardial necrosis.
- ST elevation is due to myocardial injury.
- T inversion is due to ischemia.

According to duration, MI are of 3 types:
- Hyperacute.
- Acute.
- Fully evolved phase.

ECG Criteria in Hyperacute MI (within First Few Minutes)

- ST—slope elevation.
- T—tall, pointed and upright, wide.
- R—increased amplitude.
- Q—absent.
- Ventricular activation time (VAT)—increased.

Q. What is the significance of hyperacute phase?

Ans. It is the most critical phase. Ventricular fibrillation is common in this period. There is myocardial injury, but still no infarction or necrosis. This phase may persist for few hours. If treated properly, myocardial blood supply is improved.

Q. What is the mechanism of tall T in hyperacute MI?

Ans. It is due to necrosis of myocardium (myocytes), releasing potassium which causes localized hyperkalemia, leading to tall T.

ECG Criteria in Acute MI (within Hours)

ST—elevation with upward convexity.

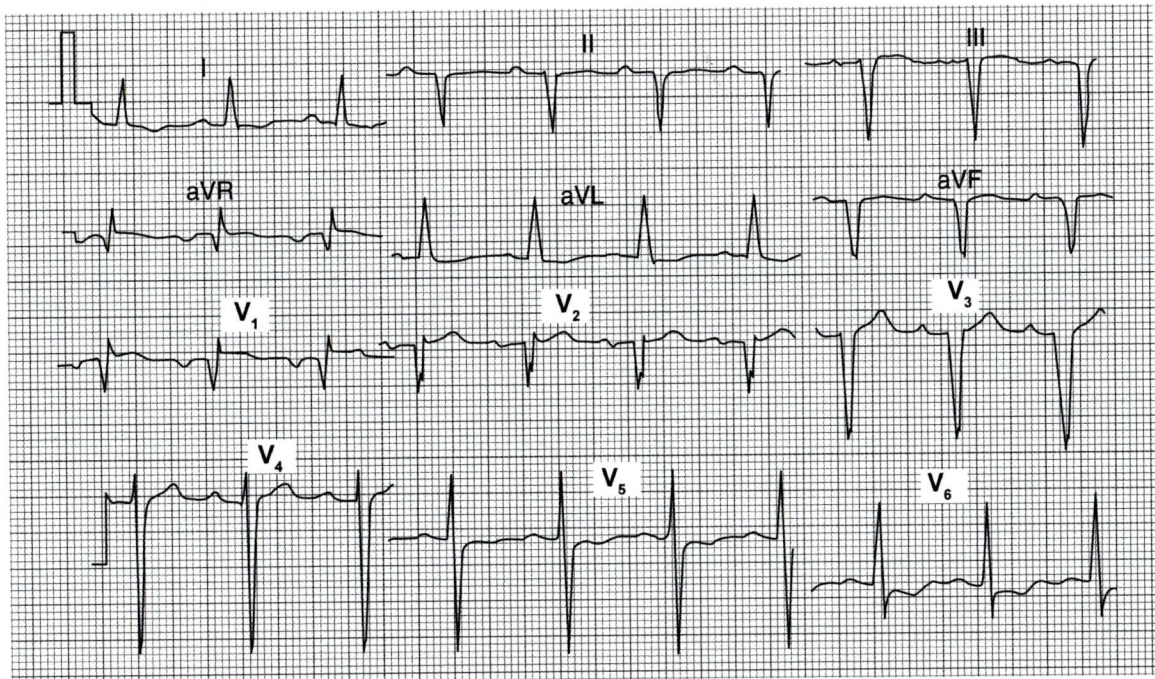

Deep Q in II, III, aVF (inferior MI), also deep Q in V_1 to V_3 (septal MI)

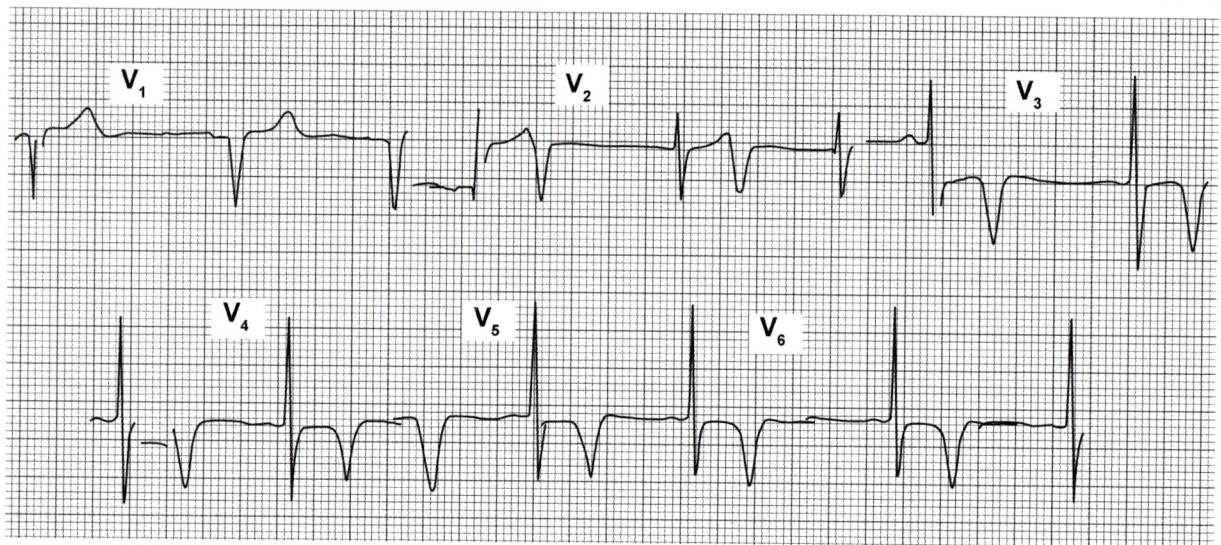

ECG Criteria in Subendocardial MI (Non-Q Wave MI or Non-ST Elevation)

- T—deeply inverted in chest leads (usually symmetrical T inversion).
- ST—depression.
- Q wave—absent.

Q. What are the differences between Q wave and non-Q wave myocardial infarction?

Ans. As follows:

- Q wave infarction means infarction of full thickness myocardium (transmural MI).
- Non-Q wave infarction means infarction of subendocardium (subendocardial MI).

Features	Q wave	Non-Q wave
1. Prevalence	47%	53%
2. Coronary occlusion	80 to 90 %	15 to 25%
3. Infarction size	Moderate to large	Small
4. Thrombolysis	Indicated	Not indicated
5. Complication	Common	Uncommon
6. Residual ischemia	10 to 20%	40 to 50%
7. Early reinfarction	5 to 8 %	15 to 25 %
8. One month mortality	10 to 15% (more)	3 to 5 % (less)
9. Two years mortality	30% (same)	30% (same)

Q. What is the clinical importance of non-Q wave MI?

Ans. As follows:

- There is no evidence that thrombolysis will improve the prognosis. So thrombolytic therapy is not indicated.
- Complications are uncommon.
- Early mortality is less.
- They are at higher risk of reinfarction.
- Frequent follow-up with adequate preventive measures are required.

NB: Remember the following points:

- MI may be STEMI (ST elevation myocardial infarction) and NSTEMI (Non-ST elevation myocardial infarction).
- Fully evolved phase is usually seen after 24 hours.
- ST elevation may not occur before 6 hours.
- Pathological Q-broad > 1 mm and deep > 2 mm or > 25% of the amplitude of R wave is suggestive of MI.
- Q wave may appear after 8 to 16 hours (commonly after 24 hours).
- ST segment returns to normal after a few days.
- T wave may remain upright for weeks to months.
- Q wave usually remains permanently in most of the cases (90% cases).
- Acute MI may be masked in presence of LBBB, WPW syndrome and pacemaker.

ECG Criteria in True Posterior MI

- R—tall and slightly wide in V_1 to V_2.
- T—upright, tall, wide and symmetrical in V_1 to V_2.
- ST—depression.
- R/S ratio—in V_1 > 1.

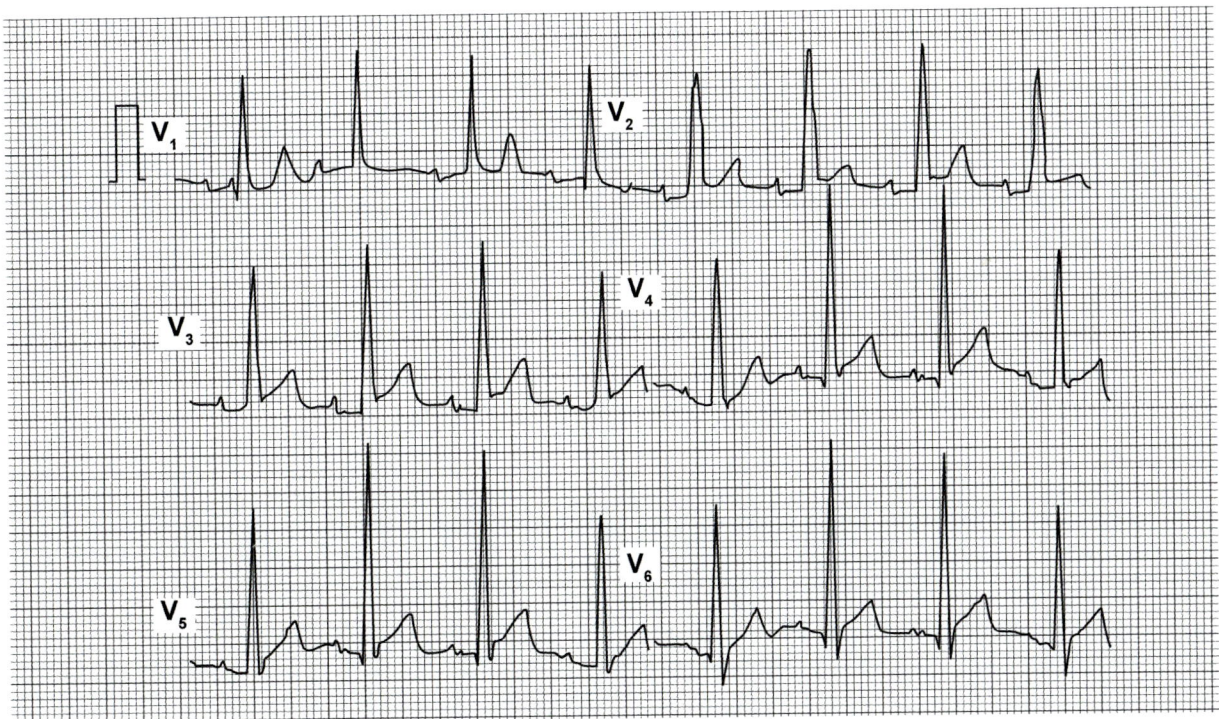

True posterior MI

Q. What are the causes of tall R in V_1?

Ans. See page no. 18.

Q. How to differentiate between RVH and true posterior MI?

Ans. As follows:
- In true posterior MI—see the ECG above.
- In RVH—tall R in V_1, T inversion and right axis deviation (may be right atrial hypertrophy).

Q. If ST remains elevated after few months of acute MI, what is the diagnosis?

Ans. Ventricular aneurysm.

Q. How to diagnose ventricular aneurysm?

Ans. As follows:
- History of myocardial infarction.
- Double apex beat, shows paradoxical movement (called **see-saw** movement).
- Heart may be enlarged.
- ECG—persistent ST elevation in repeated ECG.
- X-ray chest—heart enlarged, with a bulged or rounded protrusion from the left ventricular wall, calcification may occur at the wall of aneurysm.
- Paradoxical movement on fluoroscopy.
- Confirmed by echocardiogram (left ventriculography, radioneuclide study may be done).

Q. What are the complications of ventricular aneurysm?

Ans. As follows:
- Heart failure.
- Arrhythmia (ectopic, atrial fibrillation, occasionally serious ventricular arrhythmia, etc.).
- Systemic embolism from mural thrombus.

Q. How to treat ventricular aneurysm?

Ans. As follows:

1. Symptomatic treatment:
   - If heart failure—diuretic, ACE inhibitor, digoxin.
   - If arrhythmia—antiarrhythmic drugs.
   - Aspirin in low dose.
   - Treatment for embolism (anticoagulant, aspirin).
2. If difficult to control, surgery is indicated (aneurysectomy, but mortality is very high).

NB: Remember the following points:
- 3.5 to 20% develop aneurysm following acute myocardial infarction.
- Calcification of aneurysmal wall may develop which indicates longstanding case.

Complications of myocardial infarction: Complications may be **early** and **late**.

1. **Early complications**
   - Arrhythmia - Ventricular ectopics (more common), ventricular fibrillation, ventricular tachycardia, sinus bradycardia (common in inferior MI), sinus tachycardia, atrial fibrillation, heart block.
   - Cardiogenic shock.
   - Cardiac failure (LVF, biventricular failure).
   - Acute pericarditis (common in 2nd or 3rd day).
   - Thromboembolism (systemic and pulmonary).
   - Rupture of the papillary muscle or chordae tendineae resulting in mitral regurgitation.
   - Rupture of interventricular septum causing VSD.
   - Rupture of the ventricular wall leading to cardiac tamponade.

2. **Late complications**
   - Ventricular aneurysm (10%).
   - Postmyocardial infarction syndrome (Dressler's syndrome).
   - Frozen shoulder.
   - Postinfarct angina (may occur in up to 50% of patients).

Q. What is postmyocardial infarction syndrome (Dressler's syndrome)?

Ans. It is a late complication of myocardial infarction that occurs usually a few weeks or even months (2 to 10 weeks) after acute MI. It is characterized by **(5P's):**

- **P**ain (chest pain).
- **P**yrexia.
- **P**leurisy.
- **P**ericarditis (or pericardial effusion).
- **P**neumonitis (or pulmonary infiltrate).

Q. What is the mechanism of postmyocardial infarction syndrome?

Ans. It is due to autoimmune reaction to necrosed myocardium. Antimyocardial antibody may be found in the blood. Recurrence is common, confuses with new MI or unstable angina.

Q. How to treat postmyocardial infarction syndrome?

Ans. As follows:

- High dose aspirin (600 to 900 mg) every 4 to 6 hours or other NSAID.
- In severe or in recurrent case—corticosteroid may be given.
- Anticoagulant should be discontinued (unless strong evidence for high-risk of thromboembolism).

Q. What are the enzymatic changes of acute myocardial infarction ?

Ans. As follows:

- *Troponins:* Troponin I and troponin T are highly specific, rise in 2 to 4 hours, persist up to 7 days (may be up to 2 weeks). Minor rise may be seen in unstable angina.
- *CPK:* Starts to rise in 4 to 6 hours, peak in 12 hours. It returns to normal within 48 to 72 hours. CK-MB is cardiac specific.
- *Aspartate aminotransferase (AST / SGOT):* Increases after 12 hours, peak in 24 hours, and returns to normal in 3 to 4 days.
- *LDH:* Rises after 12 hours, peak in 3 to 4 days, becomes normal after 7 to 10 days.

Enzymatic changes with time in acute MI

Enzyme	Rise (hrs)	Peaks at (hrs)	Persists for
Troponin I and T	2 to 4	12 to 15	7 days (up to 2 weeks)
CPK	4 to 6	12	2 to 3 days
AST/SGOT	12	24	3 to 4 days
LDH	12	3 to 4 days	7 to 10 days

NB: Remember the following points:

- Troponin I and T, also CPK rise early in acute MI.
- In a patient treated with thrombolytic agent, reperfusion is accompanied by rapid rise of CPK due to wash out effect.

Q. How to treat acute MI?

Ans. As follows:

- Admission in CCU.
- Complete bed rest.
- High flow O_2 inhalation (60%)—2 to 4 L/min by nasal cannula.
- To relieve pain—injection morphine (5 to 10 mg) or diamorphine (2.5 to 5 mg) plus antiemetic (cyclizine or metoclopromide) IV. It may be repeated, if necessary.
- Chewable aspirin—300 mg.
- Thrombolytic therapy—streptokinase, provided there is no contraindication.
- Other therapy:
  - β-blocker (if no contraindication)—IV bolus atenolol, 5 to 10 mg or metoprolol 5 to 15 mg slowly over 5 minutes. Oral atenolol 25 to 50 mg BD, or bisoprolol 5 mg daily or metoprolol 25 to 50 mg BD or TDS may be given.
  - Sublingual nitroglycerin—0.3 to 1 mg (may be repeated).
  - Heparin—12,500 IU, BD, S/C.
  - ACE inhibitor.

Q. What are the criteria of thrombolytic therapy?

Ans. As follows:

- Typical history of chest pain.
- ECG change—ST elevation > 1 mm in limb leads or 2 mm in chest leads (in 2 or more contiguous leads) or new left bundle branch block.
- High cardiac enzyme.

(Diagnosis of acute MI requires at least two of these three criteria).

NB: Remember the following points:

- Thrombolysis should be started, if there is typical chest pain and high cardiac enzyme (in the absence of ECG changes).

- Streptokinase is more effective, if started particularly within 6 hours (greatest benefit within 1st 2 hours), may be given in 6 to 12 hours, unlikely to be beneficial after 12 hours. Reperfusion occurs in 50 to 70% of cases.

- Dose—1.5 million units in 100 cc normal saline given IV for 1 hour.

- Toxicity—allergic reaction, hypotension, bleeding (major hazard).

- Larger the infarction, greater the benefit with thrombolytic. Anterior infarction response better than inferior.

Q. What are the contraindications of thrombolytic therapy?

Ans. As follows:

1. **Absolute contraindications**
   - Hemorrhagic stroke or stroke of unknown origin at any time.
   - Ischemic stroke in preceding 6 months.
   - Central nervous system damage or neoplasm.
   - Recent major trauma, surgery, head injury (within preceding 3 weeks).
   - Gastrointestinal bleeding within the last month.
   - Coagulation or bleeding abnormalities.
   - Suspected dissecting aortic aneurysm.
   - Diabetic retinopathy (proliferative).

2. **Relative contraindications**
   - Transient ischemic attack in the preceding 6 months.
   - Oral anticoagulant therapy.
   - Heavy vaginal bleeding, pregnancy or puerperal bleeding.
   - Severe hypertension (malignant hypertension, systolic > 180 and diastolic > 120).
   - Previous subarachnoid or intracerebral hemorrhage.
   - High probability of active peptic ulcer.
   - Advanced liver disease.
   - Infective endocarditis.

NB: Streptokinase is avoided, if the patient had received it within 5 days to 5 years. Circulating neutralizing antibody is produced. In such case, alteplase or tPA may be given.

Other thrombolytic drugs—tenecteplase, retaplase may be used.

Q. What is the treatment of MI, if thrombolysis is failed or contraindicated?

Ans. Primary percutaneous transluminal coronary angioplasty (PTCA) can be done.

Q. What is the role of anticoagulant in MI?

Ans. Heparin (12,500 unit twice daily SC) and oral aspirin after successful thrombolysis are quite effective. These may prevent reinfarction and thromboembolism. Heparin may be used for 7 days. After heparin, warfarin should be considered, if there is persistent atrial fibrillation or extensive anterior MI or echocardiography shows mural thrombus.

Q. How would you follow-up a patient after an acute MI?

Ans. The patient should be reviewed after 6 to 8 weeks.

Risk factors should be reviewed and modified accordingly:
   - Lifestyle modification (avoid stress, heavy work, etc.).
   - Smoking should be stopped.
   - Regular exercise.
   - Diet (weight control, lipid-lowering)
   - Good control of hypertension (BP < 140/85 mm Hg) and diabetes mellitus.
   - Antiplatelet (aspirin or clopidogrel) should be continued indefinitely.
   - β-blocker (for long time) may be discontinued after 3 years in low-risk, normotensive patient.
   - ACE inhibitor should be continued indefinitely in patient with persistent LV dysfunction (EF < 40%).
   - Lipid lowering agents (target total cholesterol < 5.0 mmol/L and/or LDL < 3.0 mmol/L).
   - Rehabilitation.

NB: Myocardial infarction may be difficult to diagnose, if following diseases are present:

   - WPW syndrome.
   - LBBB and LVH.
   - Cardiomyopathy.
   - Hyperkalemia.
   - COPD with RVH.
   - Chest deformity.

ACUTE PERICARDITIS

ECG Criteria

- ST—elevated with upward concavity (chair shaped or saddle shaped)—better seen in L_I, L_{II}, aVL, aVF, V_4 to V_6.
- T—upright in acute phase.

Subsequent ECG changes:
- ST returns to baseline.
- T inversion that remains for weeks to months.

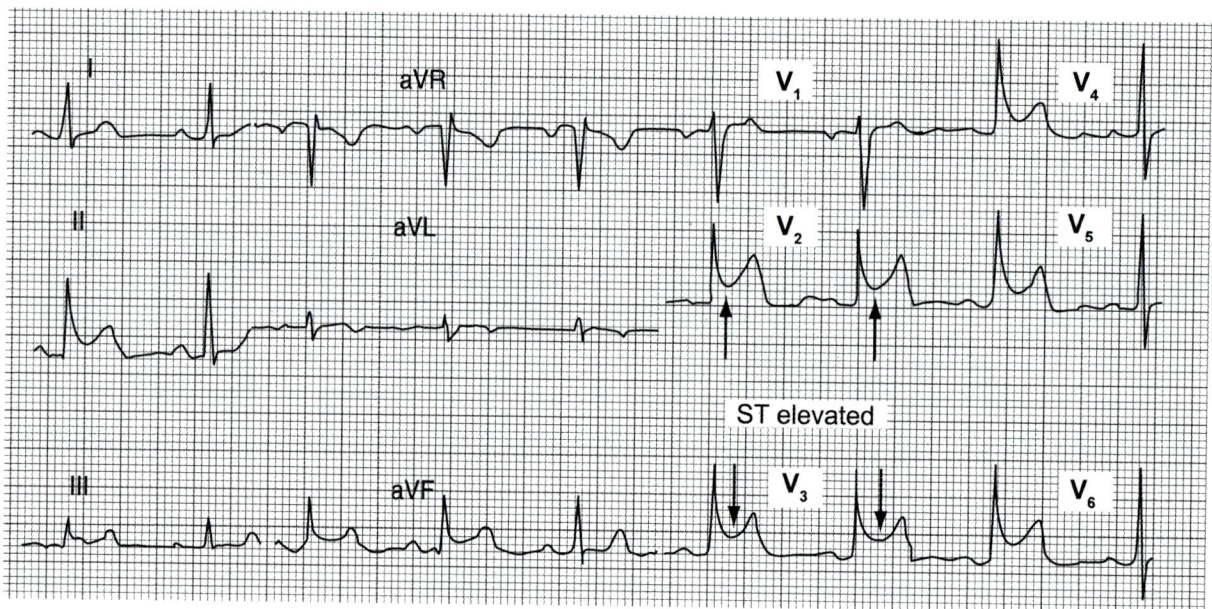

ST elevation in II, aVF, V_2 to V_6

Q. How to differentiate acute pericarditis from acute myocardial infarction by ECG?
Ans. As follows:
- In myocardial infarction—ST elevation with upward convexity.
- In pericarditis—ST elevation with upward concavity (pericardium envelops the heart, so ST changes are more generalized and seen in most leads).

Q. What is the clinical finding in acute pericarditis?
Ans. Pericardial rub. Features are:
- It is a high pitched, harsh, scratching, grating, leathery sound, to and fro in quality.
- Better heard over the left lower parasternal area with the patient leaning forward (bare area of heart—it is the part of heart which is not covered by lung).
- Augmented by pressing the stethoscope.
- It is usually heard in systole, but may be present in diastole.
- It is present after holding the breath (to differentiate from pleural rub).

ECG Changes in Pericardial Effusion

- Low voltage tracing.
- Sinus tachycardia.

Q. What are the presentations of acute pericarditis?

Ans. As follows:
- Chest pain which is retrosternal. It is usually sharp or stabbing in nature, may radiate to the shoulder and neck.
- Pain is aggravated by movement, lying down and deep breathing, exercise and swallowing.
- Pain may be relieved by sitting or bending forward.

Q. What are the causes of acute pericarditis?

Ans. As follows:
- Following acute myocardial infarction (usually in 2nd or 3rd day).
- Viral (coxsackie B, echovirus)—common cause.
- Acute rheumatic fever.
- Bacterial *(Staphylococcus aureus, Hemophilus influenzae)*.
- Tuberculous pericarditis.
- Fungal (histoplasmosis, coccidioidomycosis).
- Uremia (an indication of urgent dialysis).
- Malignancy (from carcinoma of bronchus, breast, lymphoma, leukemia).
- Trauma.
- Radiation.
- Drugs (doxorubicin, cyclophosphamide).
- Collagen disease (SLE, scleroderma).

Q. How would you treat acute pericarditis?

Ans. As follows:
- To relieve pain—NSAID (indomethacin or ibuprofen or aspirin).
- In severe or recurrent case—corticosteroid should be given.
- If no response to steroid—azathioprine or colchicine may be given.
- If recurrence with no response to medical treatment—pericardiotomy may be done.
- Treatment of primary cause—antibiotic, if bacterial infection. Anti-Koch's, if tuberculosis is suspected.

Postmyocardial Infarction Pericarditis

Occurs in 20% of patient in the first few days following MI, more commonly anterior MI and ST elevation MI with high serum cardiac enzymes. Incidence is less to 5 to 6% with thrombolysis. Pericarditis may occur as Dressler's syndrome, 2 to 10 weeks after infarction.

WOLFF-PARKINSON-WHITE (WPW) SYNDROME

ECG Criteria

- PR—short < 0.12 second.
- QRS—wide.
- Delta wave—in the upstroke of QRS (slurred QRS).
- Q wave—may be present in lead II, III and aVF (confused with inferior myocardial infarction).

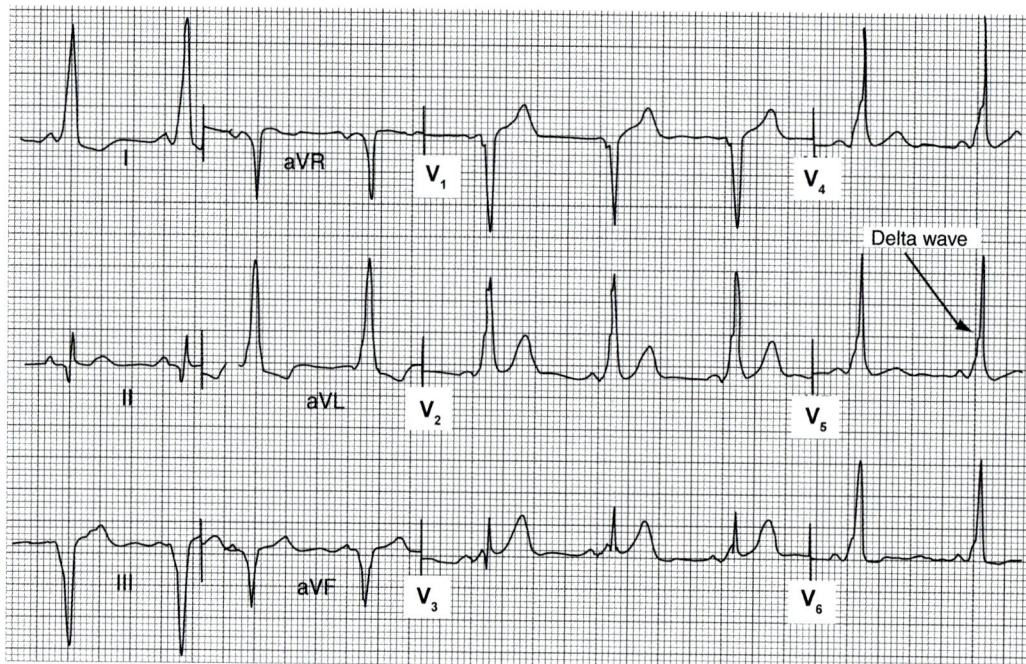

WPW syndrome type A

Q. What is WPW syndrome?

Ans. It is a syndrome in which there is an accessory pathway that bypasses the AV node and connects the atrium and ventricle (by bundles of Kent). May be associated with other congenital anomaly, commonly Ebstein anomaly.

Q. What are the types of WPW syndrome?

Ans. It is of 2 types:
- Type A—accessory pathway on the left side (in ECG, tall R in V_1 and V_2).
- Type B—accessory pathway on the right side (in ECG, deep Q in V_1 and V_2).

(The accessory pathway is called the bundle of Kent).

NB: See in V_1—Type A (deflection—**above**), type B (deflection—**below**).

Q. How to treat WPW syndrome?

Ans. As follows:
1. If asymptomatic—no treatment is required.
2. If symptomatic:
   - Transvenous radiofrequency catheter ablation of accessory pathway is the specific treatment.
   - If this is not available—prophylactic antiarrhythmic drug should be given (β-blocker, amiodarone,flecainide, propafenone). These drugs prolong refractory period of accessory pathway.
   - Previously, surgical resection of accessory pathway used to be done.

Q. What are the presentations of WPW syndrome?

Ans. As follows:
- May be asymptomatic, may present with palpitation.
- Paroxysmal attack of atrial or supraventricular tachycardia (most common) due to re-entry circuit.
- Atrial fibrillation.
- Syncope.
- Sudden death (due to atrial fibrillation).
- Rarely—ventricular tachycardia, ventricular fibrillation.

Q. Why digoxin is avoided in WPW syndrome?

Ans. Digoxin blocks the AV node and increases the conduction through the accessory pathway. So, it increases the heart rate (verapamil may cause same effect). It may precipitate ventricular fibrillation.

Q. What are the drugs contraindicated in WPW syndrome ?

Ans. Digoxin and IV verapamil. These drugs shorten the refractory period of accessory pathway.

Q. Why the PR interval is short and what is the mechanism of delta wave?

Ans. As follows:
- *Short PR interval:* Impulse is conducted rapidly from the atria to the ventricles through the accessory pathway, causing early ventricular depolarization. So, PR interval is short.
- *Delta wave:* The accessory pathway causes early depolarization of part of the ventricle, giving rise to slow upstroke (delta wave—first portion of QRS complex). Then the normally conducted impulse through the AV node causes depolarization of the rest of ventricle, giving rise to the rest of QRS complex.
  Delta wave is absent, if there is tachycardia, as the ventricle is excited by normal pathway.

Q. How to treat atrial fibrillation with WPW syndrome ?

Ans. It is a medical emergency. Sudden death may occur. Treatment is as follows:
- If troublesome symptoms—DC shock should be given. If not available, IV flecainide.
- Radiofrequency ablation of abnormal pathway.
- Drugs that slow conduction of accessory pathway may be used—Amiodarone, flecainide, disopyramide, sotalol, etc.

NB: Remember the following points:

- Hallmark of WPW syndrome in ECG is delta wave.
- When WPW syndrome is associated with tachycardia, it may be confused with ventricular tachycardia.
- Digoxin and verapamil may increase the heart rate and even precipitate ventricular tachycardia and ventricular fibrillation.

In presence of WPW syndrome, the following diseases may be difficult to diagnose.

Type A confuses with
- Right bundle branch block.
- Right ventricular hypertrophy.
- True posterior myocardial infarction.

Type B confuses with
- Left bundle branch block.
- Left ventricular hypertrophy.
- Inferior myocardial infarction.

LOWN-GANONG-LEVINE (LGL) SYNDROME

ECG Criteria

- PR interval—short.
- QRS—normal (no delta wave).

Q. What is Lown-Ganong-Levine syndrome?

Ans. It is a syndrome in which there is a congenital accessory pathway (James bypass tract) that joins the atrium to the common bundle of His.

Q. Why QRS is normal in LGL syndrome?

Ans. The accessory pathway simply connects the atrium to the common bundle of His. It does not activate the ventricle directly. So, PR is short, no delta wave and QRS is normal.

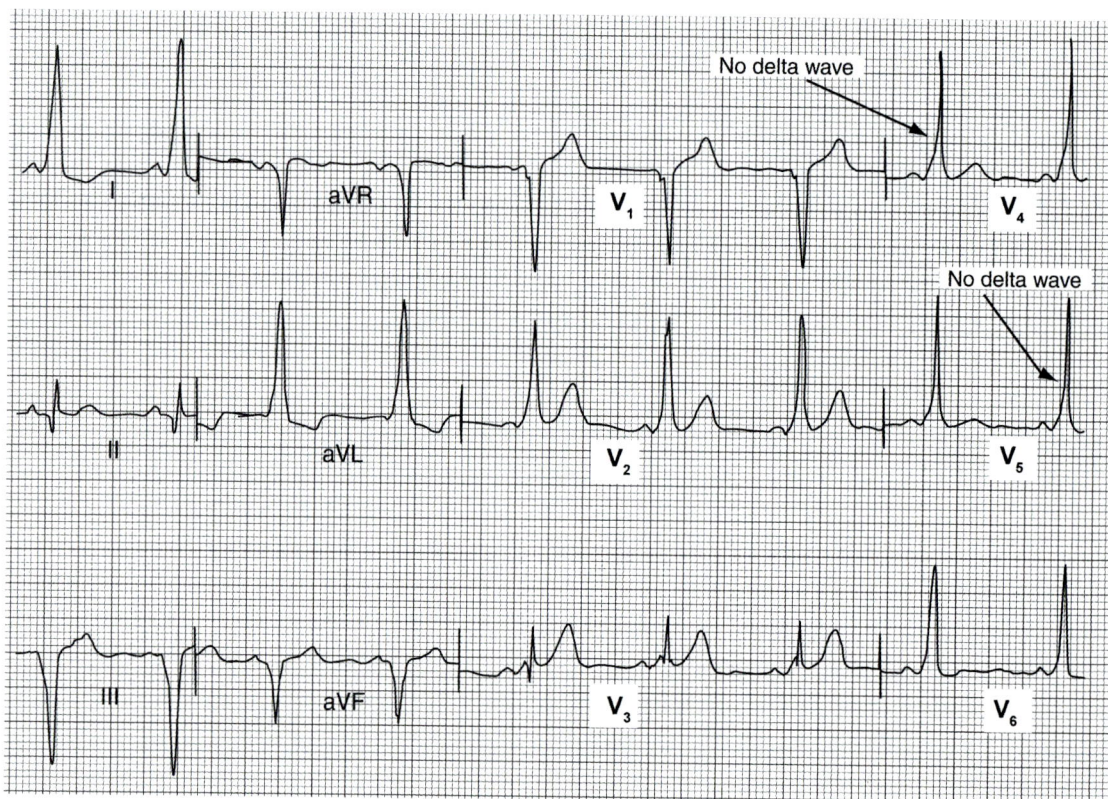

Q. What is the presentation of Lown-Ganong-Levine syndrome?

Ans. Asymptomatic usually.

Q. What is the prognosis and treatment of Lown-Ganong-Levine syndrome?

Ans. Good prognosis. No treatment is necessary.

Q. What are the types of accessory pathways ?

Ans. Three types:
- Bundles of Kent.
- Mahaim's fiber are AV bypass tract within the conduction system. PR is normal, but QRS is abnormal.
- James bypass tract.

SINUS ARRHYTHMIA

ECG Criteria

- *PP or RR interval:* Short in inspiration and long in expiration.
- *Rhythm:* Irregular (PP or RR interval is irregular).

Q. What is sinus arrhythmia?

Ans. It is an arrhythmia in which heart rate increases in inspiration and decreases in expiration.

Q. What is the mechanism?

Ans. It is the normal manifestation of autonomic activity which varies with respiration.

- In inspiration, parasympathetic activity diminishes, so heart rate increases. It reverses during expiration.
- Sinus arrhythmia is a benign condition, common in children and young adults. Sometimes, in healthy old person.
- It is absent in autonomic neuropathy.

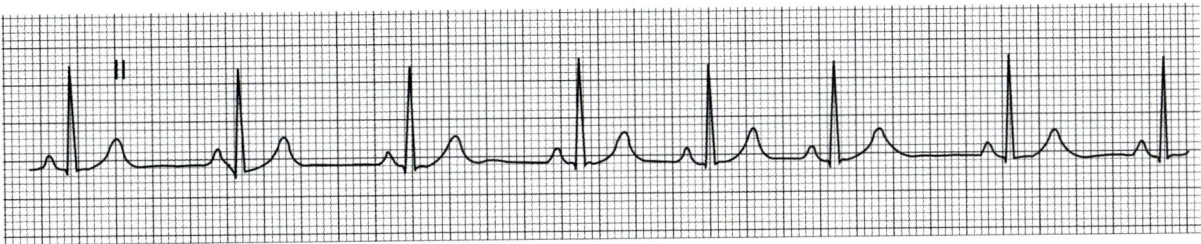

Irregular RR interval

Sinus arrhythmia may be associated with:
- Sinus bradycardia.
- Wandering pacemaker.
- Sinus tachycardia.

Sinus arrhythmia may be of 2 types:
- *Respiratory sinus arrhythmia:* Relation with respiration. Common in children and young adults. It is a benign condition.
- *Non-respiratory sinus arrhythmia:* No relation with respiration. It may be associated with any cardiac disease (myocardial infarction, heart failure), sinus bradycardia, digoxin therapy, enhanced vagal tone, etc. May be idiopathic in many cases. It is common in elderly. Full evaluation of cardiac function should be done.

SINUS TACHYCARDIA

ECG Criteria

• Heart rate— > 100 beats/minute.
• P, QRS and T—normal.
• Rhythm—regular.

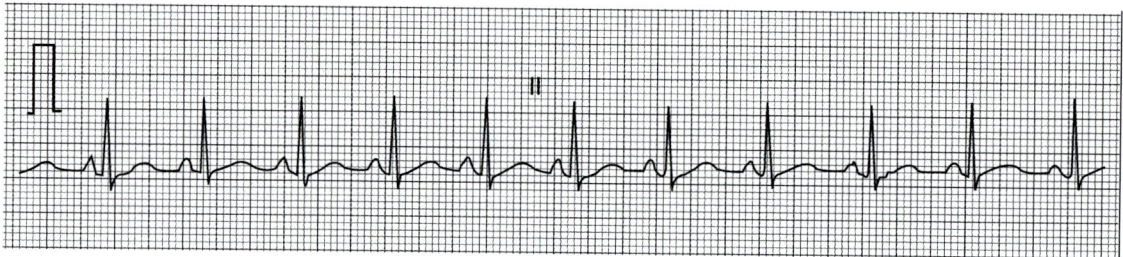

Q. What is sinus tachycardia? What are the causes of sinus tachycardia?

Ans. Sinus tachycardia is the sinus rhythm with a heart rate greater than 100/min. Causes are:

1. Physiological—anxiety, emotion, exercise, pain, pregnancy.
2. Pathological:
   • Anemia.
   • Fever.
   • Thyrotoxicosis.
   • Shock (except vasovagal attack in which bradycardia is present).
   • Heart failure.
   • Sick sinus syndrome.
   • Bleeding and hypovolemia.
   • Chronic constrictive pericarditis.
   • Acute anterior myocardial infarction (bradycardia is common in acute inferior myocardial infarction).
   • Drugs (salbutamol, atropine, adrenaline, isoprenaline, ephedrine, propantheline, thyroxine).

Q. What are the differences between sinus tachycardia and supraventricular tachycardia?

Ans. See in supraventricular tachycardia (page no. **81**).

Q. What is inappropriate sinus tachycardia ?

Ans. Persistent increase in resting heart rate unrelated to or out of proportion with the level of physical activity or emotional stress. Common in women and also in health professionals.

Q. What are the causes of narrow-complex tachycardia and broad-complex tachycardia?

Ans. Causes of narrow-complex tachycardia:

• Sinus tachycardia.
• Atrial tachycardia.
• Atrial flutter.
• Atrial fibrillation.
• AV re-entry tachycardia (SVT).

Causes of broad-complex tachycardia:

• Ventricular tachycardia.
• Supraventricular tachycardia with aberrant conduction.
• WPW syndrome.

SINUS BRADYCARDIA

ECG Criteria

- Heart rate— < 60/minute.
- P, QRS and T—normal.
- Rhythm—regular.

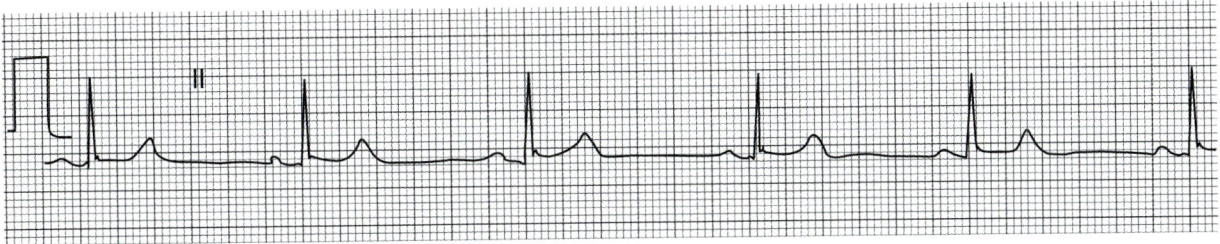

Q. What is sinus bradycardia ? What are the causes of sinus bradycardia?

Ans. Sinus bradycardia is the sinus rhythm with heart rate less than 60/min.

Causes are:

1. Physiological (due to increased vagal tone):
   - Athlete.
   - Sleep.
   - Occasionally, healthy elderly.
2. Pathological:
   - Hypothyroidism.
   - Hypothermia.
   - Raised intracranial pressure (due to inhibitory effect on sympathetic outflow).
   - Drugs (digoxin, β-blockers, verapamil).
   - Acute inferior myocardial infarction.
   - Obstructive jaundice (due to deposition of bilirubin in conducting system).
   - Sick sinus syndrome.
   - Electrolyte imbalance (hypokalemia).
   - Neurally mediated syndromes, due to a reflex (Bezold-Jarisch), which causes bradycardia and reflex peripheral vasodilatation. These are—carotid sinus syndrome, neurocardiogenic (vasovagal) syncope (syndrome), which present as syncope or presyncope.

NB: If heart rate is less than 40/min, it is less likely to be sinus bradycardia. Always think of complete heart block.

Q. What are the causes of bradycardia?

Ans. As follows:

- Sinus bradycardia due to any cause.
- Sick sinus syndrome.
- Second degree heart block (Mobitz type II).
- Complete heart block.
- Nodal rhythm.
- Idioventricular rhythm.
- Drugs (β-blocker, digoxin, etc.).

NB: Sinus bradycardia may be associated with sinus arrhythmia.

SUPRAVENTRICULAR TACHYCARDIA

ECG Criteria

- P—absent.
- QRS—narrow.
- Rhythm—regular.
- Heart rate—high (150 to 250/minute).

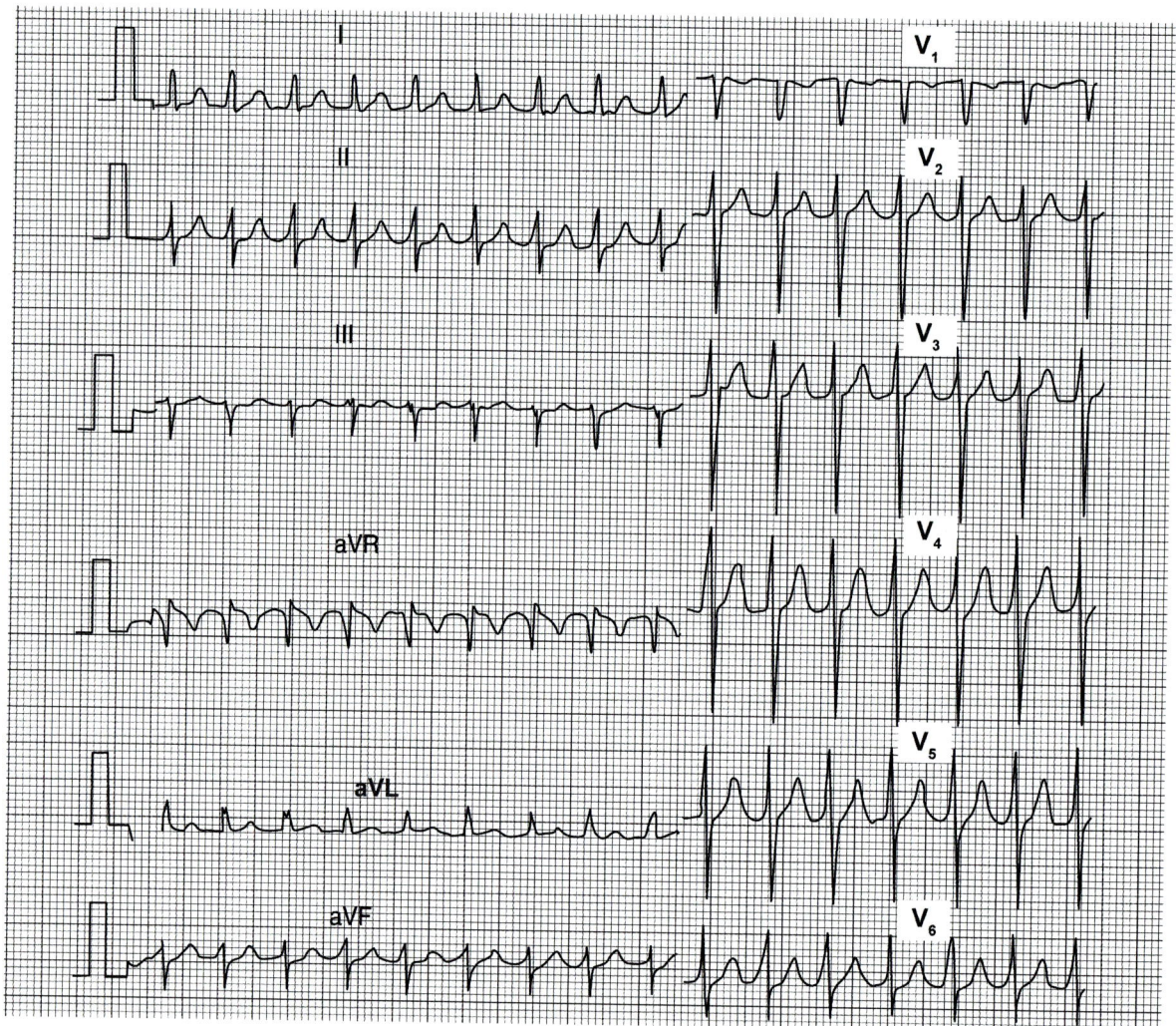

Q. What are the causes of supraventricular tachycardia (SVT)?

Ans. As follows:

1. Physiological—anxiety, tension, tea, coffee, alcohol.
2. Pathological:
    - Thyrotoxicosis.
    - Ischemic heart disease.
    - WPW syndrome.
    - Digitalis toxicity.

Q. What are the differences between sinus tachycardia and supraventricular tachycardia?

Ans. As follows:

Points	Sinus tachycardia	Supraventricular tachycardia
1. Onset	Gradual	Sudden
2. Pulse	<160/minute	>160/minute (140 to 220)
3. ECG	P, QRS, T-Normal	P absent (buried in QRS), QRS is narrow
4. Carotid sinus massage or valsalva maneuver	No or little response	May respond abruptly
5. Symptoms	Palpitation, usually present	Sudden palpitation, dizziness, syncope, breathlessness. There may be polyuria after attack (due to release of atrial natriuretic peptide)
6. Prognosis	Not serious	Hemodynamic instability is common

Q. What is the complication of SVT?

Ans. In SVT, because of rapid heart rate, there is short diastolic filling time. This results in reduction of stroke volume and precipitate heart failure.

Q. How to treat SVT?

Ans. As follows:
- Rest and reassurance.
- Carotid sinus massage or valsalva maneuver. It acts by increasing the vagal tone.
- If no response:
  — IV adenosine—3 mg over 2 seconds. If no response in 1 to 2 minute, then 6 mg IV.
  — If still no response in 1 to 2 minutes, then 12 mg (maximum dose).
  — Or IV verapamil 10 mg slowly over 5 to 10 minutes may be given (Verapamil should be avoided if QRS > 0.12 second or history of WPW syndrome or if the patient is on β-blocker).
- Other drugs—β-blocker, disopyramide or digoxin may be used.
- If the patient is hemodynamically unstable (hypotension, pulmonary edema) then DC shock should be given.
- If the attack is frequent or disabling—prophylactic oral therapy with β-blocker, verapamil, disopyramide or digoxin may be given.
- In WPW syndrome—transvenous radiofrequency catheter ablation is the treatment of choice.
- In some cases, if there is no response—antitachycardial pacing is done (overdrive atrial pacing).

Q. What is the mode of action of adenosine? What are the side effects and contraindications of adenosine therapy?

Ans. As follows:
1. *Mode of action of adenosine:* It causes transient AV block, lasting for few seconds (half-life is 8 to 10 seconds).
2. *Side effects (all are transient):*
   - Chest pain.
   - Dyspnea.
   - Bronchospasm.
   - Choking sensation.

- • Transient flushing.
- • Hypotension.
3. Contraindications:
   - • H/O bronchial asthma.
   - • Second or third degree heart block.
   - • Sick sinus syndrome.

Q. What are the types of supraventricular tachycardia?

Ans. As follows:
- • Sinus tachycardia.
- • AV nodal re-entry tachycardia (AVNRT).
- • AV reciprocating tachycardia (AVRT).
- • Atrial tachycardia.
- • Atrial flutter.
- • Atrial fibrillation.
- • Multifocal atrial tachycardia.
- • Accelerated junctional tachycardia (due to accessory pathway).

NB: Remember the following points:

- • SVT is a misnomer. The types mentioned above are all SVT, but the part written here is actually AV re-entry tachycardia with absent P wave (also it looks like nodal tachycardia with absent P wave).

- • Sinus tachycardia neither starts abruptly nor stops abruptly.

- • If SVT is associated with WPW syndorme, verapamil should not be given intravenously. Adenosine is safe in such case.

- • Look for carotid bruit before carotid sinus massage. Otherwise, thrombus may be dislodged and may cause cerebral embolism.

NODAL RHYTHM (JUNCTIONAL RHYTHM)

ECG Criteria

- Heart rate—40 to 60/minute.
- P—small, inverted (P may not be seen, buried in QRS or after QRS).
- PR interval—short.

Nodal rhythm may be of 3 types:

- *High nodal:* Small inverted P before QRS (simulate low atrial ectopic).
- *Mid nodal:* P is not seen (buried in QRS).
- *Low nodal:* P after QRS.

Q. What is nodal rhythm?

Ans.   When the impulse originate from AV node, it is called nodal or junctional rhythm. If the rate is high, it is called **junctional tachycardia**.

Usually, it occurs due to depressed activity of SA node.

Nodal rhythm may be transient or permanent.

1. Transient—may occur in normal people.
2. Also transient or permanent nodal rhythm may occur in:
   - Digitalis toxicity.
   - Ischemic heart disease (commonly, inferior myocardial infarction).
   - Rheumatic myocarditis.
   - Myocarditis due to any cause.

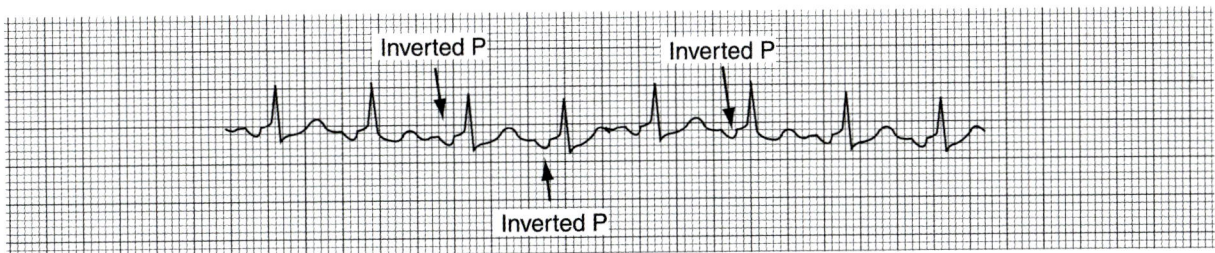

High nodal rhythm

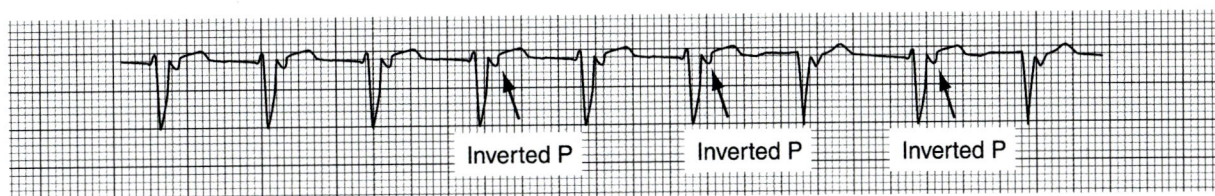

Low nodal rhythm

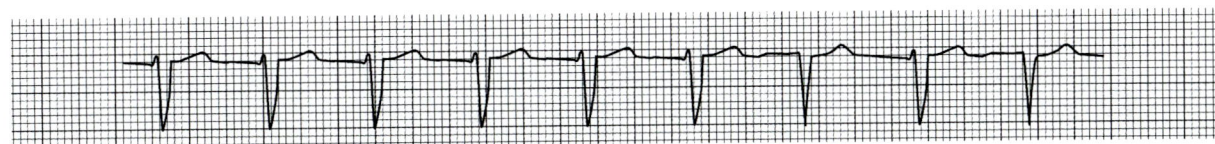

Mid nodal rhythm (P buried in QRS)

ATRIAL TACHYCARDIA

ECG Criteria

- P—Small, abnormal shape (may be upright or inverted).
- Atrial rate—140 to 220/minute.
- QRS—normal.
- Rhythm—normal.

(There may be 2:1, 3:1 or variable AV block. Atrial tachycardia with AV block is common in digoxin toxicity).

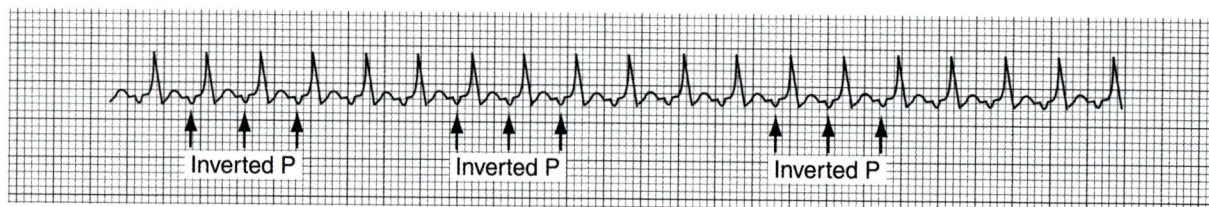

Inverted P   Inverted P   Inverted P

Q. What is the mechanism of atrial tachycardia? What are the causes of atrial tachycardia?

Ans. It is due to the ectopic focus that arise from any part of atrial myocardium.

Causes are:

- Ischemic heart disease.
- Rheumatic heart disease.
- Cardiomyopathy.
- Sick sinus syndrome.
- Digoxin toxicity.

Q. How to treat atrial tachycardia?

Ans. As follows:

1. If due to digoxin—it should be stopped.
2. If not due to digoxin:
   - To control the heart rate—digoxin, β-blocker, verapamil may be used. Amiodarone, flecainide also may be used.
   - If no response—DC cardioversion may be done.
   - Atrial overdrive pacing may also be done in selected cases.
   - Occasionally, transvenous radiofrequency catheter ablation may be done (specially with persistent and troublesome symptoms).

NB: Remember the following points:

- Carotid sinus massage will not terminate atrial tachycardia. However, it increases the AV block, thereby facilitate the diagnosis.
- Atrial tachycardia is usually paroxysmal, so it is called paroxysmal atrial tachycardia (PAT).

Q. What is multifocal atrial tachycardia (MAT)?

Ans. It is a rapid and irregular conduction rhythm originating from two or more sites of atrium. ECG shows two or more ectopic P wave of different configuration and PR is variable. It is common in COPD (due to hypoxemia).

PACEMAKER

ECG Criteria (Atrial Pacing)

- There is a spike followed by P wave.
- QRS—normal.

ECG Criteria (Ventricular Pacing)

- There is a spike followed by QRS.
- QRS—wide (looks like LBBB).

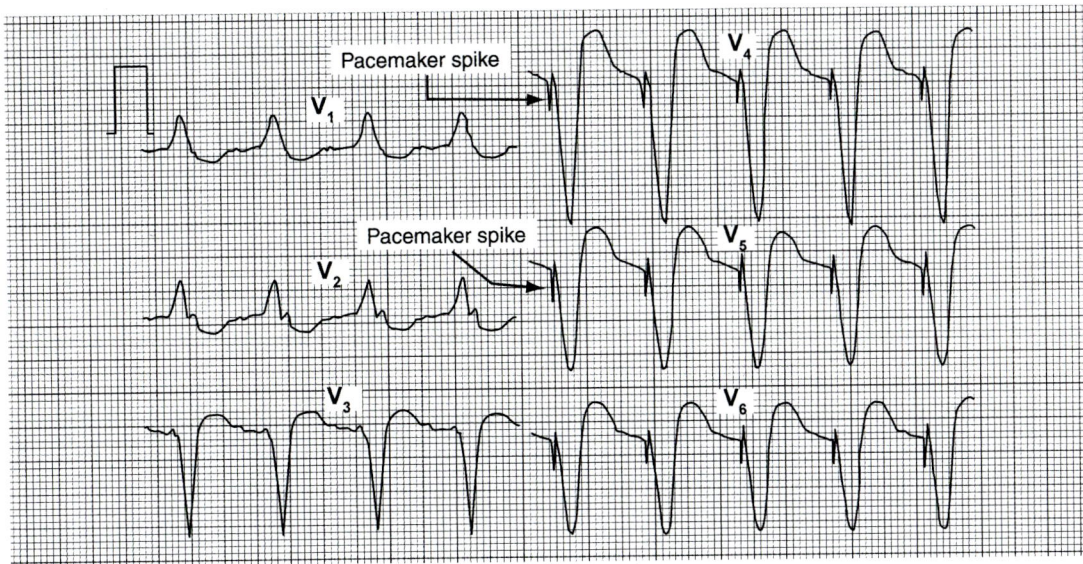

Ventricular pacemaker

NB: Remember the following points:

- *In atrial pacing:* Spike is followed by P and normal QRS.
- *In dual chamber pacing:* One spike is followed by P and another is followed by wide QRS.
- *In right ventricular pacing:* Wide QRS looks like LBBB pattern.
- *In atrial or ventricular pacing:* Spike may not be seen (in demand pacemaker).
- Diagnosis of MI may be difficult in presence of pacemaker.

Q. What are the indications of permanent pacemaker?

Ans. Most common—complete heart block with syncope or Stokes Adam's syndrome and sick sinus syndrome.

Others

- Symptomatic or asymptomatic Mobitz type 2 second degree AV block.
- Symptomatic Mobitz type 1 second degree AV block.
- Bifascicular or trifascicular block with syncope.
- Carotid sinus syndrome with bradycardia.
- Repeated vasovagal syndrome with bradycardia.
- In some cases of permanent atrial fibrillation (when other treatment fails, radiofrequency ablation followed by permanent pacemaker).

NB: After myocardial infarction, permanent pacemaker is indicated in the following conditions:

- Inferior infarction with complete heart block persisting over 2 weeks.
- Anterior infarction with persistent type 2 or complete heart block or newly acquired bundle branch or bifascicular block with transient type 2 second degree heart block or complete heart block.

Indications of Temporary Pacemaker

- Acute inferior myocardial infarction with second or third degree AV block or severe bradycardia with hemodynamic change.
- Acute extensive anterior MI with second or third degree AV block or new bifascicular block (LBBB or RBBB with left anterior hemiblock, RBBB with left posterior hemiblock).
- Patient awaiting for permanent pacing.
- Some tachycardia, such as AV re-entry tachycardia and ventricular tachycardia can be terminated by overdrive pacing.
- After open heart surgery.
- Some cases of cardiac arrest.
- Severe digitalis toxicity.

DETAILS ABOUT PACEMAKER

Pacemaker is an artificial device used to electrically stimulate the heart.

It is composed of two parts:
- Battery powered generator.
- Wire electrode - which is attached to the heart chamber to be stimulated (atrium or ventricle or both).

Two types of pacemaker—temporary and permanent.

Temporary pacemaker: They are two types:
- *Transcutaneous pacing:* Administered by delivering an electrical stimulus sufficient to induce cardiac contraction through two large adhesive gel pad electrodes placed over the apex and upper right sternal edge or over the precordium and back. It is easy and quick to set-up, but cause significant discomfort, because it induces forceful pectoral and intercostal muscle contraction. It is the preferred method in selected patient with asymptomatic bradycardia or conduction abnormality. May be life saving for patient in whom cardiac arrest is precipitated by bradycardia.
- *Transvenous pacing:* The pacing wire is introduced through a peripheral vein (internal jugular, or anticubital or subclavian or femoral) and placed in the apex of right ventricle, under fluoroscopic imaging. The electrode is connected to a portable battery-operated external pulse generator. It is withdrawn, when cardiac function is improved (usually after 7 to 10 days). Preferred method in patient with symptomatic bradycardia. A temporary pacemaker is always set to work "on demand", usual rate is 60 to 80/min.

Complications of temporary pacing—pneumothorax, brachial plexus or subclavian artery injury, local infection or septicemia *(Staph. aureus)* and pericarditis.

Permanent pacemaker: The battery-powered generator is placed subcutaneously in the chest wall or axillary region and the electrode is placed through a vein in the cardiac chamber. They are two types—dual chambered or single chambered (atrial or ventricular).

There are **two modes** of pacemaker function:
- *Fixed rate:* It fires specific preset rate, regardless of patient's own heart rate.
- *Demand pacemaker:* It works when the patient's heart rate falls below a preset rate. Currently, all pacemakers that are used are demand type.

Demand pacemaker has two components:
- *A sensing mechanism:* Designed so that the pacemaker will be inhibited, when the heart rate is adequate.
- *A pacing mechanism:* Designed to trigger the pacemaker when no intrinsic QRS complex occurs within a predetermined time period.

There are commonly **3-letter** code that describes pacemaker function, designated as:
- *First:* Chamber paced.
- *Second:* Chamber sensed.
- *Third:* Mode of response.

Letter code of pacing modes and functions

First: Chamber paced	Second: Chamber sensed	Third: Mode of response
V = Ventricle	V = Ventricle	T = Triggered
A = Atrium	A = Atrium	I = Inhibited
D = Double	D = Double	D = Double
O = None	O = None	O = None

Single Chamber Pacing (AAI, VVI)

VVI is commonly used. Ventricular pacing is only suitable for patients with continuous atrial fibrillation and bradycardia.

AAI is less reliable, but it is commonly used in sinoatrial disease (sick sinus syndrome) with intact atrioventricular conduction.

Tip of the electrode is placed in right ventricle or atrium.

Main problems are:
- It is unable to maintain normal pacemaker function, as the rate of pacemaker is fixed.
- Cannot adapt the different need of rate during exercise.
- Also the normal sequence of atrial and ventricular contraction is lost, i.e. atrioventricular synchrony is not maintained.
- VVI pacemaker may be associated with pacemaker syndrome.

Dual Chamber Pacing (DDD)

One electrode is placed in right atrium and one is placed in right ventricle.

It has some advantages:
- It maintains the atrioventricular synchrony. So, there is improved exercise performance of the patient.
- Prevents pacemaker syndrome, which is common in single chamber pacing.
- There is also lower incidence of atrial arrhythmia in a patient with sinoatrial disease.

Main problems of DDD:
- If sinus node function is abnormal—the paced rate does not increase with activity.
- Pacemaker mediated tachycardia—if they sense a retrogradely conducted P wave after ventricular depolarization, they trigger another ventricular beat, which may in turn cause another retrogradely conducted P wave. It leads to pacemaker mediated tachycardia. This can be overcome by reprogramming atrial refractory period (by increasing refractory period or by shortening atrioventricular delay).

Q. What are the complications of pacemaker?

Ans. As follows:

Early complications:

- Pneumothorax.
- Infection.
- Lead displacement.
- Cardiac tamponade.
- Pocket hematoma.

Late complications:

- Infection.
- Erosion of generator or lead.
- Chronic pain at implant site.
- Lead fracture.
- Malfunction.
- Perforation of ventricular wall.
- Ventricular arrhythmia (PVC).
- Electromagnetic interference.
- Pacemaker failure.
- Pacemaker mediated tachycardia (by dual chamber pacing).
- Pacemaker syndrome (by single chamber pacing).

Pacemaker Malfunction

Pacemaker malfunction may occur due to:

- Dislodgement of pacemaker wire.
- Or by fibrosis around the tip of pacemaker wire.

ECG Changes in Pacemaker Malfunction

- ECG shows pacemaker spikes, but no QRS.
- In other case (specially with a broken electrode wire or a short circuit in pacing circuit or electrical interference from muscles of chest wall), no pacemaker spike is seen in ECG. Failure to sense may occur in which pacemaker spike is inappropriate that may fall on T wave.

NB: If there is malfunction in temporary pacemaker, always search for loose connection between the battery and pacing wire. There may be faulty battery or dislodged wire.

Q. What is pacemaker syndrome?

Ans. It is a disorder characterized by transient hypotension, fatigue, dizziness, syncope, and distressing pulsation in the neck and chest. This occurs at the onset of ventricular contraction due to loss of atrioventricular synchrony. It occurs in single chamber pacing, which can be prevented by dual chamber pacing or by reducing the pacemaker rate so that, sinus rhythm predominates.

DIGITALIS (DIGOXIN) EFFECT

ECG Criteria
- ST—depression (sloping or scooping depression, reverse tick mark, may be rounded concave that looks like thumb impression, mostly in V_4 to V_6).
- QT—short.

NB: This effect is not due to digitalis toxicity, rather indicates digoxin effect.

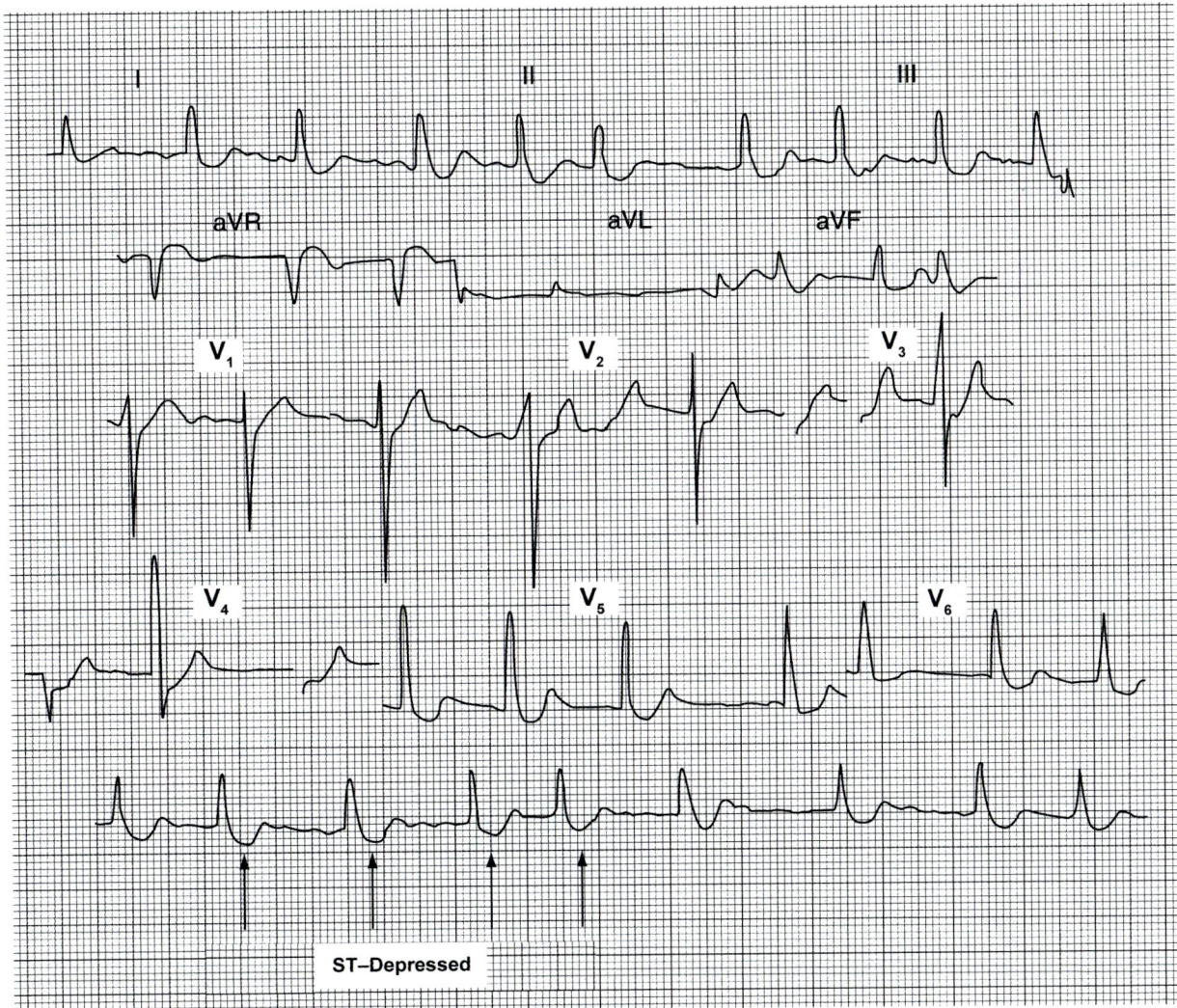

Digoxin effect with atrial fibrillation

Q. What are the toxicity of digoxin?
Ans. As follows:
1. Extracardiac:
   - Anorexia, nausea, vomiting, diarrhea, abdominal pain.
   - Visual disturbance, drowsiness, confusion, delirium, depression, hallucination, gynecomastia.

2. Cardiac:
   - Any arrhythmia—ventricular ectopic, ventricular bigeminy, paroxysmal atrial tachycardia with AV block, sinus bradycardia, nodal rhythm.
   - All types of heart block (First degree, second degree and complete heart block), bidirectional ventricular tachycardia (successive QRS alternate in direction—one upward and one downward).
   - Atrial fibrillation and atrial flutter rarely occur.

Q. How to treat digoxin toxicity?

Ans. As follows:
- Digoxin should be stopped.
- Correction of electrolyte imbalance, specially hypokalemia.
- Treatment of underlying arrhythmia.
- In severe bradycardia or complete heart block with hemodynamic change—temporary pacemaker may be given.
- In severe life threatening case or in digoxin poisoning—digoxin specific antibody may be given.

HYPOKALEMIA

ECG Criteria

- U—prominent in chest leads (most common).
- Others—ST depression, T is small or inverted, prolonged PR interval.

Q. What are the effects of hypokalemia on heart?

Ans. As follows:
- Arrhythmia—atrial and ventricular including ventricular tachycardia, ventricular fibrillation.
- Aggravates digoxin toxicity.
- Cardiac arrest (in diastole).

Q. How to treat hypokalemia?

Ans. As follows:
- If serum potassium is > 2.5 mmol/L—oral potassium therapy.
- If severe or serum potassium is < 2.5 mmol/L—potassium is given in infusion (with dextrose or normal saline).
- Treatment of primary cause.

NB: Potassium should never be given in direct IV. Failure to correct hypokalemia may be due to concurrent hypomagnesemia. So, it should be measured and corrected).

Q. What are the causes of hypokalemia?

Ans. As follows:
- Diuretics (specially thiazide, frusemide)—most common cause.
- Gastrointestinal loss—diarrhea, vomiting, purgative abuse, villous adenoma, ileostomy.
- Renal loss—RTA type I and II, renal tubular necrosis (diuretic phase), Bartter's syndrome, Liddle's syndrome, Gitelman's syndrome.
- Endocrine cause—Cushing's syndrome, Conn's syndrome.
- Others—heart failure, liver failure, nephrotic syndrome, drug (salbutamol, fenoterol), insulin therapy (in diabetic ketoacidosis), alkalosis, hypokalemic periodic paralysis, Chronic hypokalemia is associated with interstitial renal disease.

Q. What are the effects of hypokalemia?

Ans. As follows:
- May be asymptomatic (if serum potassium > 2.5 mmol/ L).
- If severe hypokalemia (if serum potassium < 2.5 mmol/L)—muscular weakness, paralysis, loss of tendon reflex, paralytic ileus, arrhythmia, increase digoxin toxicity.

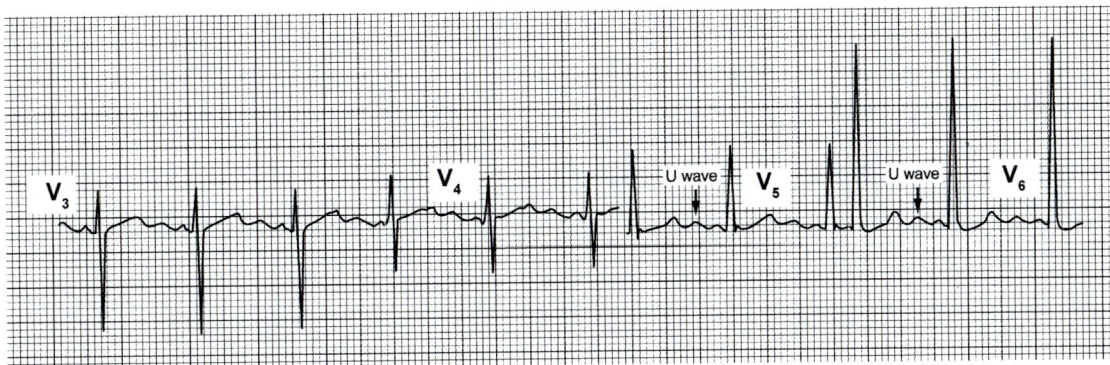

U wave

HYPERKALEMIA

ECG Criteria

- T—tall, peaked and tented (in chest leads).
- P—wide, small, ultimately absent.
- PR interval—prolonged.
- QRS—wide, slurred and bizarre.

Q. What are the causes of hyperkalemia?

Ans. As follows:

1. High potassium intake (oral or IV fluid with potassium, food or drugs containing potassium).
2. Renal diseases:
   - Acute and chronic renal failure.
   - Impaired tubular secretion of K^+ (renal lupus, amyloidosis, transplanted kidney).
3. Endocrine diseases:
   - Addison's disease.
   - Diabetic ketoacidosis.
   - Primary hypoaldosteronism.
4. Drugs:
   - Potassium sparing diuretics (spironolactone, amiloride, triamterine).
   - ACE inhibitor.
   - NSAID.
   - Cyclosporin.

NB: Combination of ACE inhibitor and K^+ sparing diuretic or NSAID is dangerous.

5. Pseudohyperkalemia (due to abnormal release of K^+ from abnormal or damaged cells), also called spurious hyperkalemia, causes of which are:
   - Blood kept at room temperature for longtime before analysis.
   - Acute leukemia.
   - Hemolysis.
   - Thrombocytosis
   - Infectious mononucleosis.
6. Miscellaneous:
   - Acidosis.
   - Rhabdomyolysis.
   - Tumor lysis syndrome.
   - Digoxin poisoning.
   - Vigorous exercise.
   - Hyperkalemic periodic paralysis.
   - Hyporeninemic hypoaldosteronism (Type IV RTA).
   - Gordon's syndrome.
   - Transfusion of stored blood.

Q. What are the effects of hyperkalemia on heart?

Ans.   As follows:

- Any arrhythmia, even ventricular tachycardia, ventricular fibrillation.
- Hyperkalemia causes hyperpolarization of cell membranes, leading to decreased cardiac excitability, hypotension, bradycardia, and eventual asystole or cardiac arrest.

Q. What are the features of hyperkalemia?

Ans.   As follows:

- May be asymptomatic.
- Muscular weakness, which may be severe causing flaccid paralysis, loss of tendon jerk.
- Paralytic ileus (abdomen may be distended).
- Tingling around the lip or finger.
- Sudden death due to cardiac arrest or arrhythmia.

Q. How to treat hyperkalemia?

Ans.   As follows:

- Withdrawal of potassium, potassium containing food and offending drug.
- Injection 10% calcium gluconate 10 to 20 cc IV slowly over 10 minutes. It may be repeated (it protects the myocardium and also reduces the risk of cardiac arrest).
- Injection 50 ml of 50% glucose IV + Inj. insulin 10 units (specially if there is hyperglycemia). This can be repeated if necessary (glucose can be given without insulin, it stimulates endogenous insulin secretion).
- Correction of acidosis—by IV sodibicarb (1.26%), 500 ml 6 to 8 hourly (until serum HCO_3 is normal).
- Treatment of primary causes.
- In some cases, exchange resins (calcium resonium 15 to 30 gm orally).
- If all fail—hemodialysis or peritoneal dialysis.

NB: Hyperkalemia is dangerous, if K^+ is > 7 mmol/L. It may cause cardiac arrest in systole.

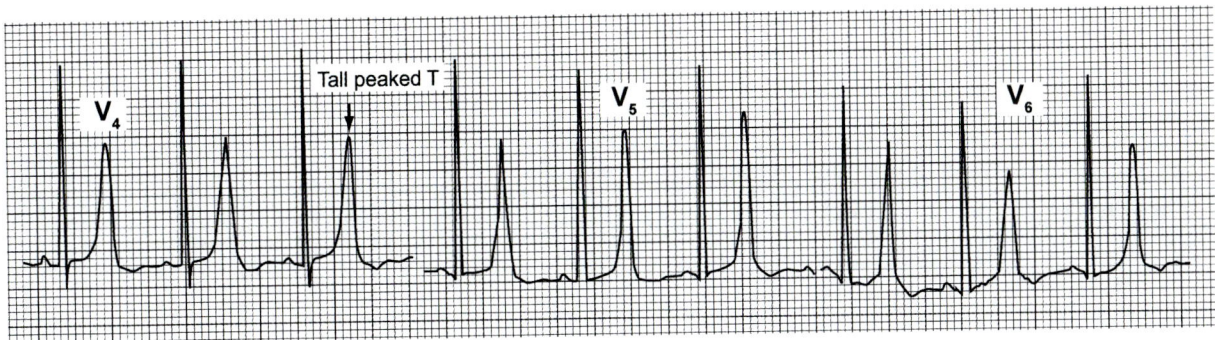

Tall peaked T

PULMONARY EMBOLISM

ECG Criteria

- Sinus tachycardia (common).
- P pulmonale (tall P wave in L_{II}, L_{III} and aVF).
- RBBB (incomplete or complete).
- ST depression and T wave inversion in right precordial leads (V_1 and V_2).
- Right axis deviation.
- S_I, Q_{III}, T_{III} pattern (S in L_I, Q and T inversion in L_{III}).
  (This is a classic combination of ECG findings in pulmonary embolism).

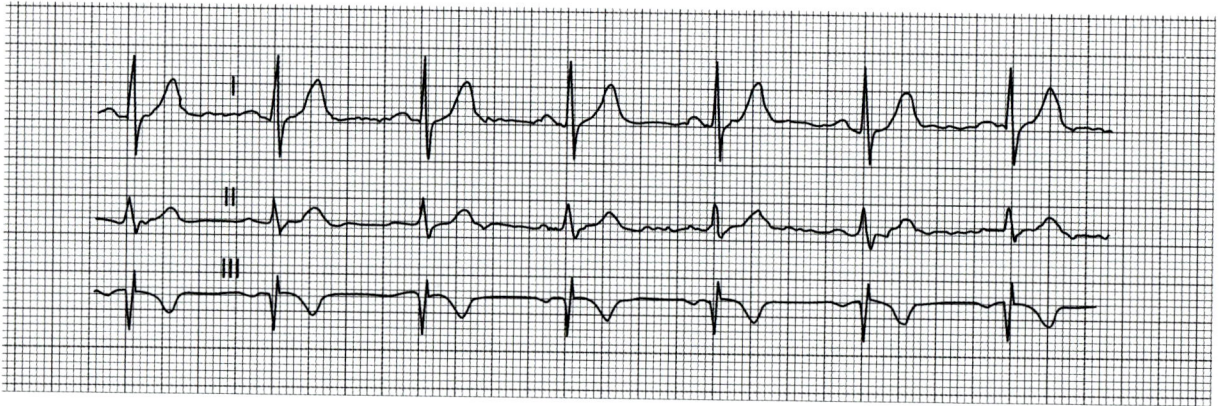

$S_1 Q_3 T_3$

Q. What are the arrhythmias that may be found in pulmonary embolism?

Ans. As follows:
- Sinus tachycardia (most common).
- Atrial fibrillation.
- Atrial flutter.
- Ventricular ectopics.

Q. What are the features of acute massive pulmonary embolism?

Ans. As follows:
- Severe central chest pain.
- Severe dyspnea.
- Faintness or syncope.
- On examination:
  — Tachycardia.
  — Tachypnea.
  — Cyanosis.
  — Wide splitting of second heart sound.
  — Right ventricular gallop.
  — Features of shock.

Q. What investigations are done to diagnose pulmonary embolism?

Ans.   As follows:
- Chest X-ray P/A view (oligemic lung fields, enlarged pulmonary artery, wedge shaped opacity due to pulmonary infarction, linear atelactasis, focal infiltration, raised hemidiaphragm. May be normal X-ray in many cases).
- ECG—see above.
- Blood gas analysis—low PaO_2 and low $PaCO_2$.
- If pulmonary infarction—neutrophil leukocytosis, high ESR, high LDH.
- Echocardiogram—vigorously contracting left ventricle and a clot in right heart or main pulmonary artery.
- Ventilation and perfusion scan (V/Q scan)—reduction of perfusion in major lung area.
- Spiral CT angiography—it is sensitive and specific for medium size embolism.
- MRI (if CT is contraindicated).
- Plasma D-dimer—if it is low or undetectable, it excludes pulmonary embolism.
- Pulmonary angiography (may be done in some cases). It is definitive.

Q. How to treat pulmonary embolism?

Ans.   As follows:
- High flow oxygen (60 to 100%).
- Relief of pain by opium (morphine or pethidine).
- Anticoagulant-inj. heparin 10,000 units IV as a bolus dose, followed by continuous infusion 1000 to 2000 units/hour. Or low molecular heparin given subcutaneously.
- Oral anticoagulant (warfarin)—started after 48 hours of heparin therapy. Heparin is usually stopped after 5 days.
- Warfarin is continued for 6 weeks to 6 months. In recurrent pulmonary embolism, it may be required to continue for lifelong.
- Fibrinolytic therapy—streptokinase (2,50,000 units by IV infusion over 30 minute followed by streptokinase 1,00,000 units IV hourly for up to 12 to 72 hours). Or alteplase (60 mg IV over 15 minutes) is used following a major embolism. Heparin should be given subsequently.
- In massive pulmonary embolism with severe hemodynamic compromise—surgical embolectomy is necessary.
- In case of recurrent pulmonary embolism—insertion of a filter in inferior vena cava above the level of renal veins may be done.

NB: Remember the following points:

- Signs and symptoms of small and medium sized pulmonary emboli may be non-specific, diagnosis is delayed or missed.
- Pulmonary embolism should be considered, if the patient presents with symptoms of unexplained cough, chest pain, hemoptysis, new-onset atrial fibrillation or other tachycardia or signs of pulmonary hypertension, if no other cause found.

DEXTROCARDIA

ECG Criteria

- *P wave:* Inverted in L_I, (upright in L_{III}).
- *R wave:* Tall in V_1, diminishing progressively in V_5 and V_6.
- *Right axis:* Deviation.

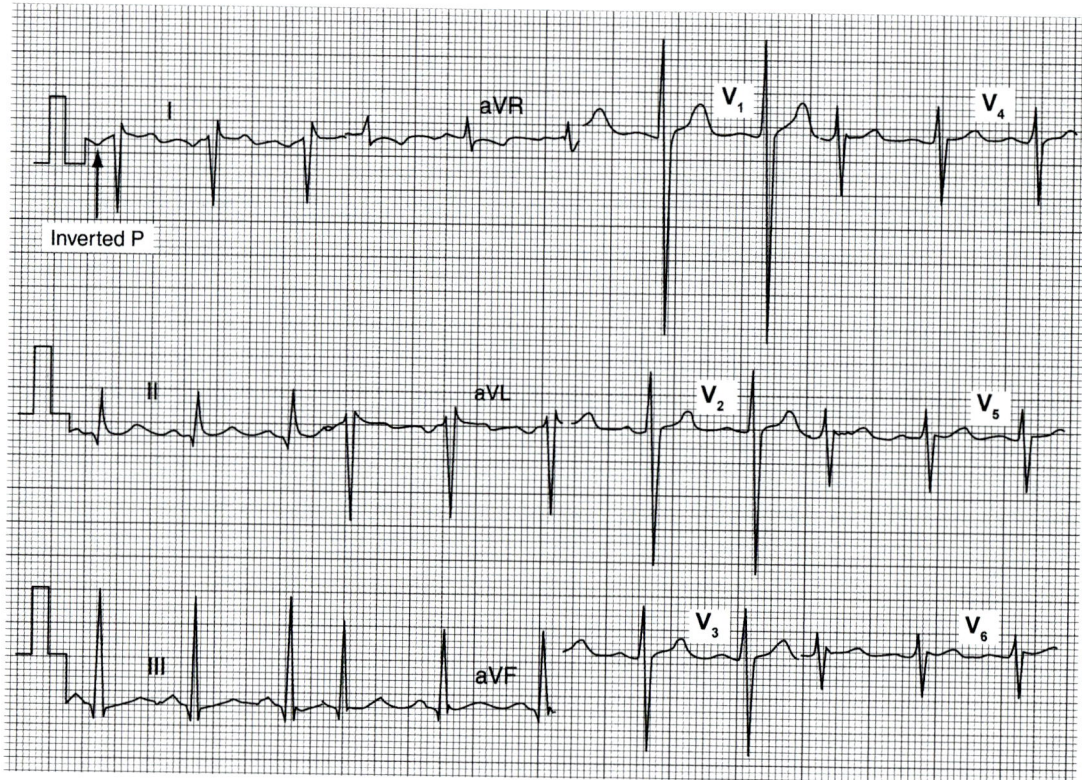

Q. What is the differential diagnosis of dextrocardia?

Ans. Incorrectly placed or reversed arm electrodes. In this case, P wave is inverted in L_I, but QRS in chest leads will remain normal (tall R in V_5 and V_6).

Q. What is dextrocardia?

Ans. It is a congenital disorder in which the heart is located in the right side of chest, but other organs are in their usual positions.

Q. If the patient has dextrocardia, what else do you want to see?

Ans. I want to see the evidence of Kartagener's syndrome, characterized by:
- Dextrocardia.
- Bronchiectasis.
- Frontal sinusitis or frontal sinus agenesis.

Q. What other investigations would you suggest?

Ans. As follows:
- CXR (heart on the right side of chest, features of bronchiectasis).
- X-ray PNS—evidence of frontal sinusitis or frontal sinus agenesis.

Q. What is situs inversus?

Ans.   When there is dextrocardia with reversal of the sites of other visceras (stomach on right side, liver on the left side, right lung is on the left and left lung is on the right).

Q. What is levocardia?

Ans.   When the heart is on the left side of chest, but there is reversal of the sites of other visceras, it is called levocardia (stomach on right side, liver on the left side, right lung is on the left and left lung is on the right).

Q. What is mesocardia?

Ans.   When the cardiac apex is in the midline, it is called mesocardia.

NB: Remember the following points:

- If dextrocardia is associated with situs inversus, the heart is usually otherwise normal.
- In case of isolated dextrocardia or levocardia, there may also be multiple cardiac anomalies.

Q. What is the clinical importance of situs inversus ?

Ans.   As follows:
- Diagnosis of acute appendicitis may be missed, as appendix is on the left side.
- As the liver is on the left side, during liver biopsy, care should be taken, so that the biopsy needle is not mistakenly given on right side.

ELECTROMECHANICAL DISSOCIATION

ECG Criteria

- P, QRS, T all normal.
- Evidence of the cause.

Q. What is electromechanical dissociation?

Ans. When the heart continues to work electrically, but unable to contract. So, there will be no cardiac output, no pulse, no blood pressure and the patient is unconscious.

Causes are:
- Cardiac tamponade.
- Hypovolemia.
- Hypothermia.
- Hypoxia.
- Tension pneumothorax.
- Cardiac rupture.
- Massive pulmonary embolism.
- Electrolyte imbalance—hypokalemia.
- Drug overdose—cardiodepressant drug, e.g. β-blocker.

Q. How to treat EMD?

Ans. Treatment depends on underlying causes.
- Specific treatment of underlying cause.
- Intubate and IV access.
- Inj. Adrenaline (1 mg IV).
- CPR.
- Other therapy—pressor agents, calcium, etc.

NB: Electromechanical dissociation is frequently a late event in cardiac arrest and indicates a poor prognosis. When electromechanical dissociation is the presenting feature, it suggests the possibility of underlying ventricular rupture and it is unlikely that the patient will be resuscitated.

However, potentially treated causes should not be overlooked.

HYPOTHERMIA

ECG Criteria

- J wave (at the junction of distal limb of QRS).
- Other findings:
  — Sinus bradycardia.
  — First and second degree heart block.
  — Prolongation of QT interval.
  — Ectopics.
  — Atrial fibrillation (if temperature < 29°C).
  — May be ventricular tachycardia, ventricular fibrillation (if temperature < 30°C).
  — Tracing may be low voltage.

COPD

Following ECG changes may occur:
- Low voltage tracing.
- P-pulmonale (right atrial hypertrophy).
- Tall R in V_1 (right ventricular hypertrophy).
- Right axis deviation.
- Poor R wave progression.
- Occasionally, multifocal atrial tachycardia.

HYPERMAGNESEMIA
(Serum magnesium > 2.5 mEq/L)

ECG Criteria

ECG change like hyperkalemia.

HYPOMAGNESEMIA
(Serum magnesium < 1.5 mEq/L)

ECG Criteria

ECG change like hypokalemia.

ATRIAL SEPTAL DEFECT

Two types of atrial septal defects: (1) Ostium primum (10%) and (2) ostium secundum (90%).

ECG Criteria in Ostium Primum Defect

- Incomplete or complete RBBB.
- Left axis deviation.

ECG Criteria in Ostium Secundum Defect

- Incomplete or complete RBBB.
- Right axis deviation.

HYPOTHYROIDISM

ECG Criteria

- Low voltage tracing.
- Sinus bradycardia.
- T inversion.

HYPERTHYROIDISM

ECG Criteria

- Sinus tachycardia (most common).
- Arrhythmia—atrial fibrillation, ectopic beat.

HYPOCALCEMIA

ECG Criteria

- Prolongation of QT interval.
- Prolongation of ST segment.

Hypocalcemia may cause atrial or ventricular arrhythmia, even torsades de pointes).

HYPERCALCEMIA

ECG Criteria

- Short QT interval.
- May be prominent U wave.
- Shortening of ST segment.
- May be prolongation of PR interval and QRS complex.

Hypercalcemia may cause atrial or ventricular arrhythmia, specially if the patient is taking digoxin.

PERICARDIAL EFFUSION

ECG Criteria

- Low voltage tracing.
- T inversion.
- Sinus tachycardia.

(There may be electrical alternans, in which height of R and T wave alternates from beat to beat. The combination of small QRS, tachycardia and electrical alternans is highly suggestive of pericardial effusion).

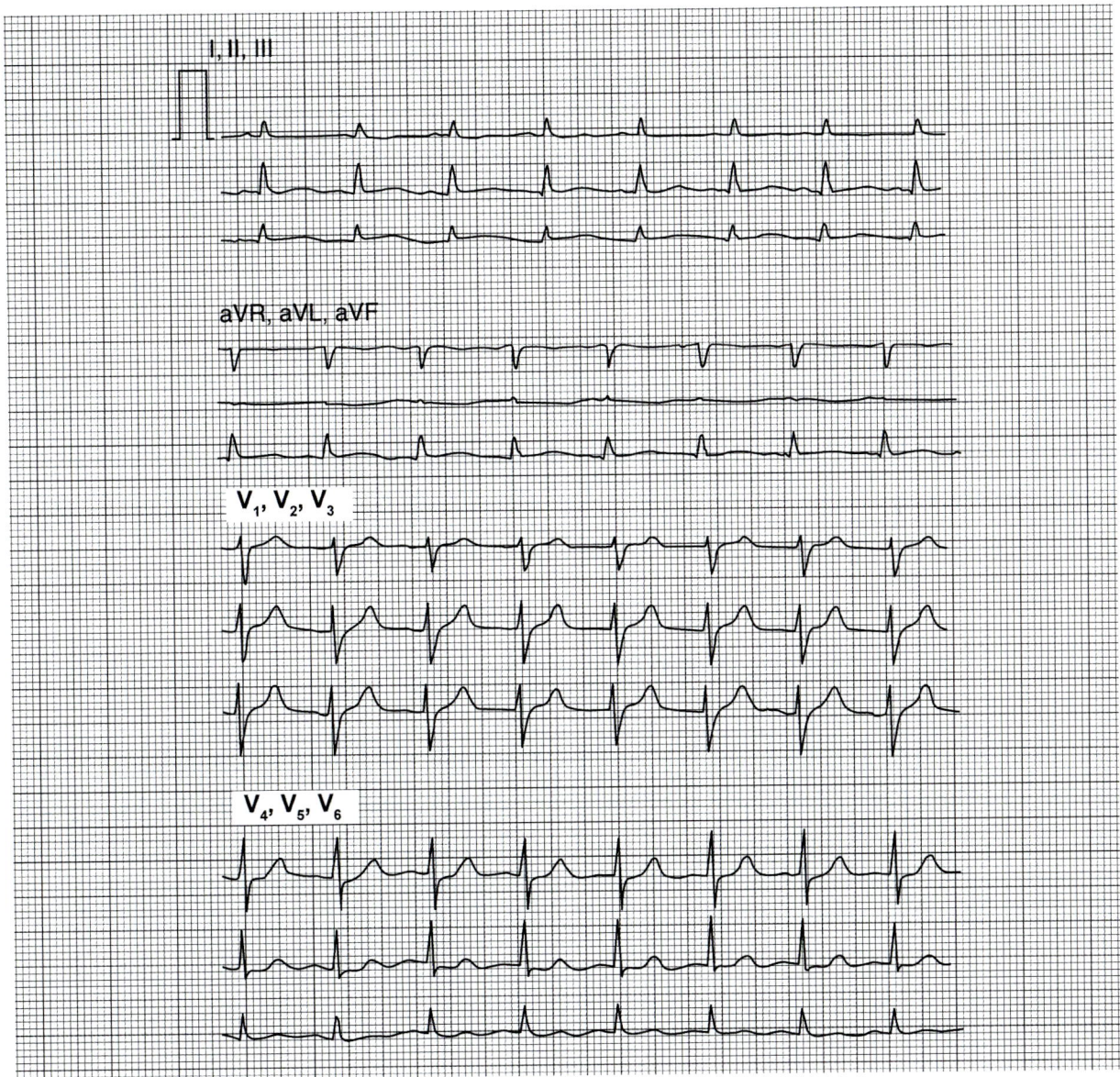

Low voltage tracing

WANDERING PACEMAKER

ECG Criteria

* P-variable configuration (some inverted, some small, some upright).
* PR interval—variable.
* QRS—normal.

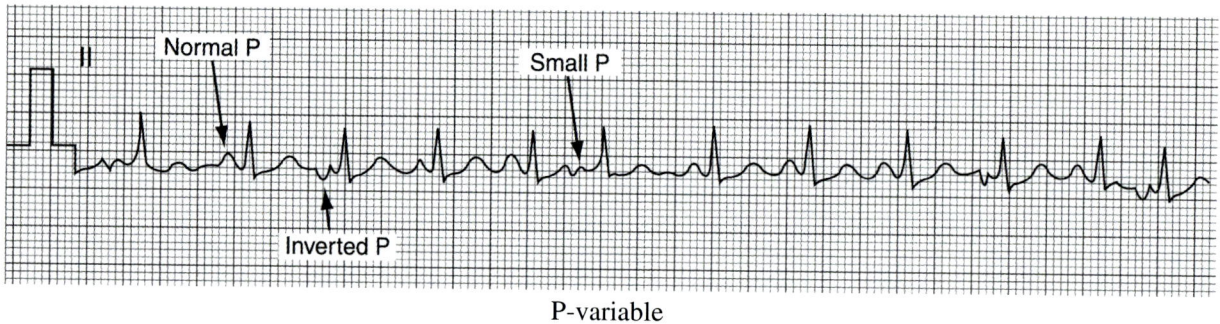

P-variable

Q. What is wandering pacemaker?

Ans. It is an arrhythmia in which there is multiple pacemaker impulses originating from two or more sites in SA node, atrium or AV junction. So, P wave configuration is variable and PR interval is also variable.

Q. What are the causes of wandering pacemaker?

Ans. As follows:
* Normal individual (due to increased in vagal tone).
* Digitalis toxicity.
* Rheumatic carditis.
* Chronic lung disease.
* Valvular disease (mitral and tricuspid valve disease).

NB: Wandering pacemaker may be associated with sinus arrhythmia.

ATRIAL ECTOPIC

ECG Criteria

- P—small or inverted (abnormal shape).
- PR interval—short (followed by wide pause).
- PP interval—irregular.

(When atrial ectopic is associated with tachycardia, it is called chaotic or multifocal atrial tachycardia. Atrial ectopic may not be followed by QRS. It is called blocked or nonconducted atrial ectopic).

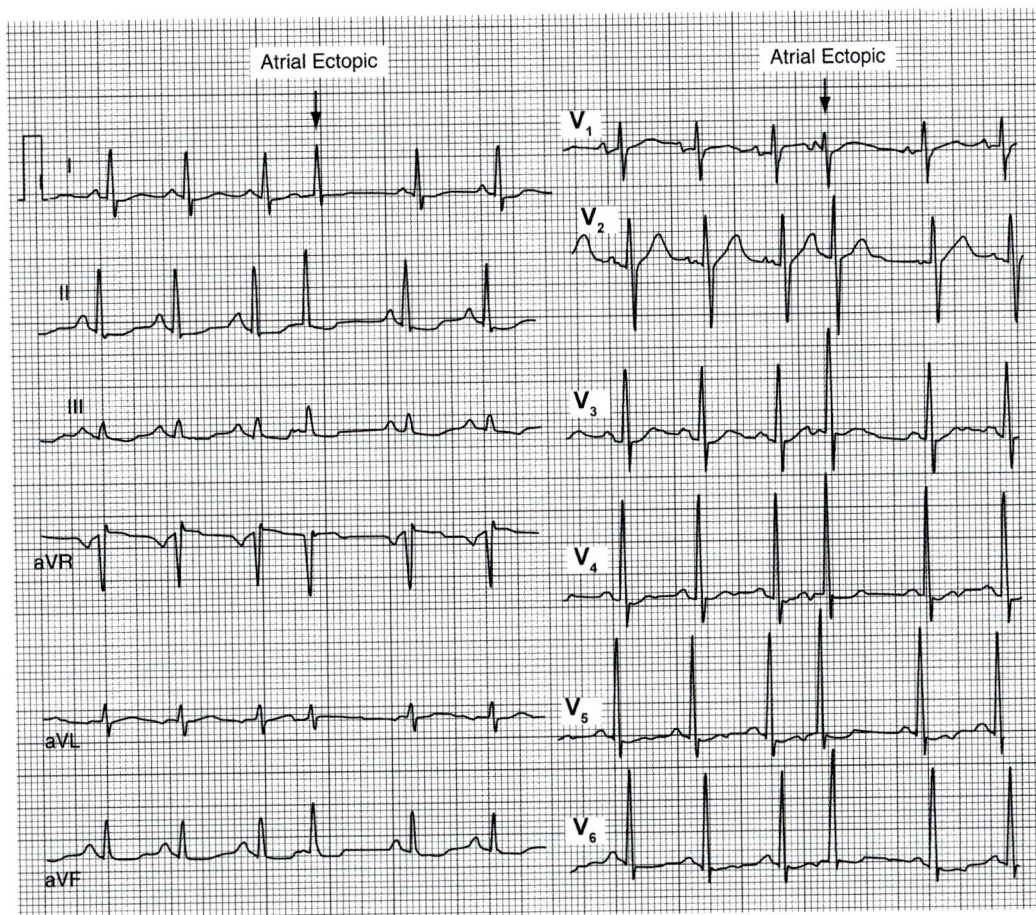

Q. What are the causes of atrial ectopics?

Ans. As follows:
- Normal people, excess tea, coffee, smoking.
- Any organic heart disease (myocarditis, cardiomyopathy).
- Electrolyte imbalance.
- COPD (usually multifocal atrial tachycardia, due to hypoxemia).

Q. What are the types of atrial ectopics?

Ans. Two types:
- *High atrial:* P is upright in L_I and aVF.
- *Low atrial:* P is inverted in L_{II}, L_{III} and aVF (confuses with high nodal ectopic).

Q. What is ectopic beat ? What is the ECG criteria?

Ans. Ectopic beat or extrasystole is a premature extra beat that comes earlier than the normal beat. It arises from abnormal focus from atria, AV node or ventricle.

ECG Criteria of Ectopic

In ECG, sequence is as follows:

- There is **Normal** beat - **Short** pause - **Ectopic** beat - **Long** pause - **Strong** beat.

Q. How many types of ectopic beat?

Ans. They are three types:

- Atrial.
- Nodal.
- Ventricular.

Atrial ectopics may be:

- High atrial.
- Low atrial.

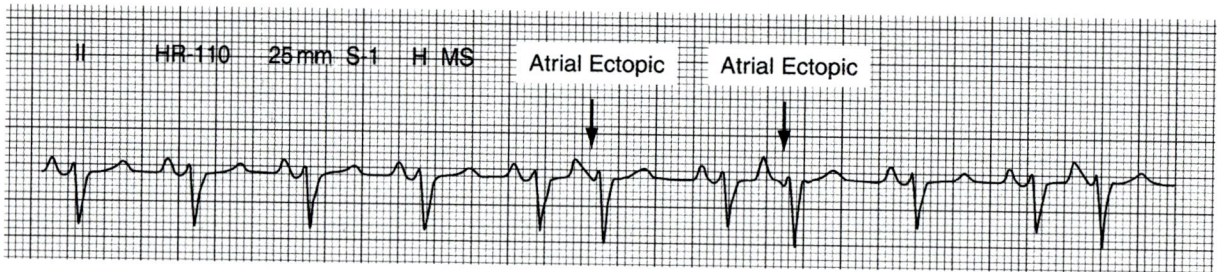

Nodal ectopics may be 3 types:

- High nodal (P inverted).
- Mid nodal (P is not seen, buried in QRS).
- Low nodal (P after QRS).

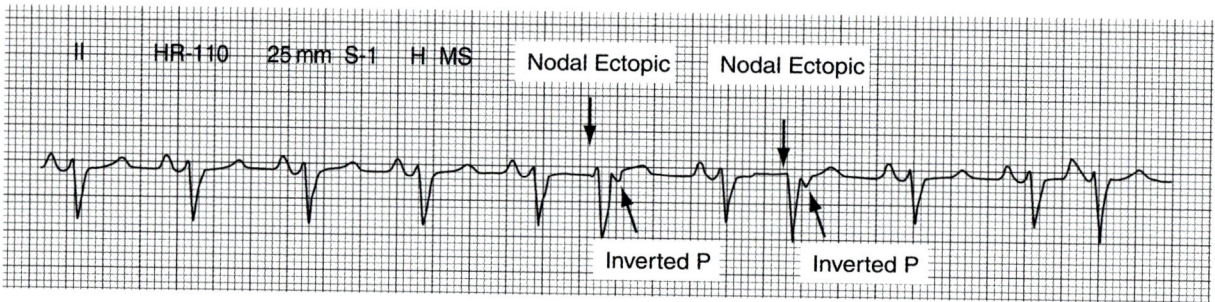

Low nodal ectopic

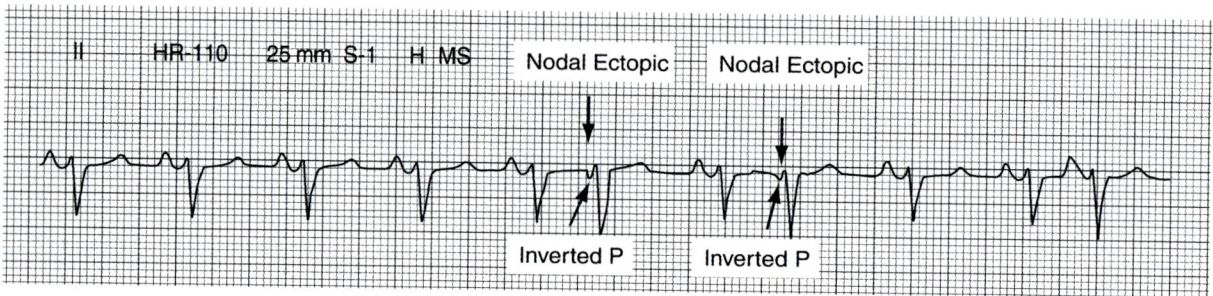

High nodal ectopic

VENTRICULAR BIGEMINY

ECG Criteria

- Every normal beat is followed by an ectopic beat.

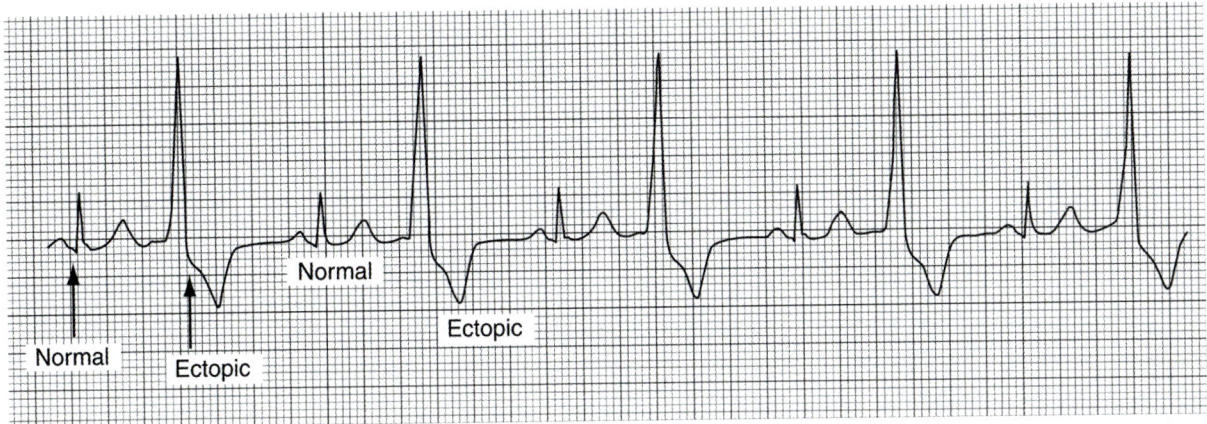

Q. What are the causes of bigeminy?

Ans. As follows:
- Digoxin toxicity.
- Myocarditis.
- Cardiomyopathy.
- After acute myocardial infarction.
- Electrolyte imbalance (hypokalemia).
- Hypoxemia.

Q. How to treat ventricular bigeminy?

Ans. As follows:
- If on any offending drug—it should be stopped.
- Correction of electrolytes, specially hypokalemia. (Also hyperkalemia, hypomagnesemia).
- Treatment of primary cause or any organic heart disease.
- If asymptomatic—no other treatment.
- If symptomatic—β-blocker. Antiarrhythmic drugs should be avoided, may worsen the prognosis.

VENTRICULAR TRIGEMINY

ECG Criteria

Every two normal beat is followed by an ectopic beat.

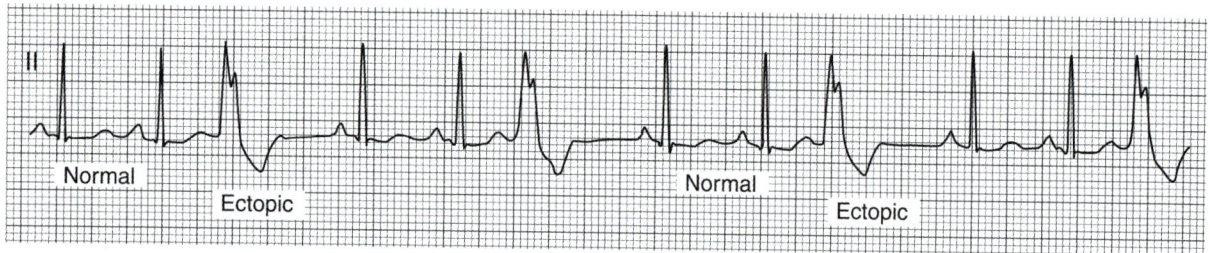

Q. What are the causes of ventricular trigeminy?
Ans. Causes are same like bigeminy.

VENTRICULAR QUADRIGEMINY

ECG Criteria

Every three normal beat is followed by an ectopic beat.

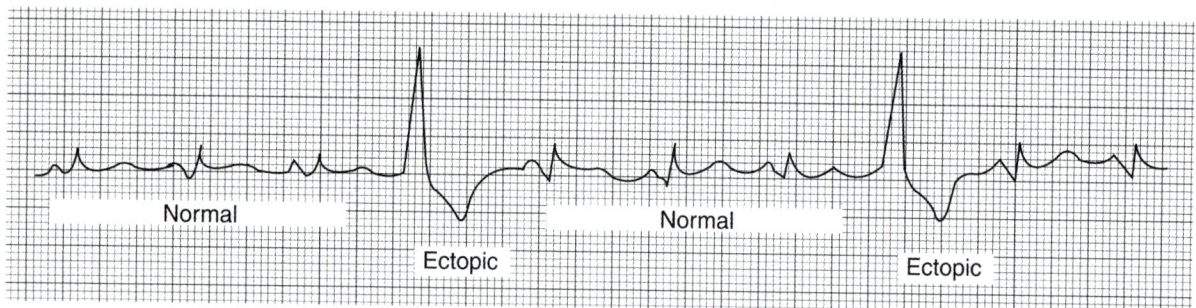

Q. What are the causes of ventricular quadrigeminy?
Ans. Causes are same like bigeminy.

CHAPTER
III

150 Tracings of ECG

"Most of the doctors can competently interpret ECG
without getting submerged in its complexities"

Remember "there is no need for the ECG to be daunting:
Just as most people drive car without knowing much
about the engines and the gardeners do not
necessarily need to be a botanist"

150 ECG tracings are included here.
The reader should interpret by himself and then
compare the findings given in the last pages.
In this way, it will offer a good
self-learning and exercise in ECG.

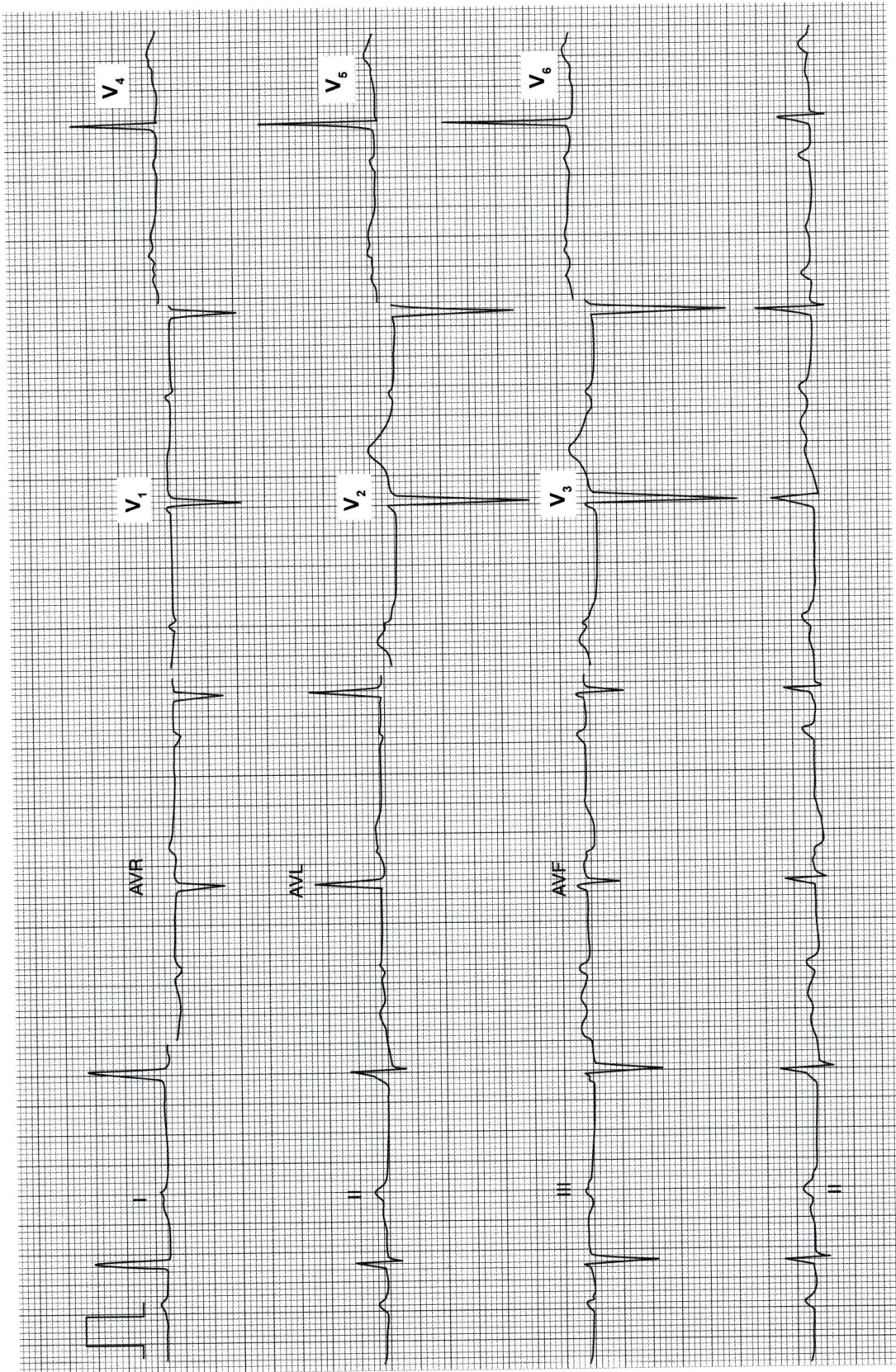

ECG NO. 1

ECG NO. 2

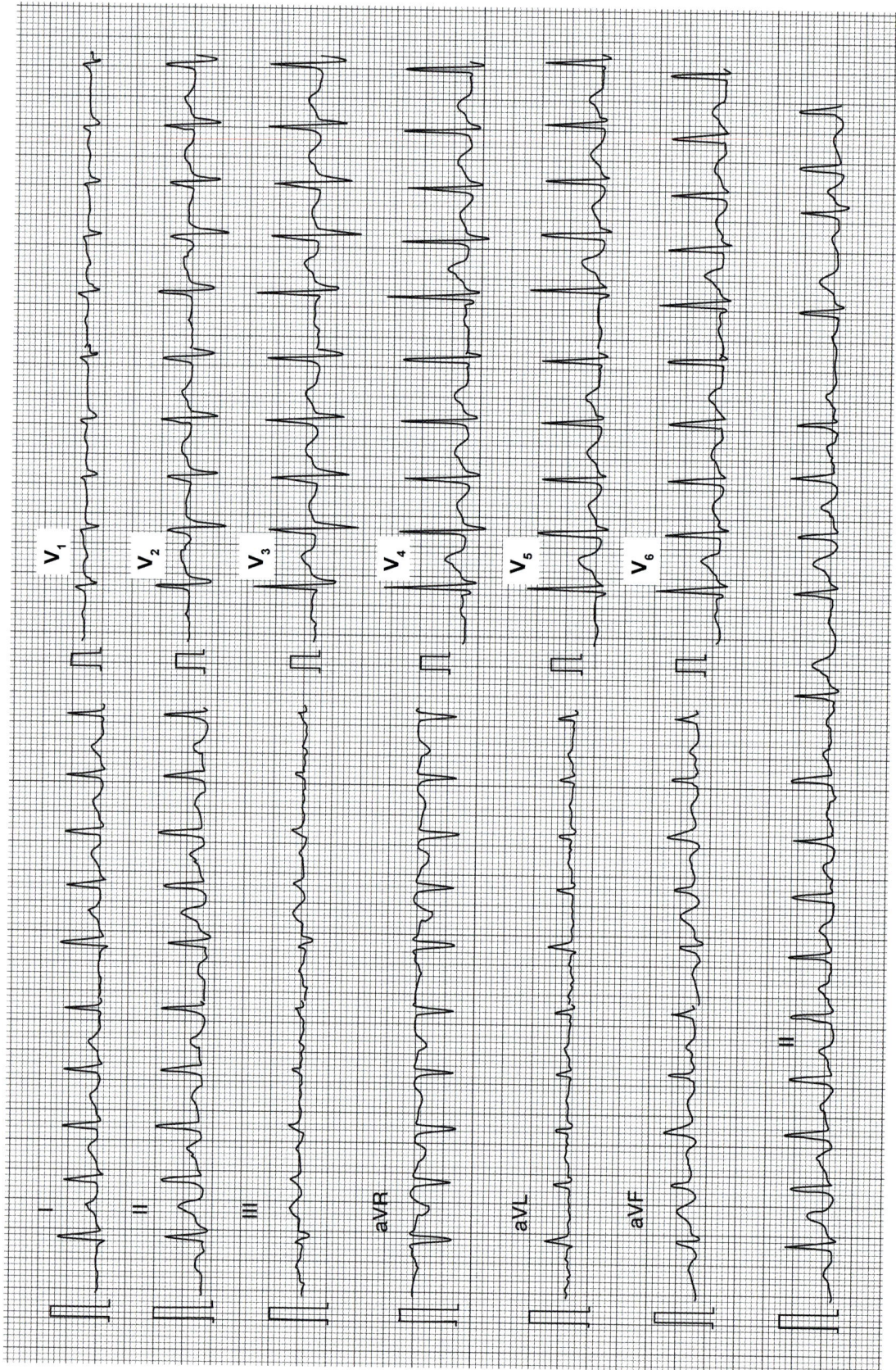

ECG NO. 3

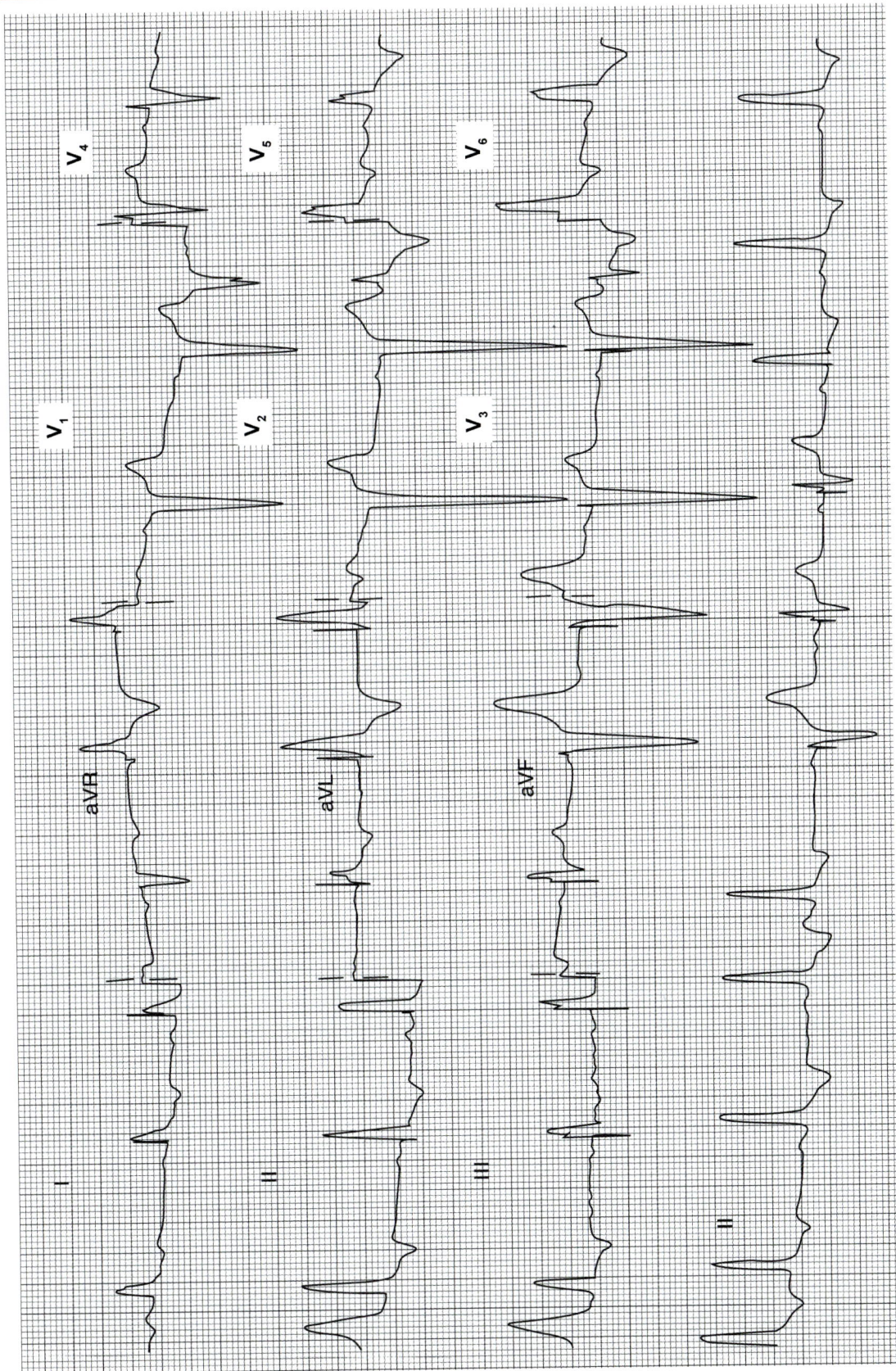

I

II

III

aVR

aVL

aVF

V₁

V₂

V₃

V₄

V₅

V₆

II

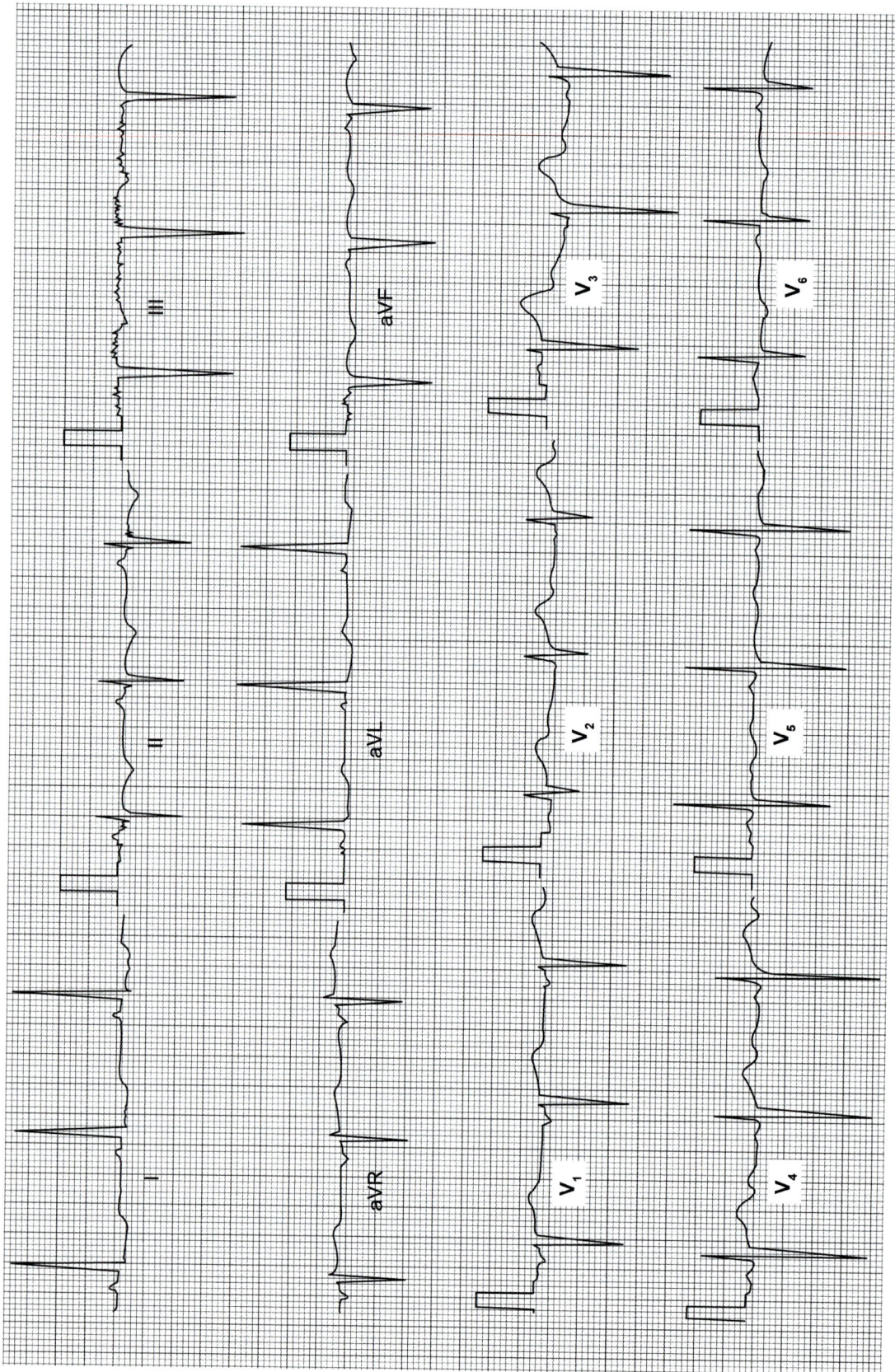

ECG NO. 4

ECG NO. 7

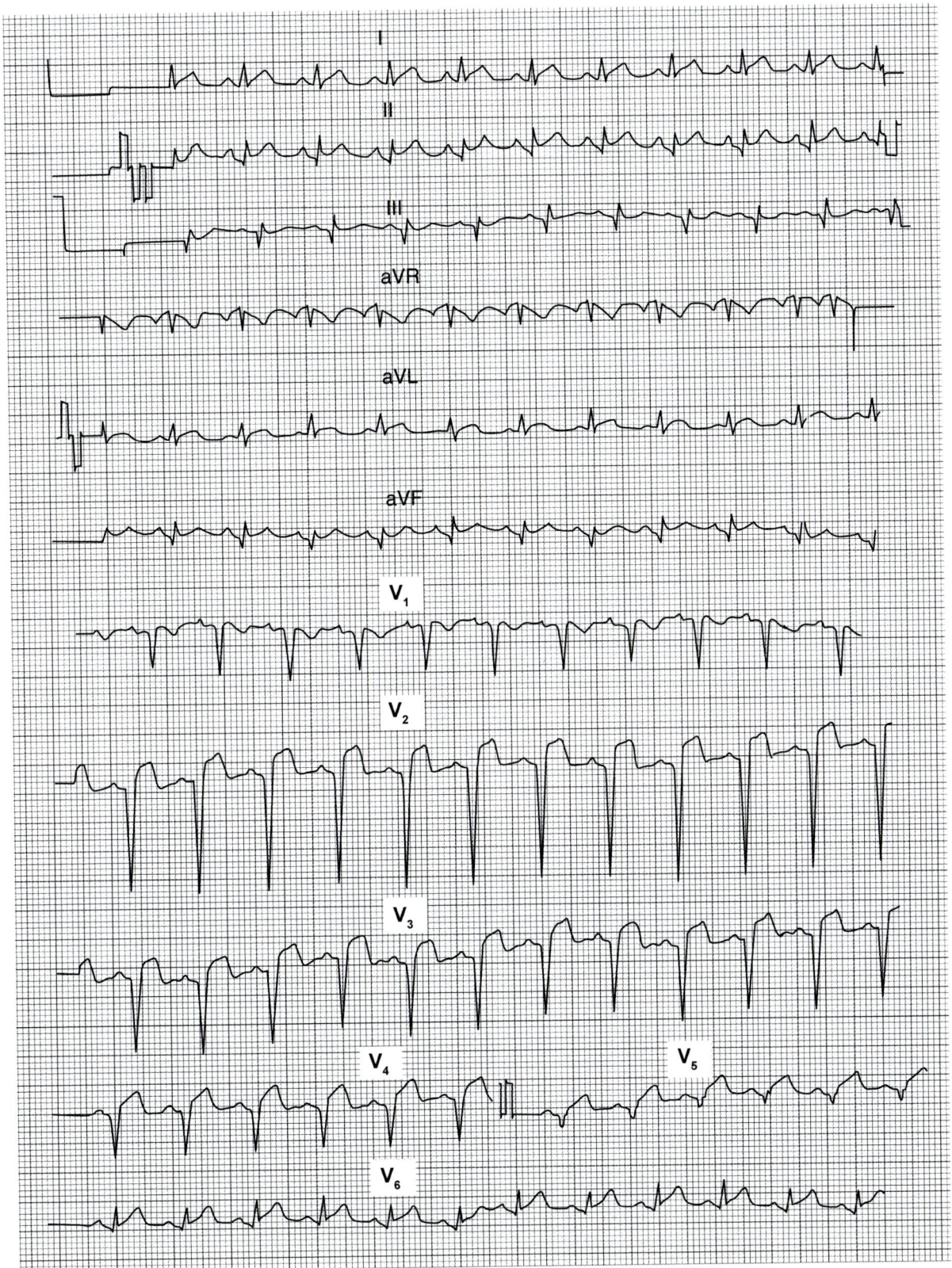

ECG NO. 8

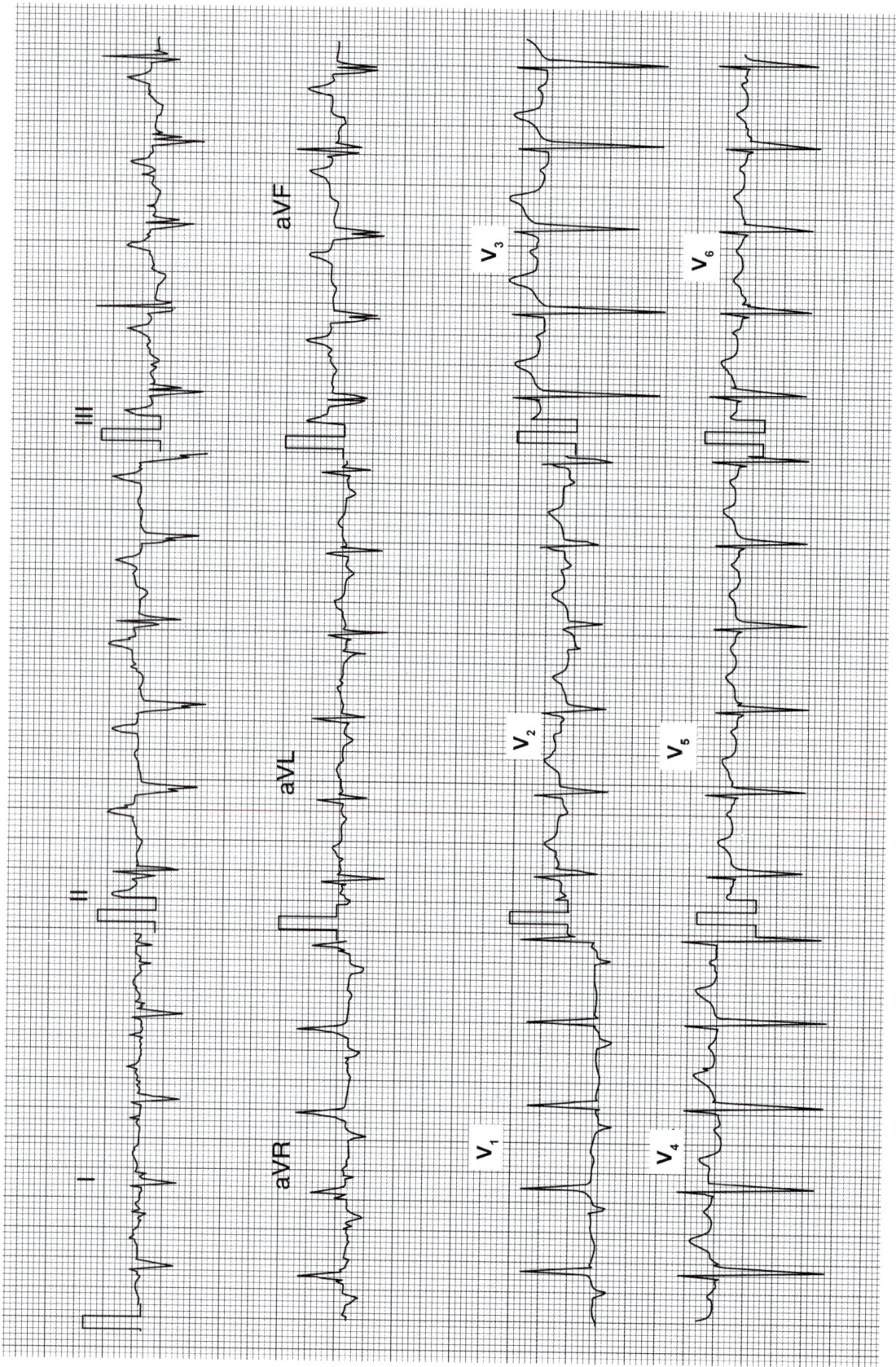

ECG NO. 9

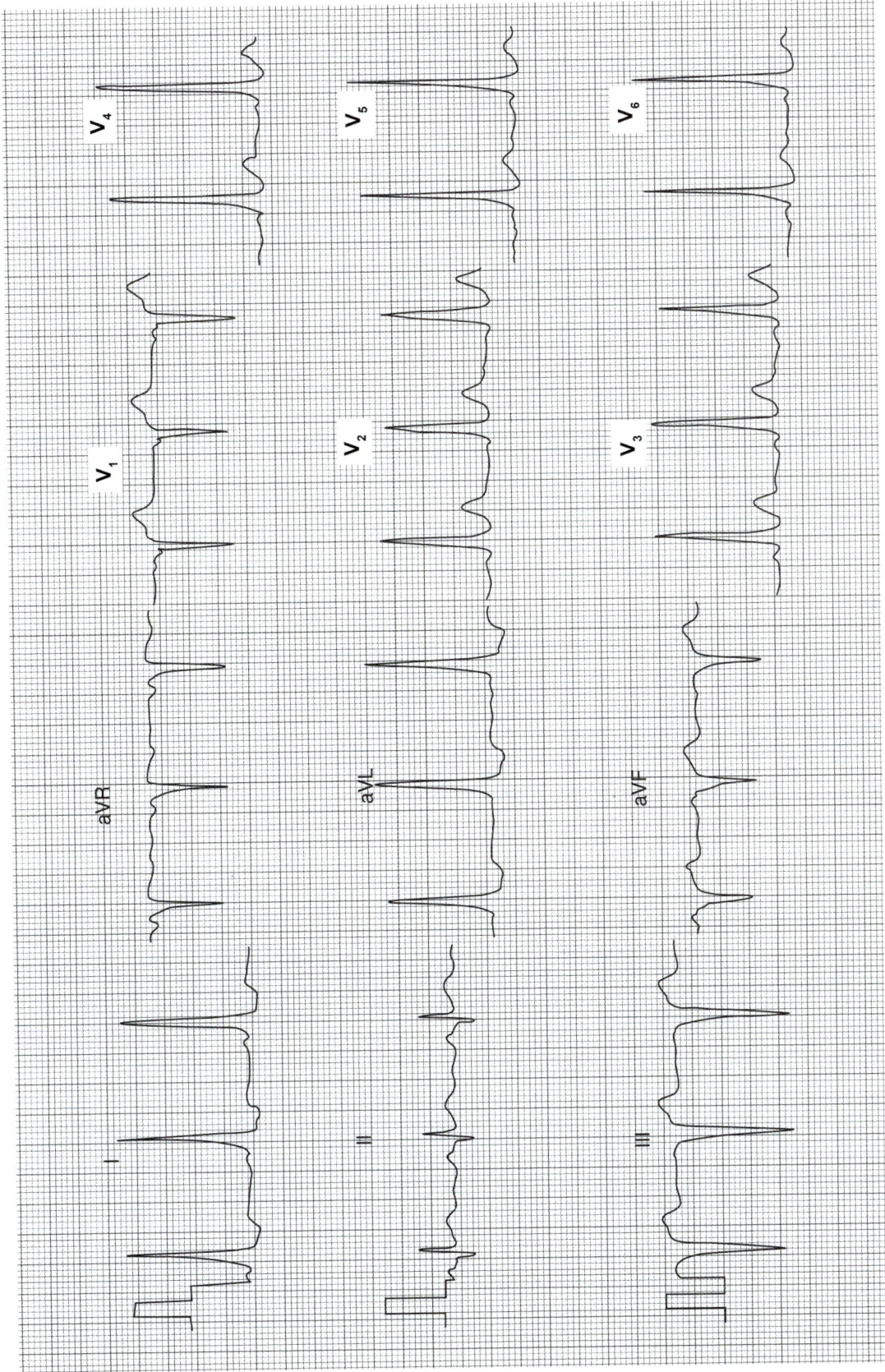

ECG NO. 10

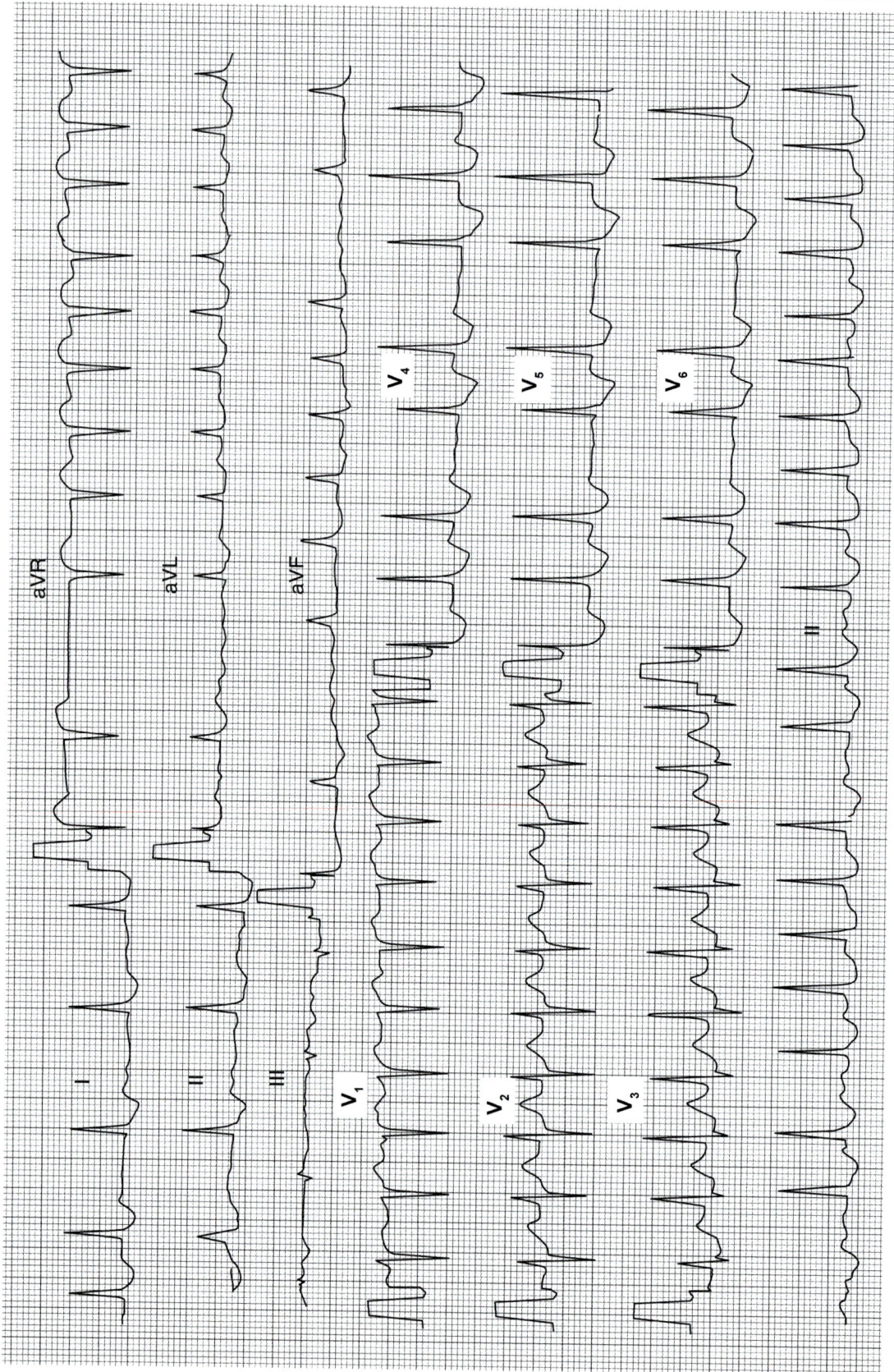

ECG NO. 11

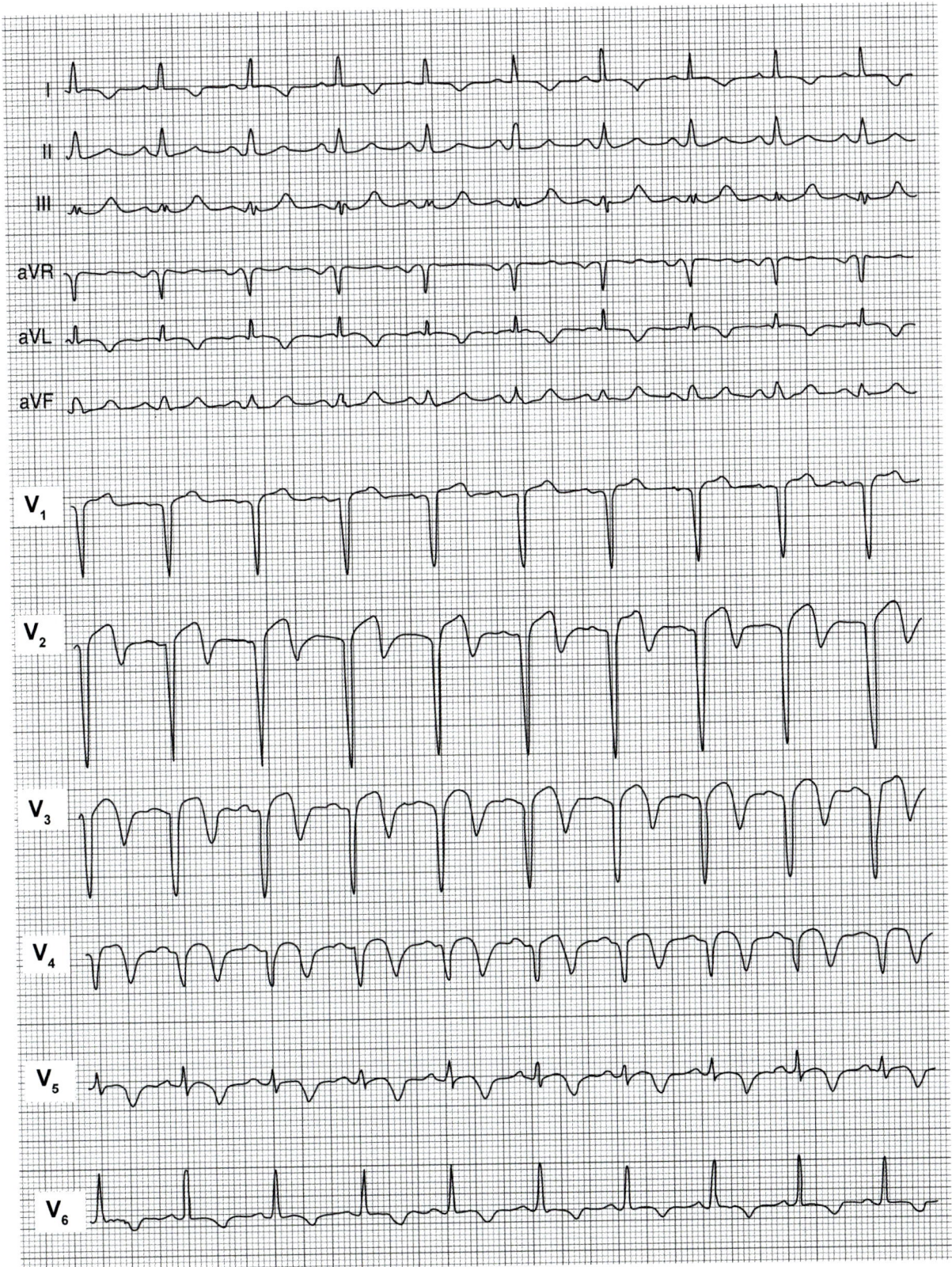

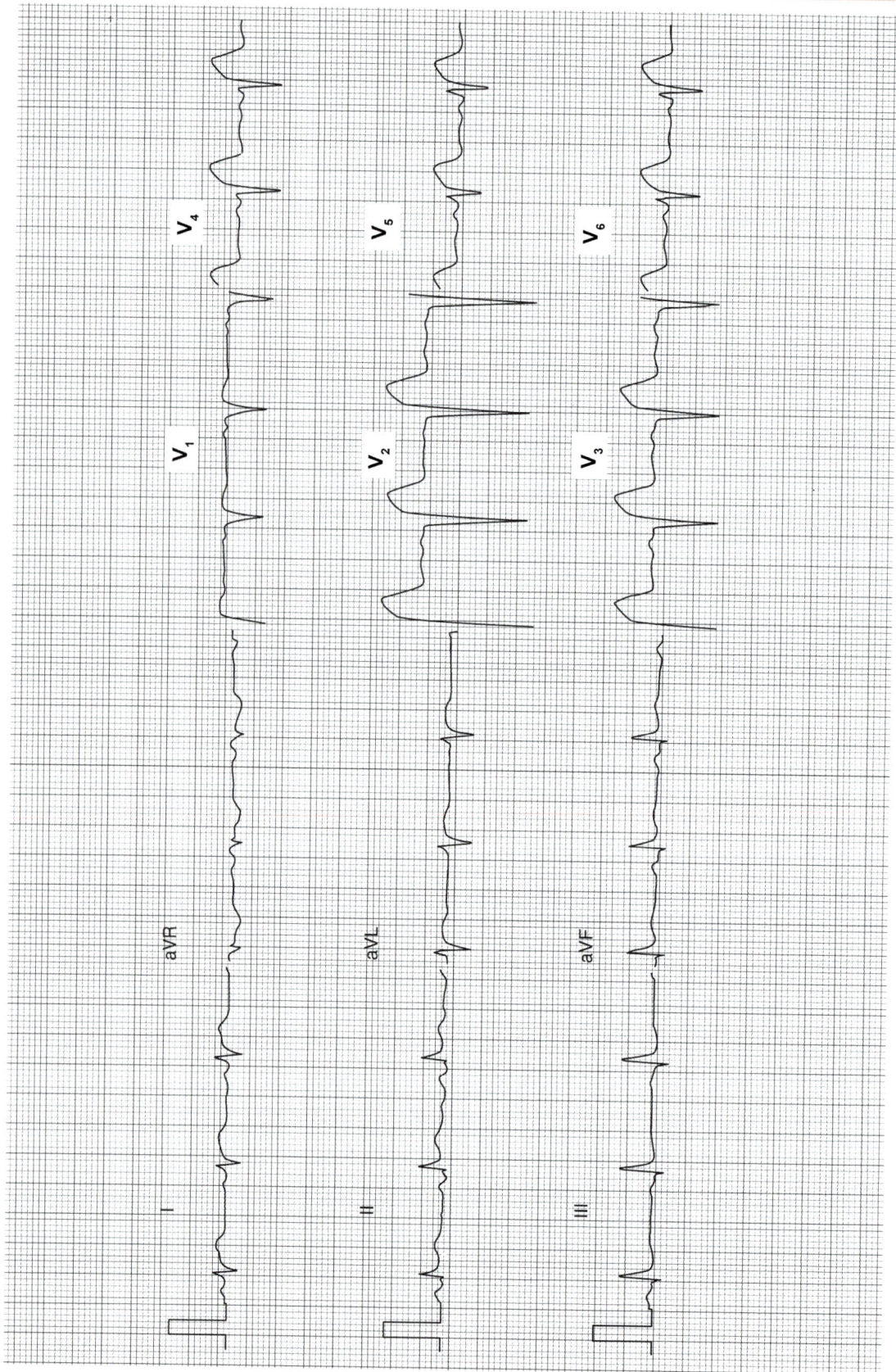

ECG NO. 13

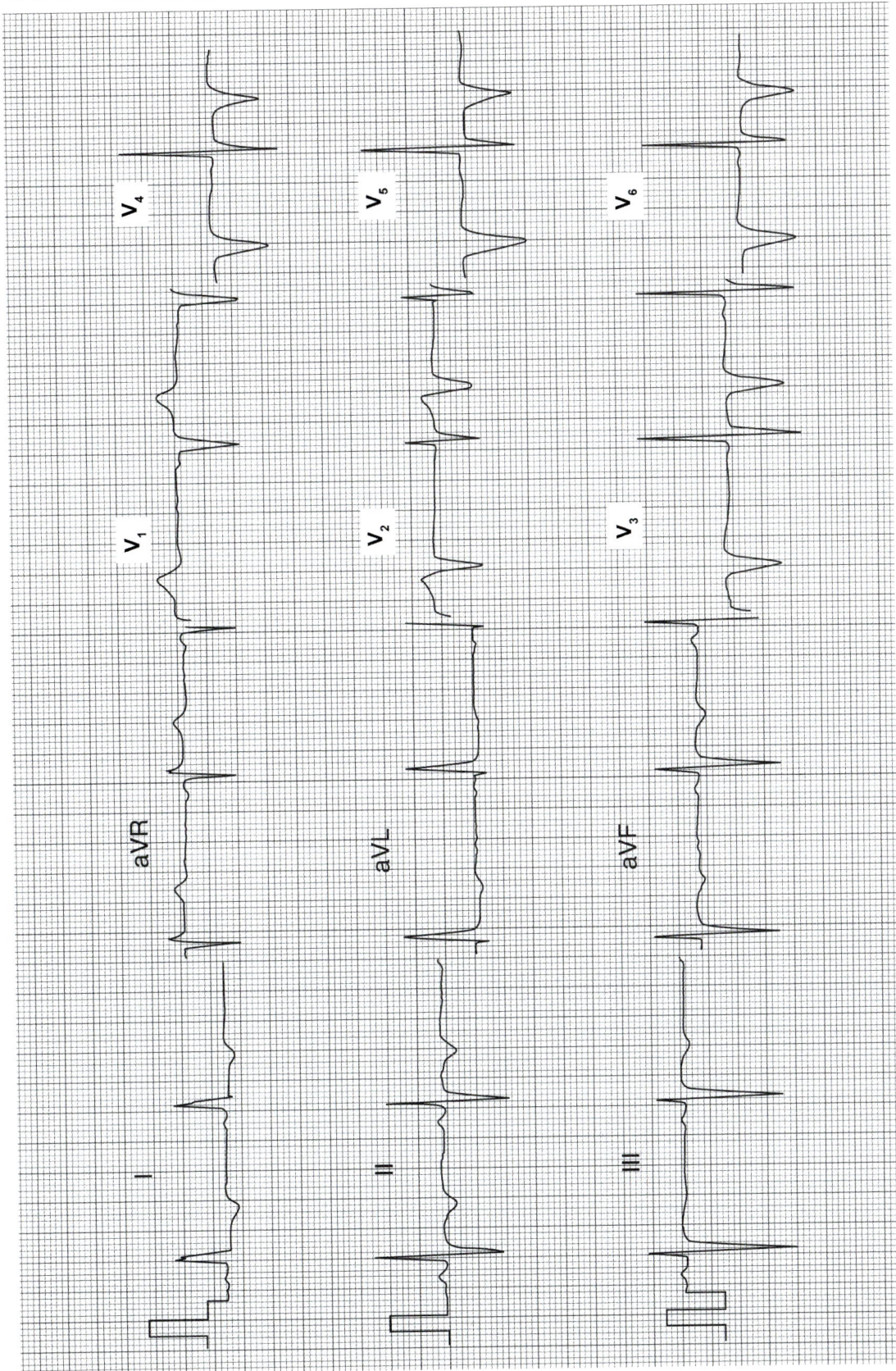

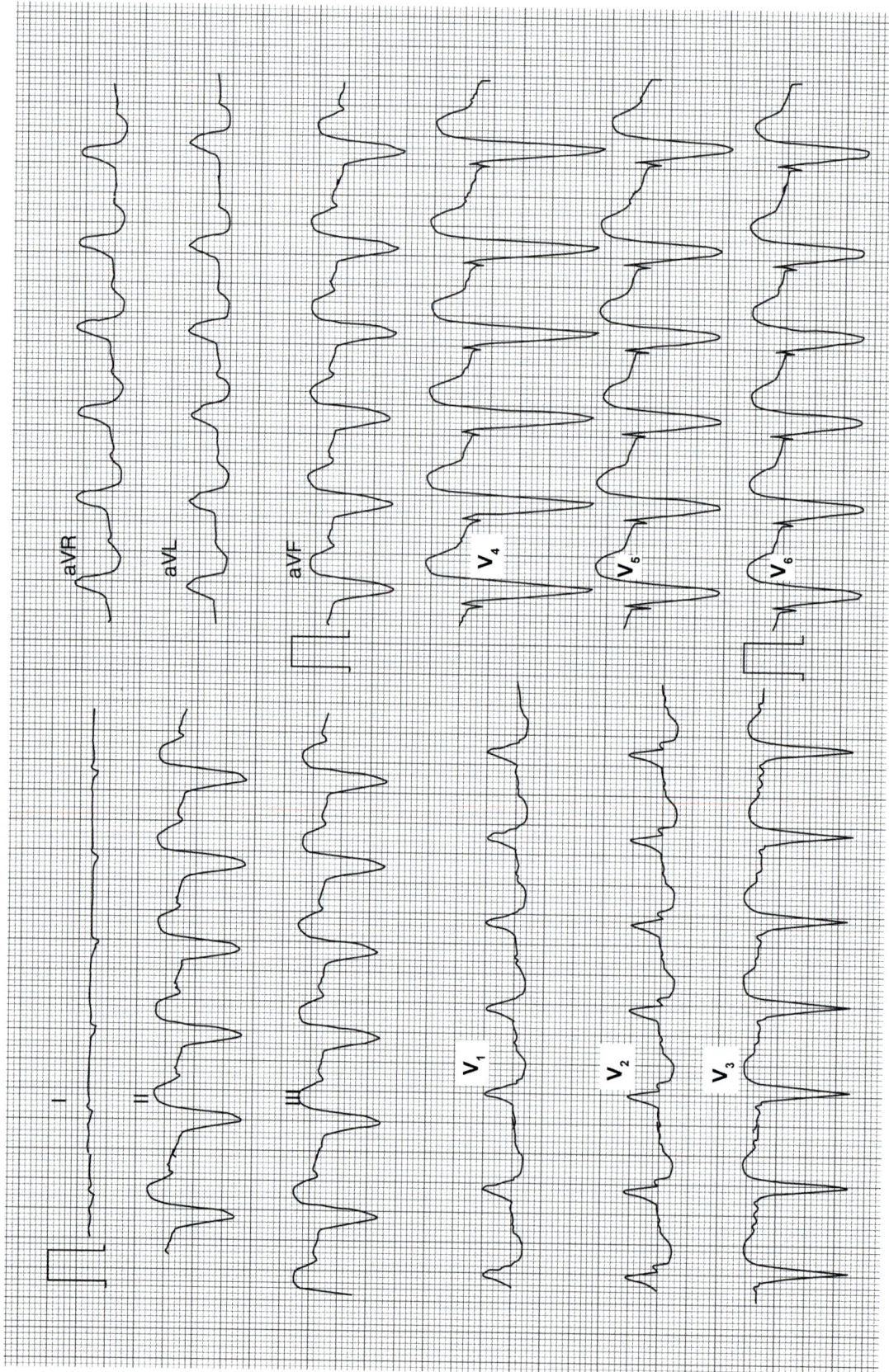

ECG NO. 14

aVR

aVL

aVF

V4

V5

V6

I

II

III

V1

V2

V3

ECG NO. 15

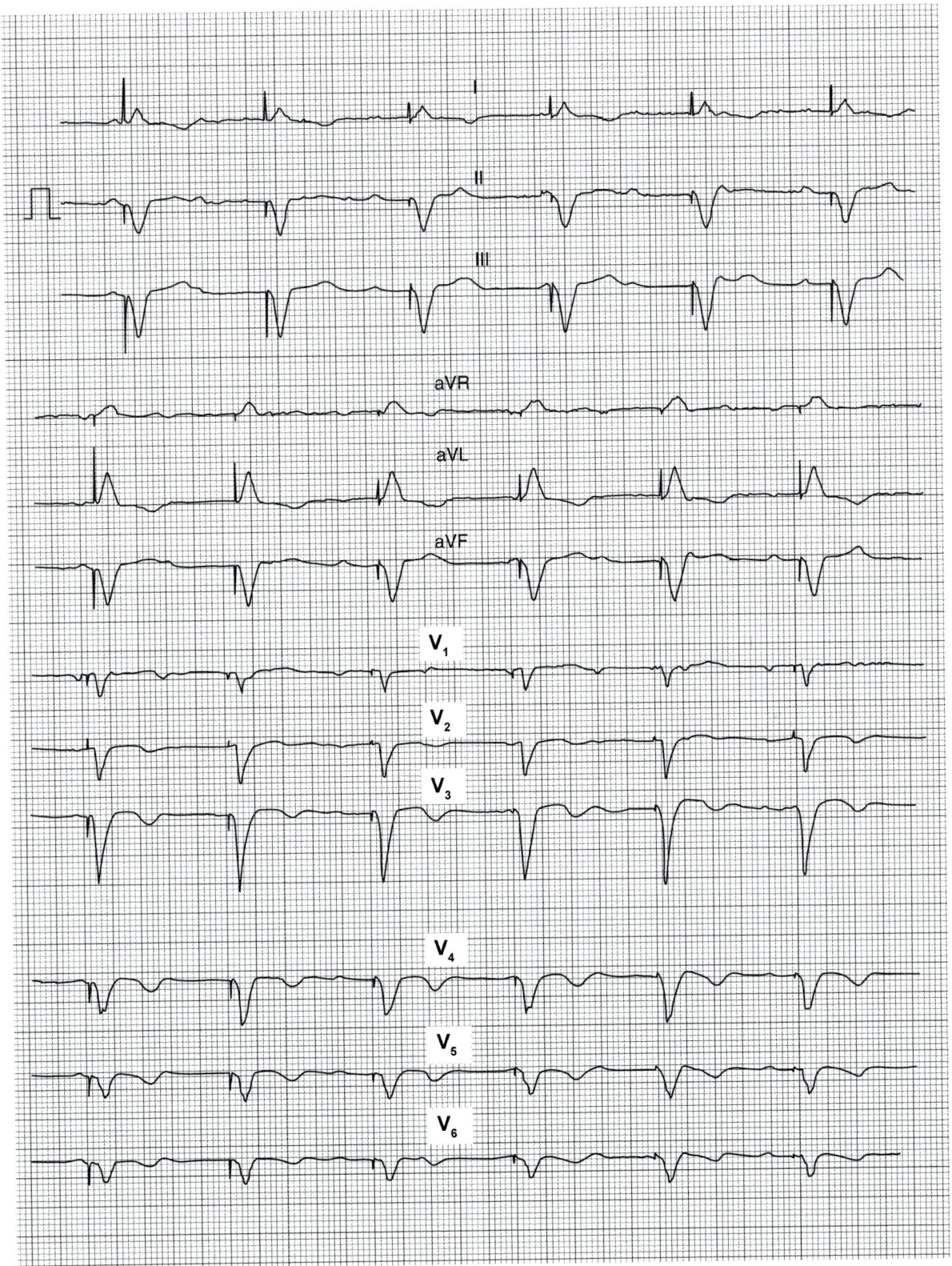

ECG NO. 16

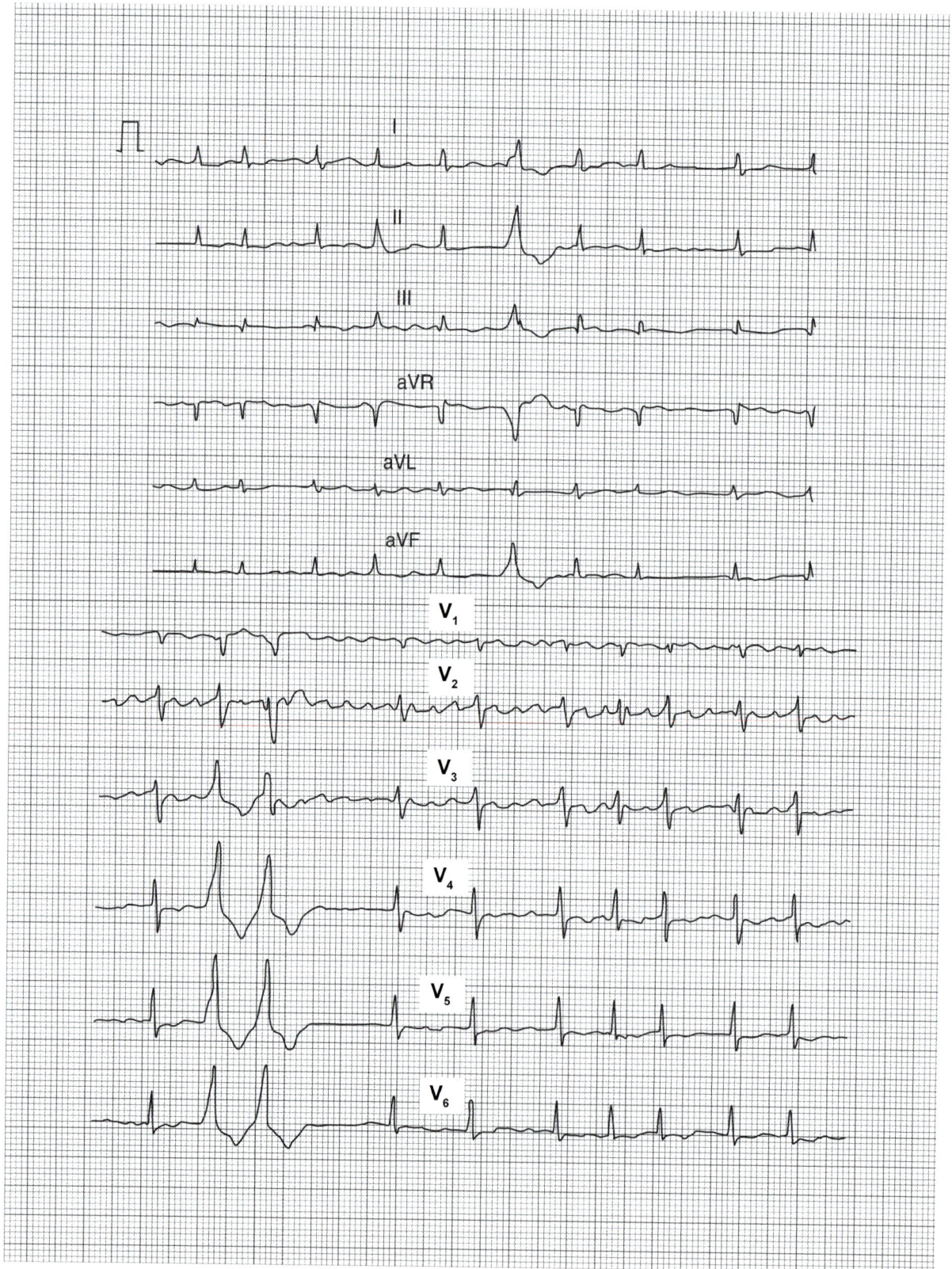

ECG NO. 17

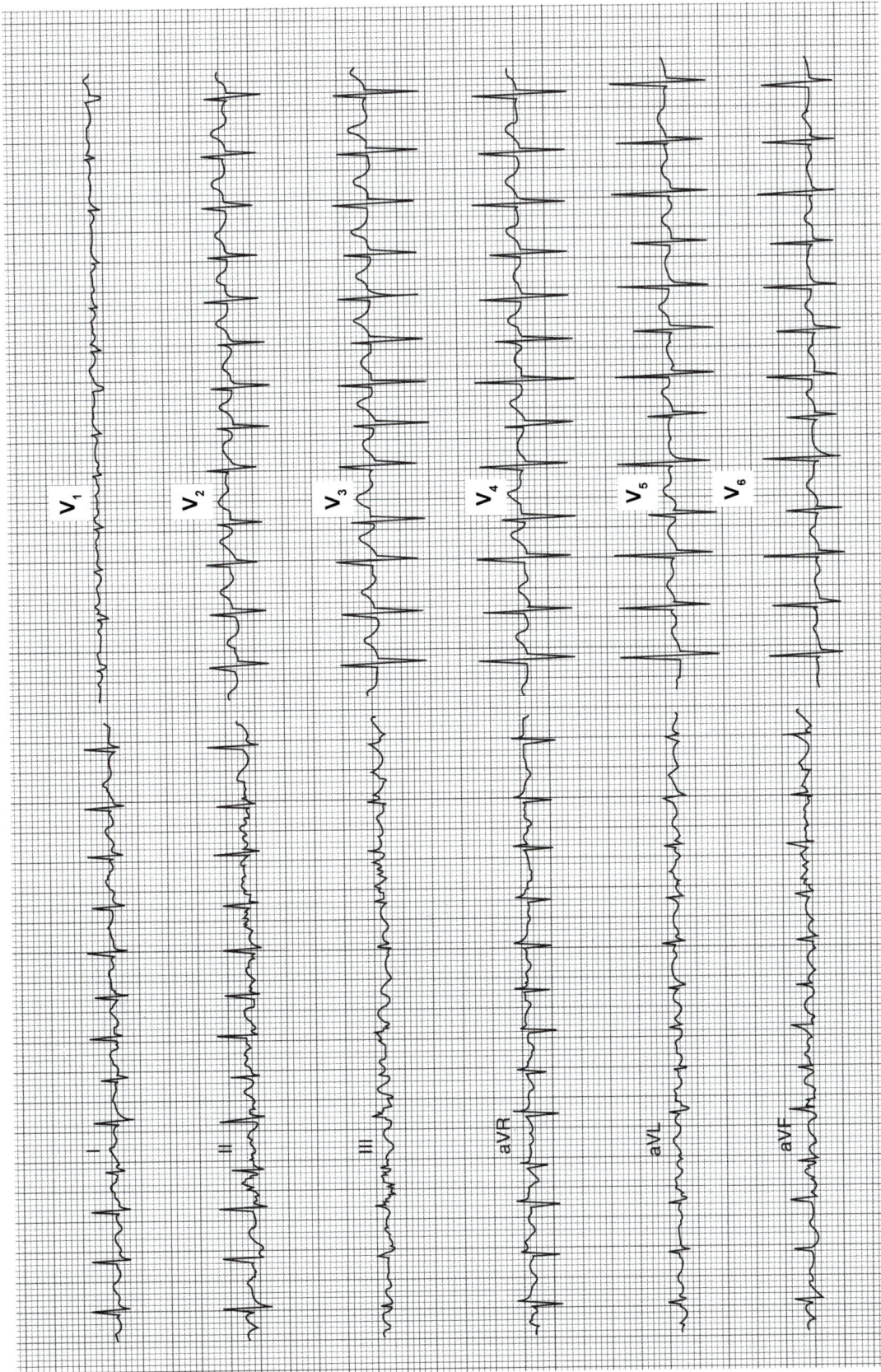

V₁
V₂
V₃
V₄
V₅
V₆

I
II
III
aVR
aVL
aVF

ECG NO. 18

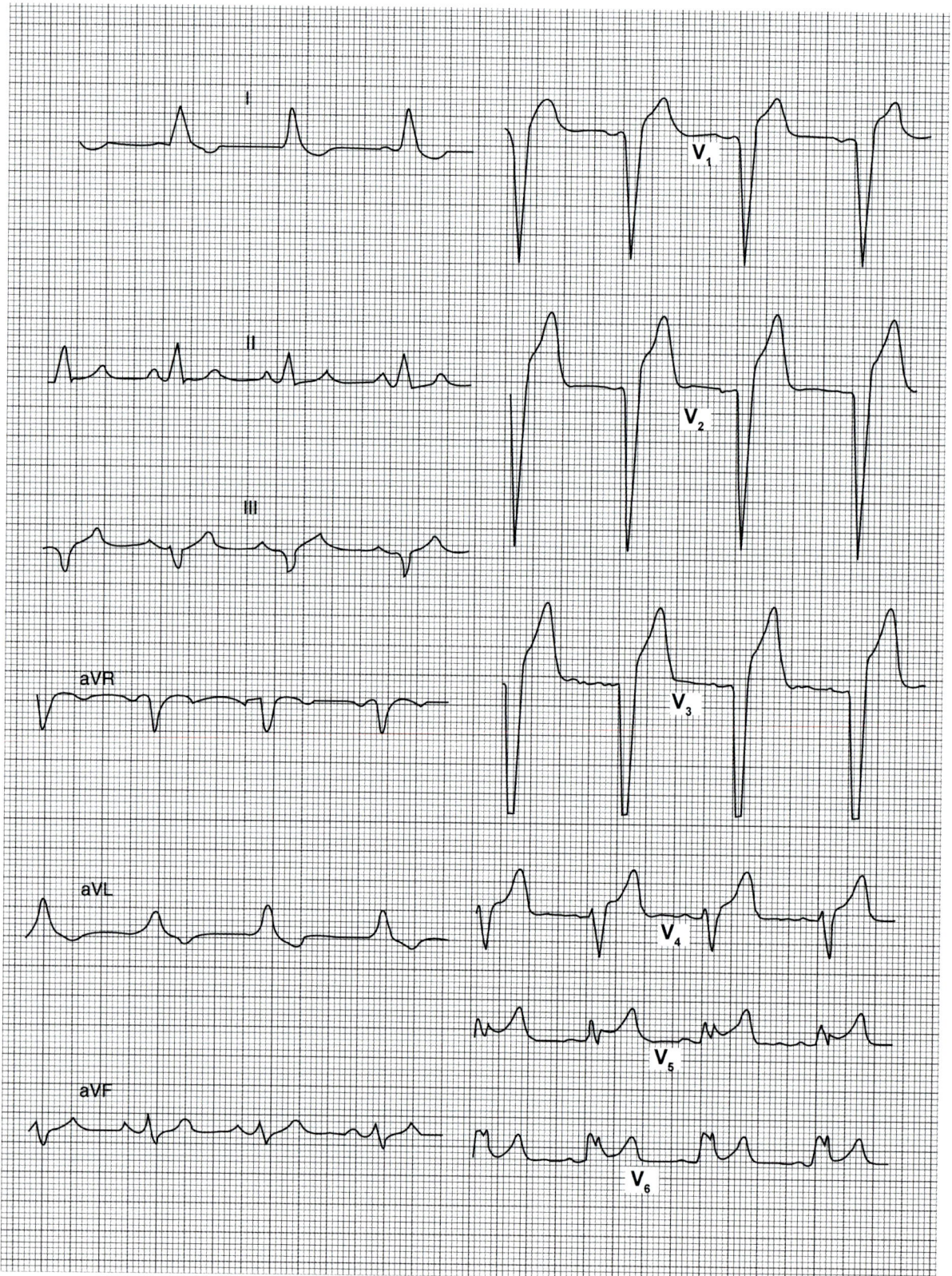

ECG NO. 19

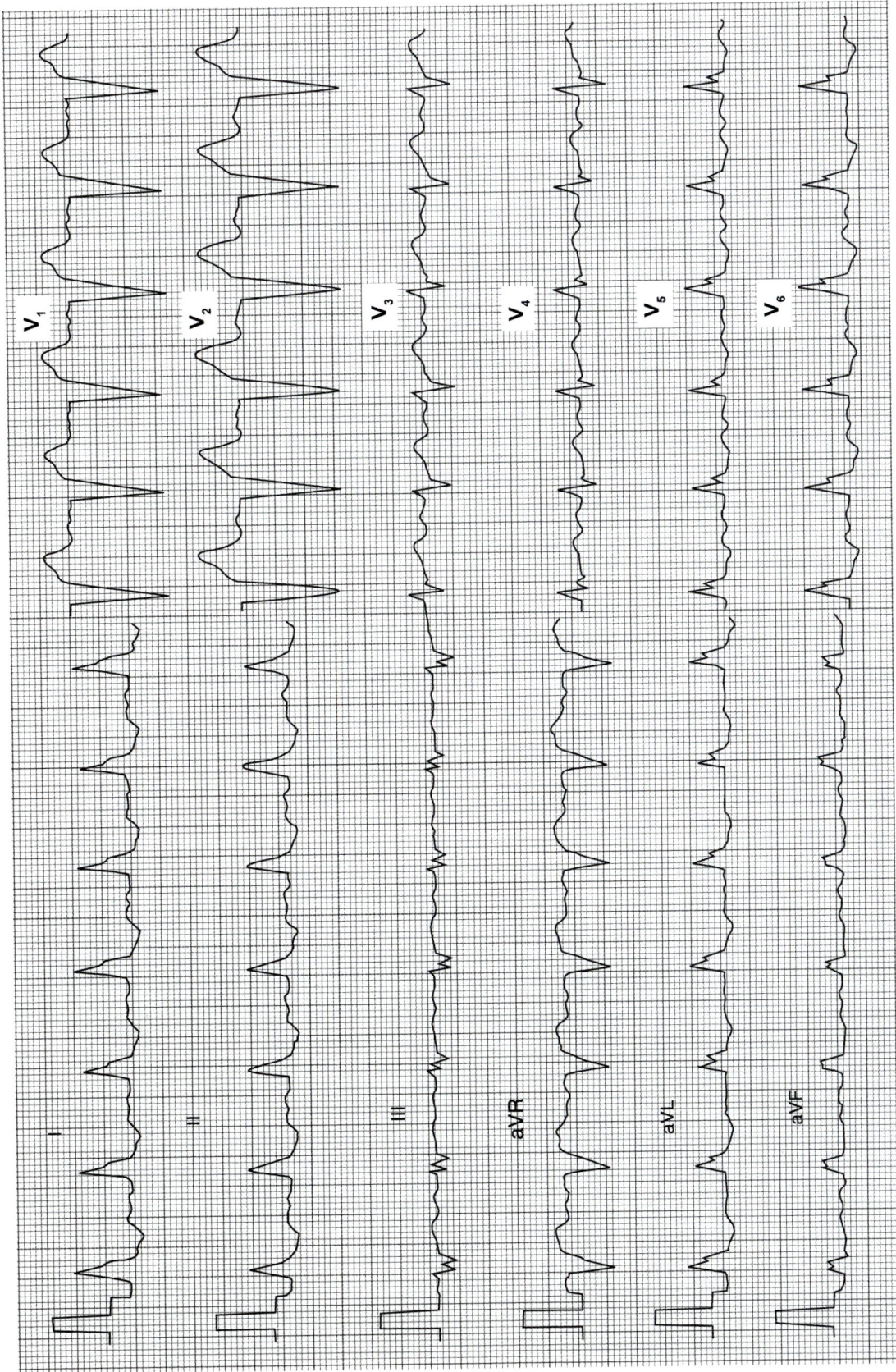

I

II

III

aVR

aVL

aVF

V₁

V₂

V₃

V₄

V₅

V₆

ECG NO. 20

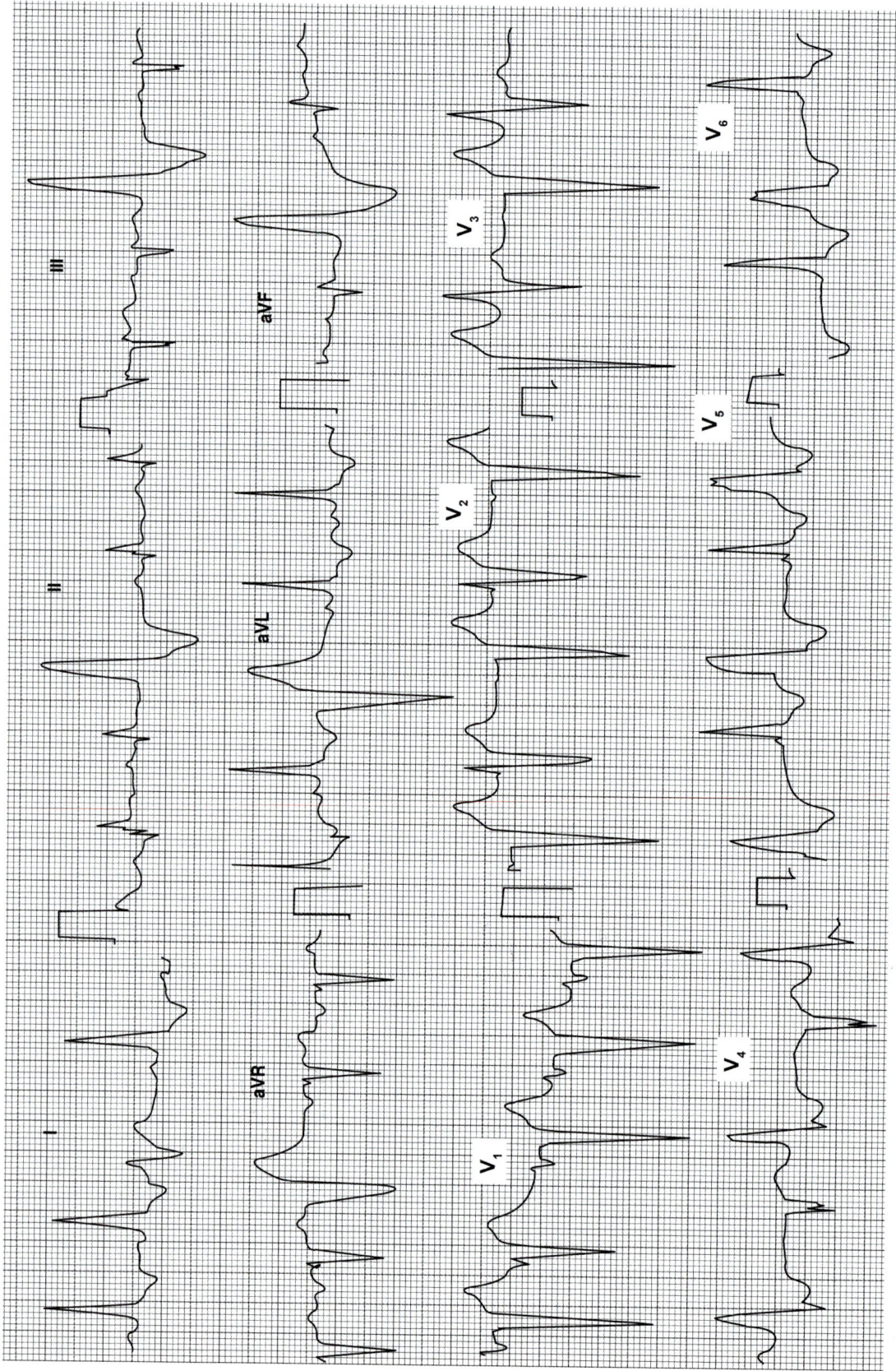

ECG NO. 21

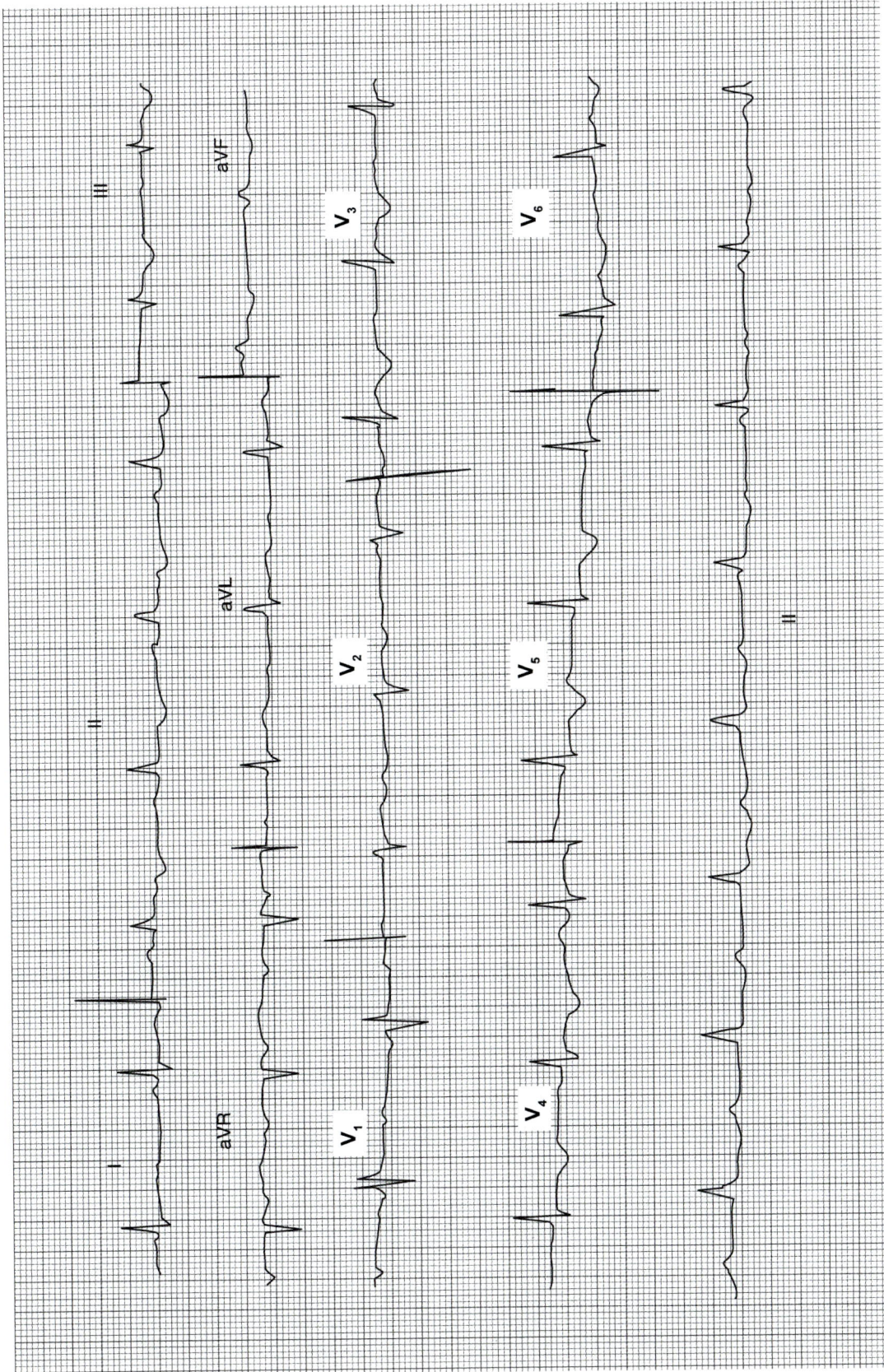

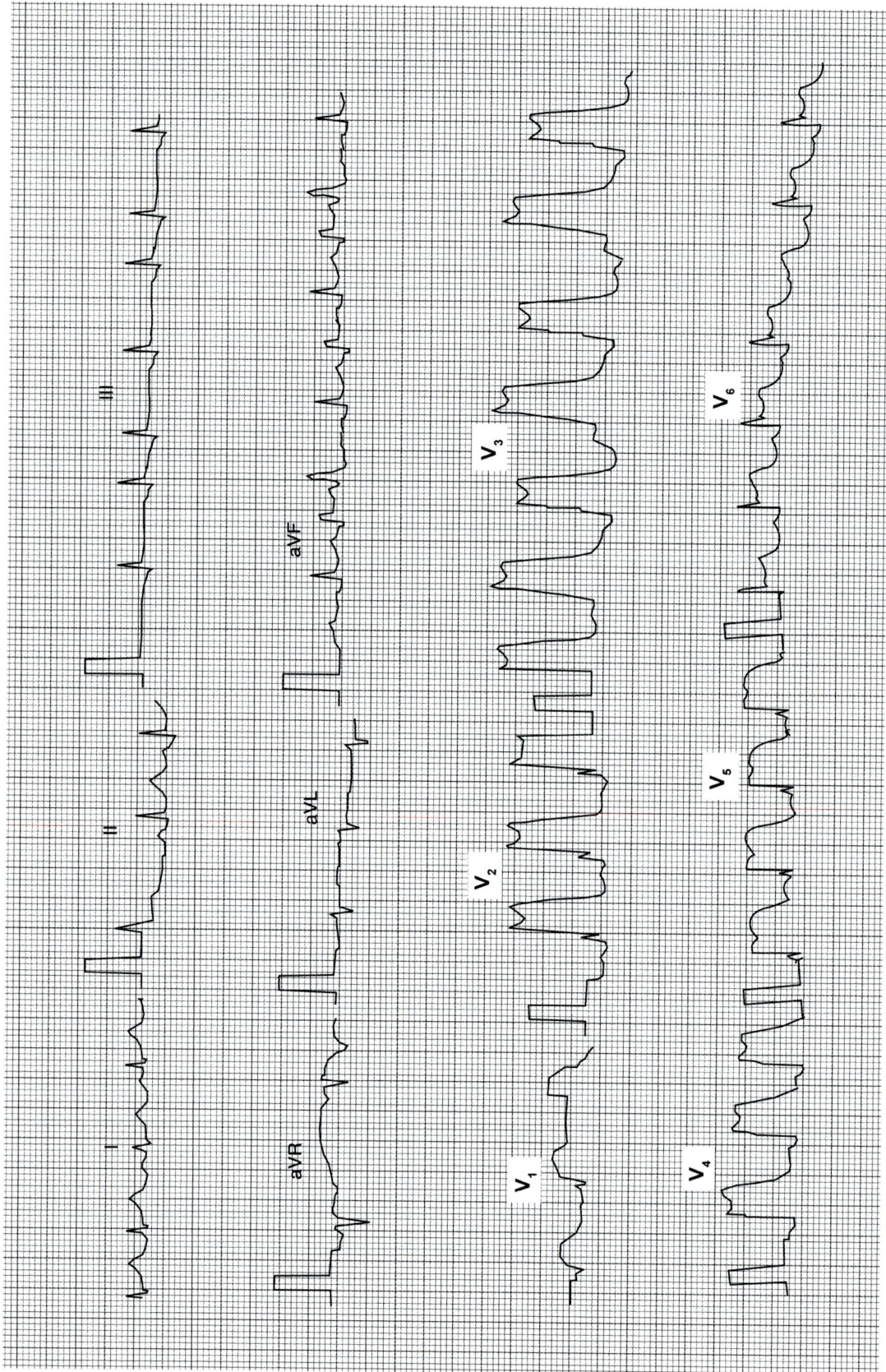

ECG NO. 23

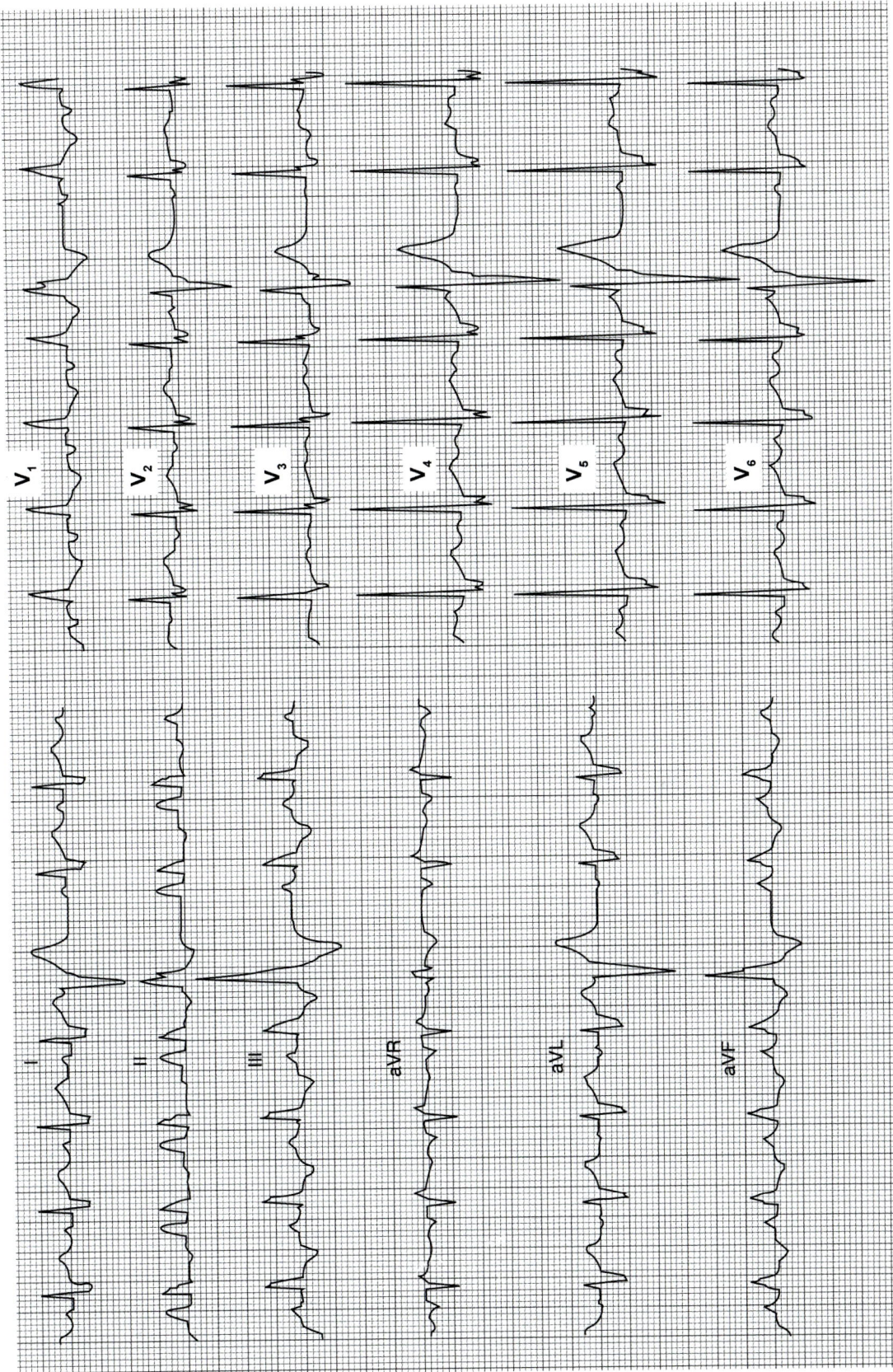

V₁
V₂
V₃
V₄
V₅
V₆

I
II
III
aVR
aVL
aVF

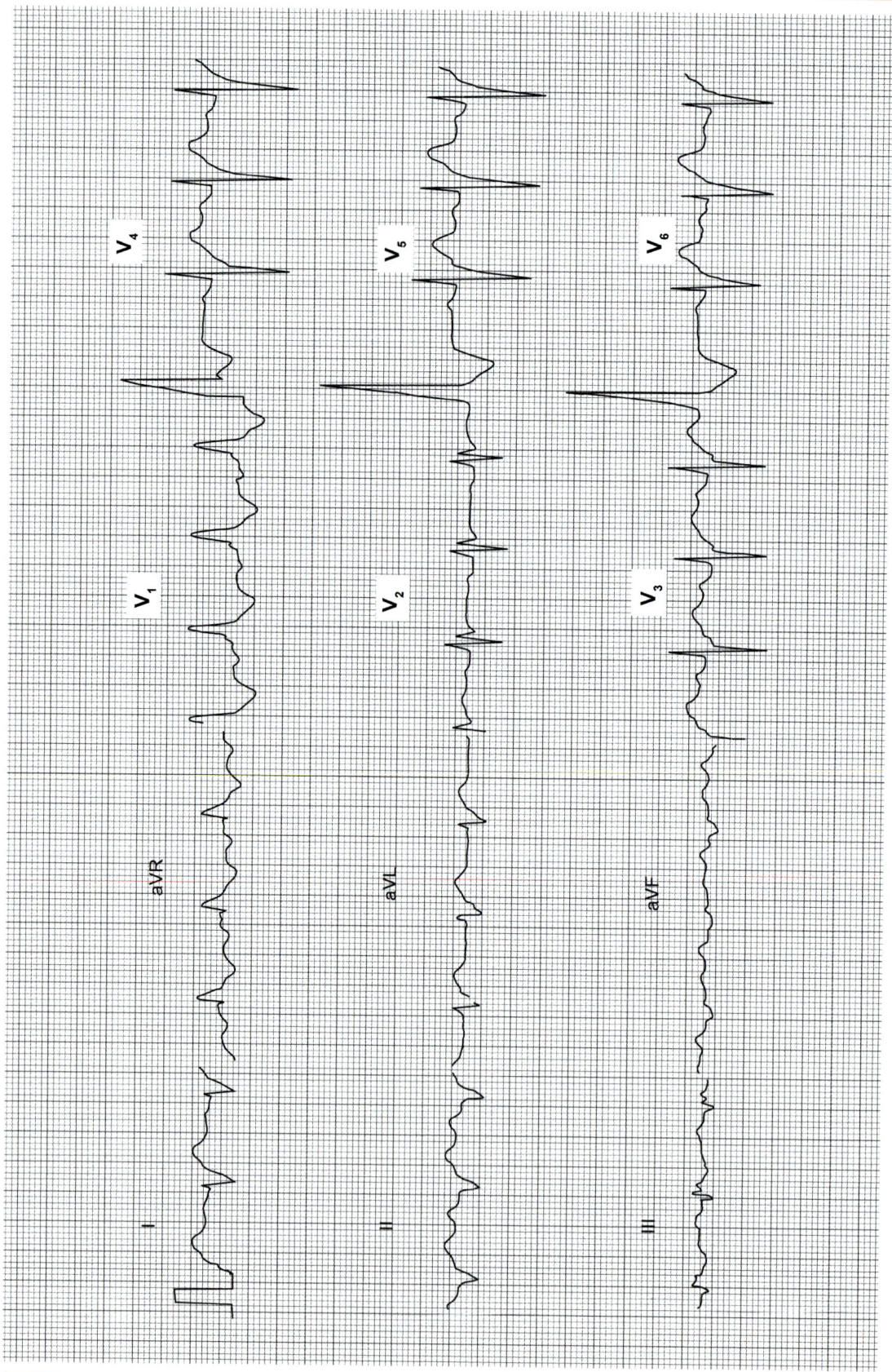

ECG NO. 25

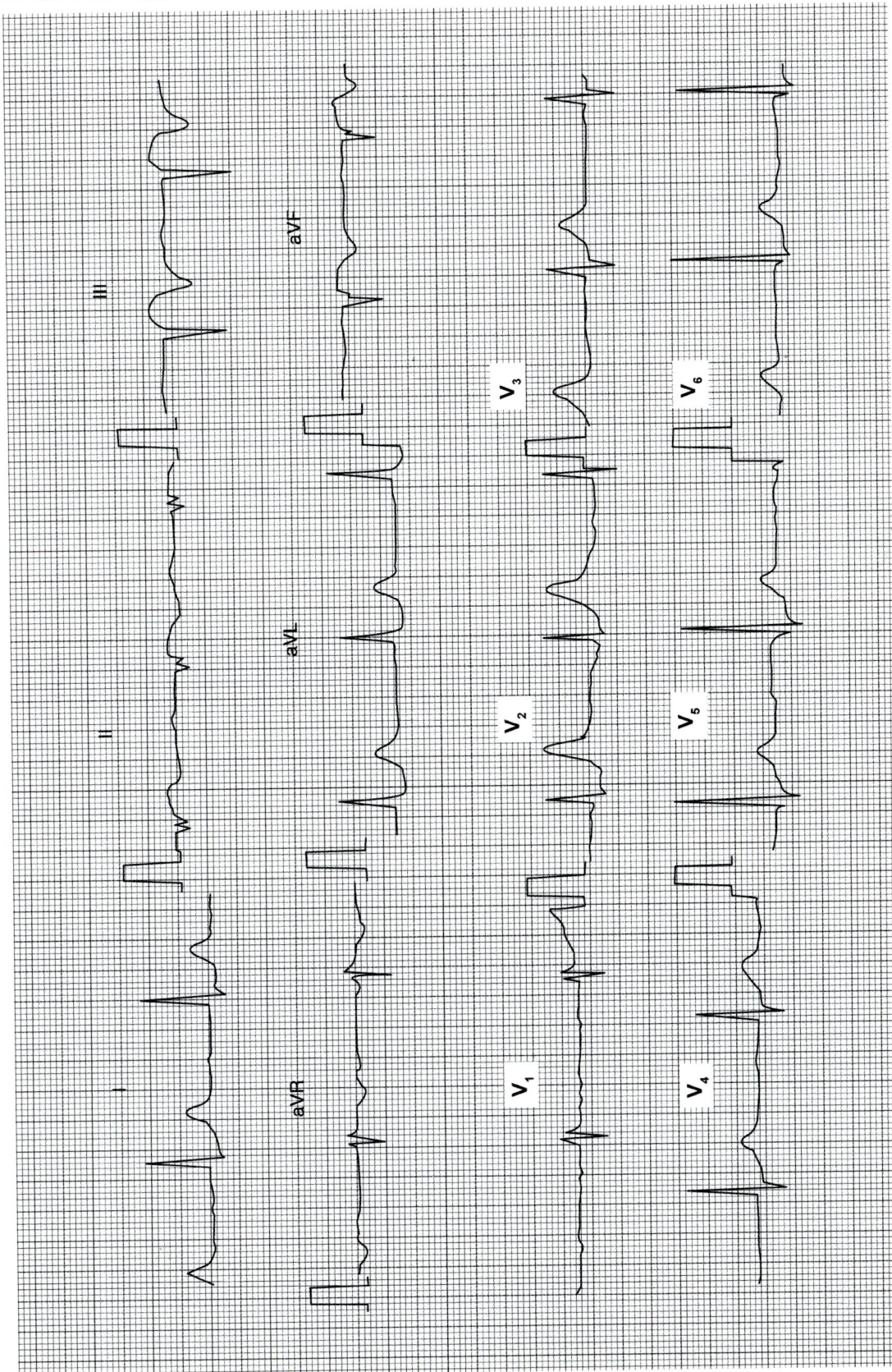

ECG NO. 26

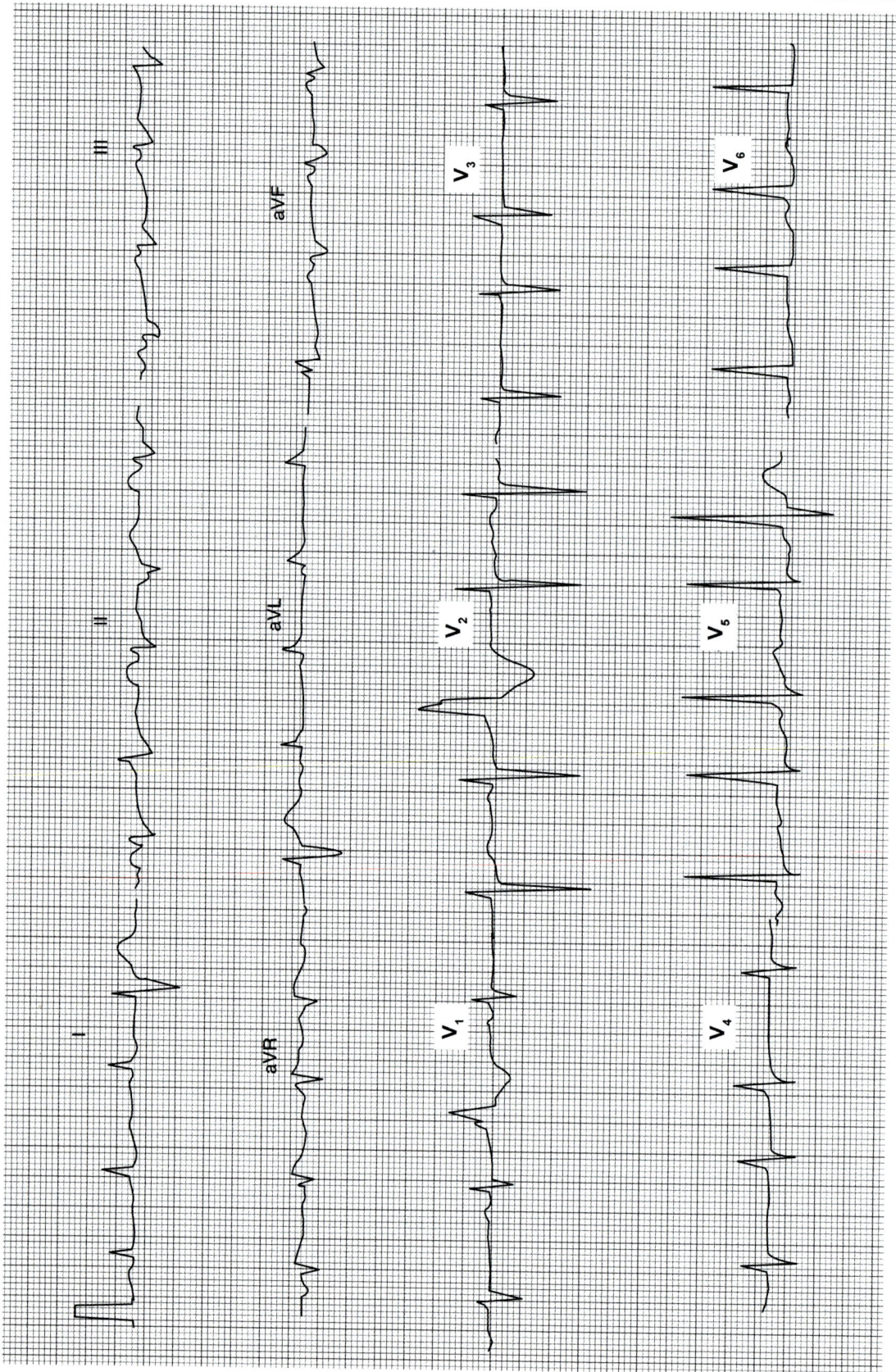

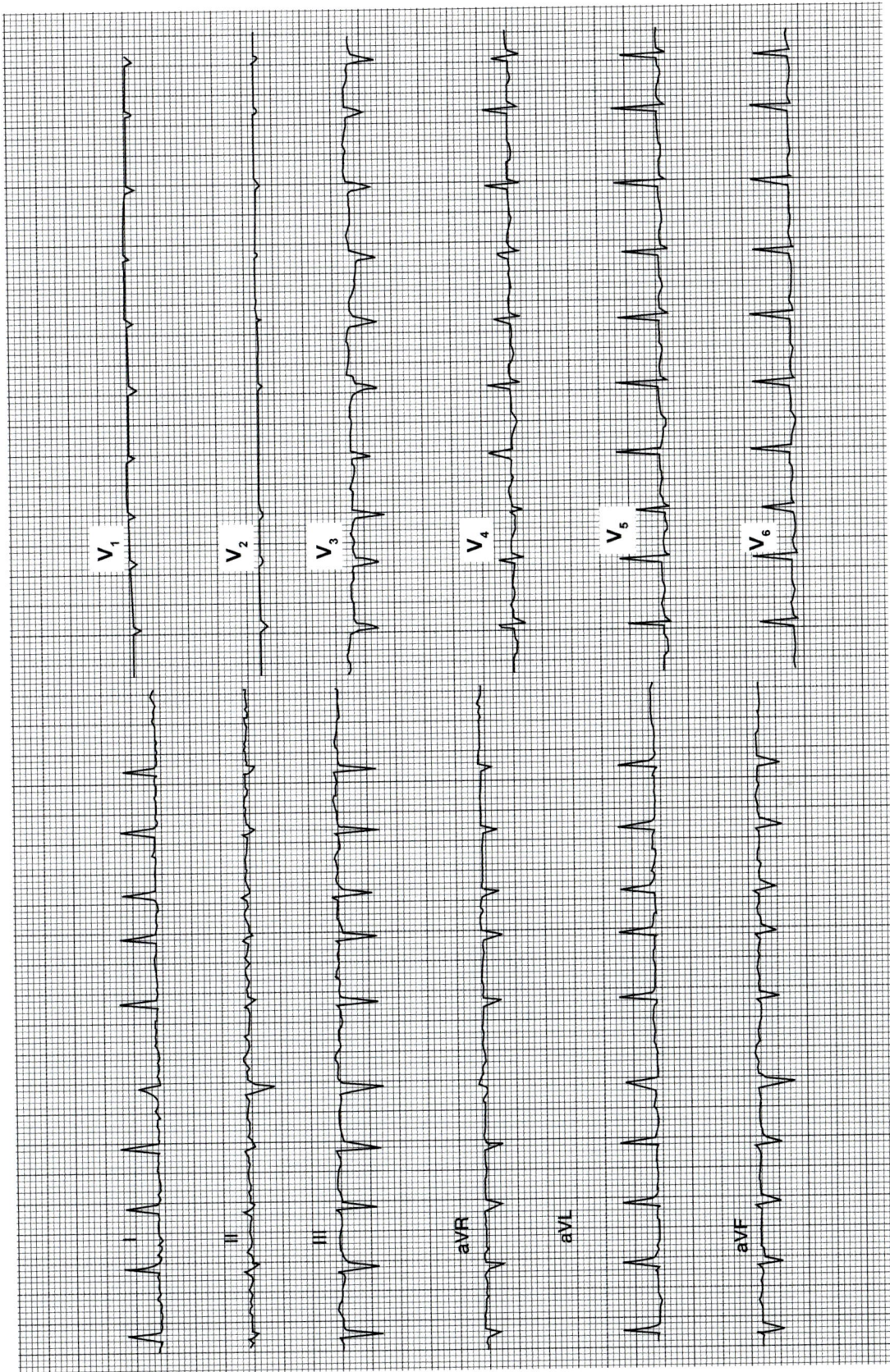

ECG NO. 27

I

II

III

aVR

aVL

aVF

V₁

V₂

V₃

V₄

V₅

V₆

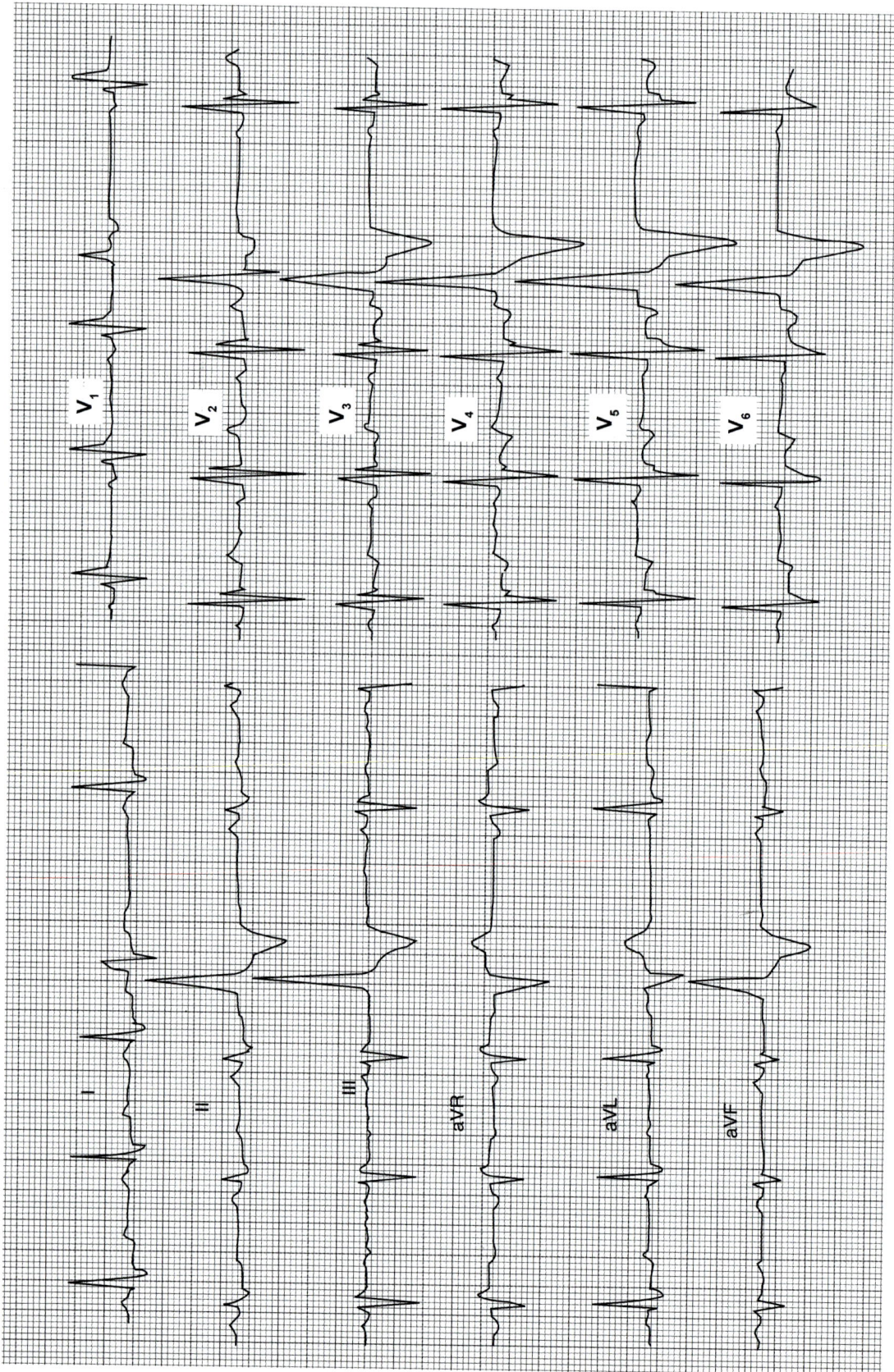

ECG NO. 29

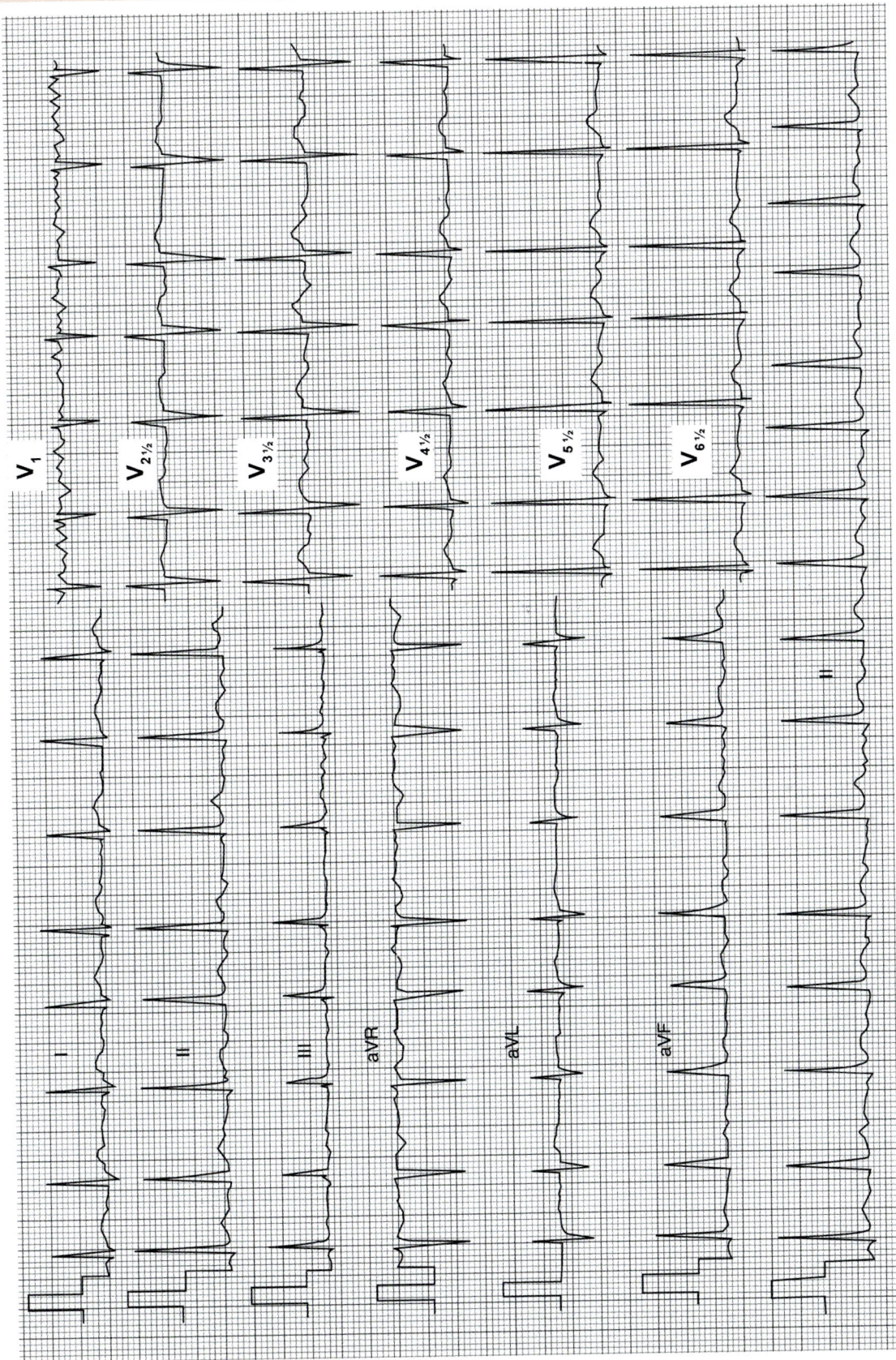

V₁   V₂½   V₃½   V₄½   V₅½   V₆½

I   II   III   aVR   aVL   aVF

ECG NO. 30

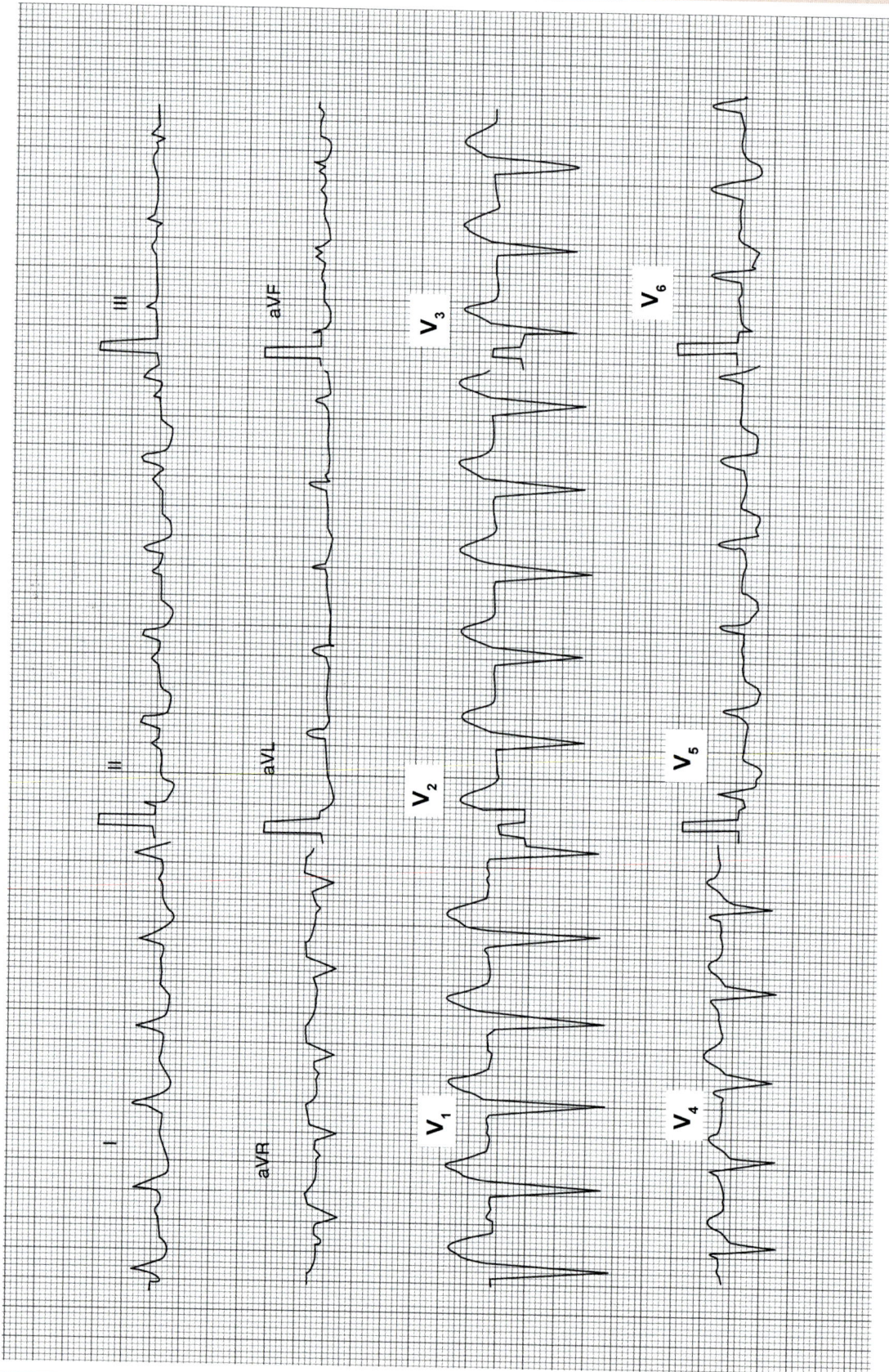

I
II
III
aVR
aVL
aVF
V_1
V_2
V_3
V_4
V_5
V_6

ECG NO. 31

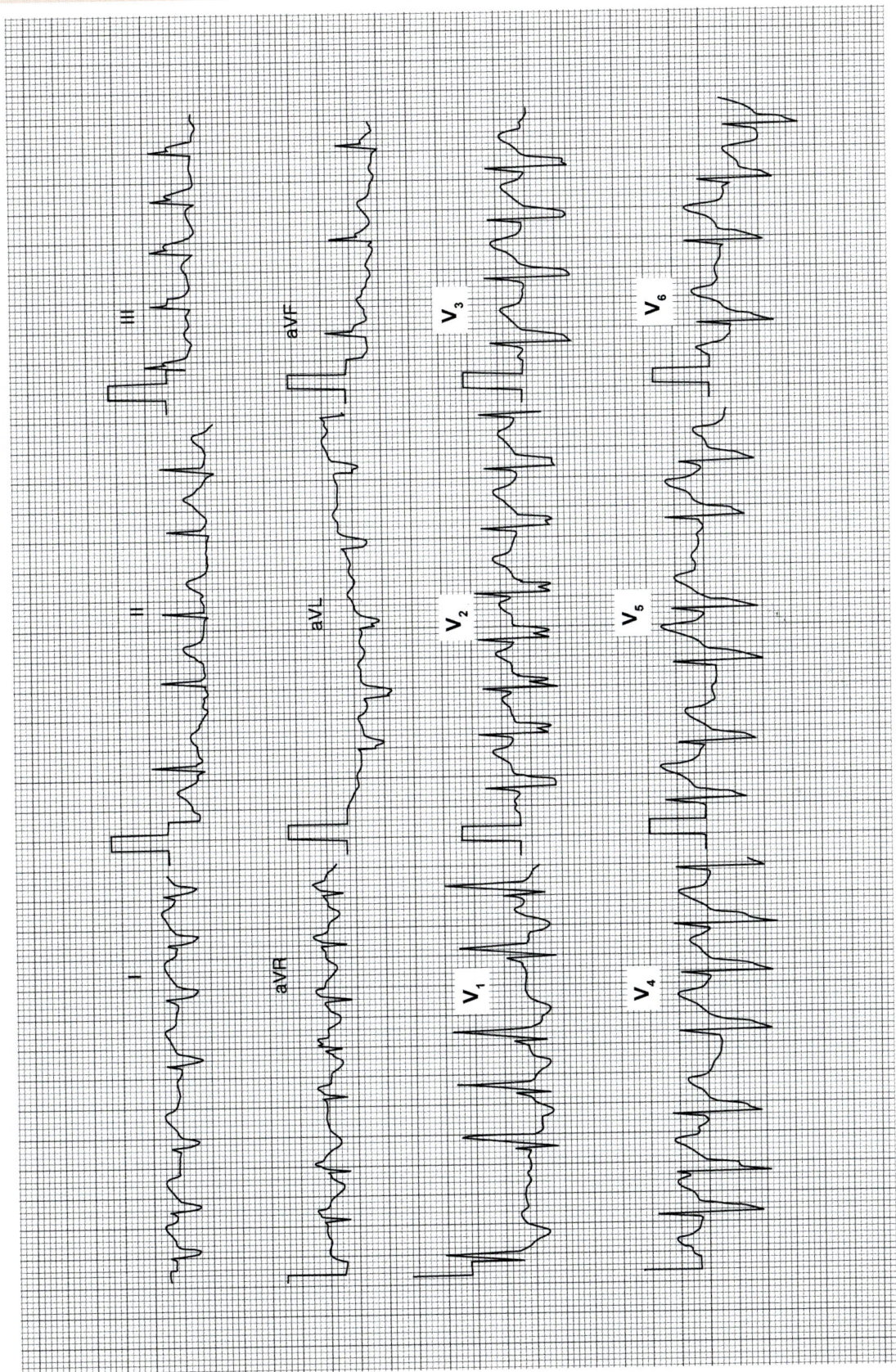

ECG NO. 32

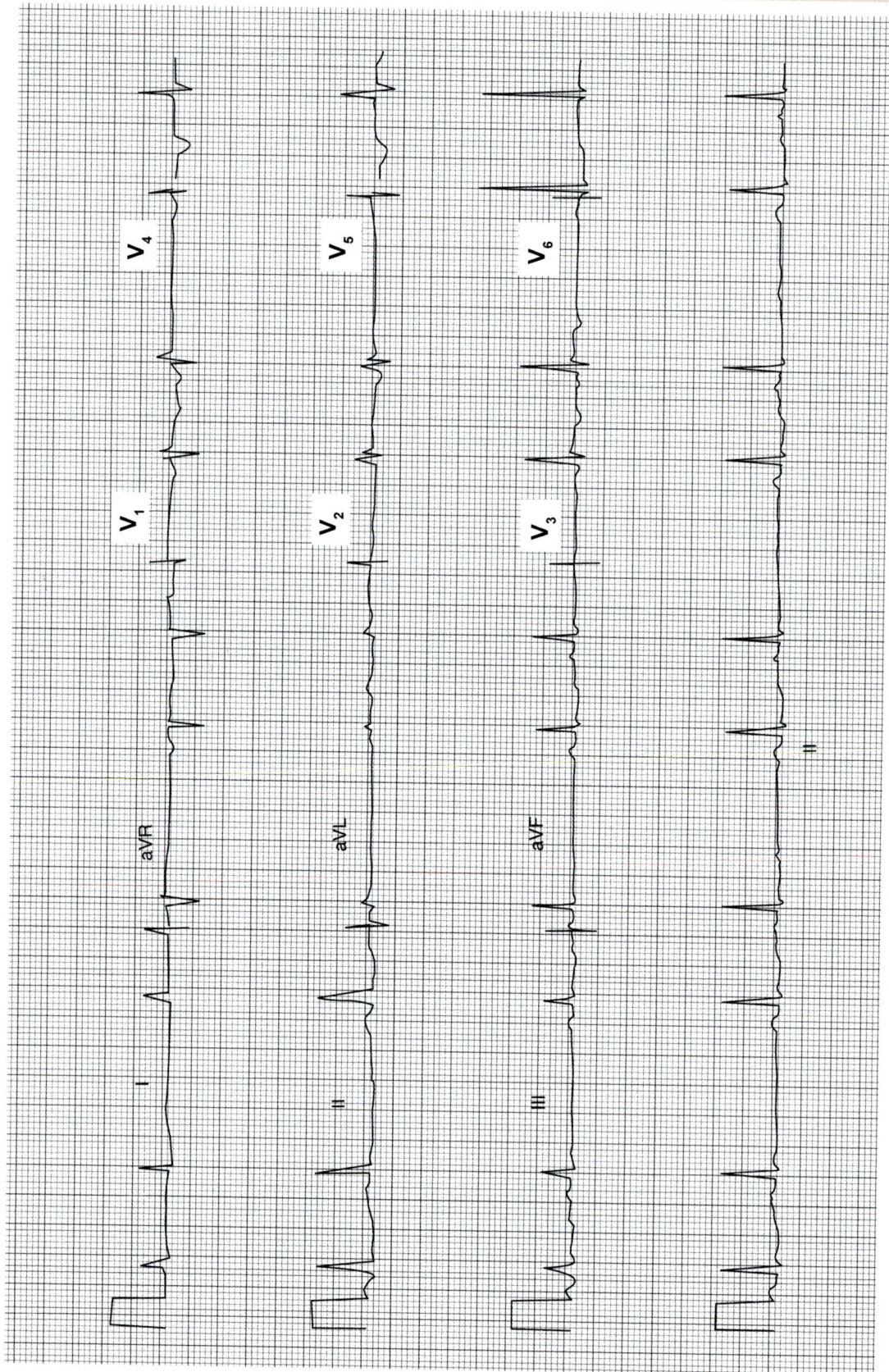

ECG NO. 33

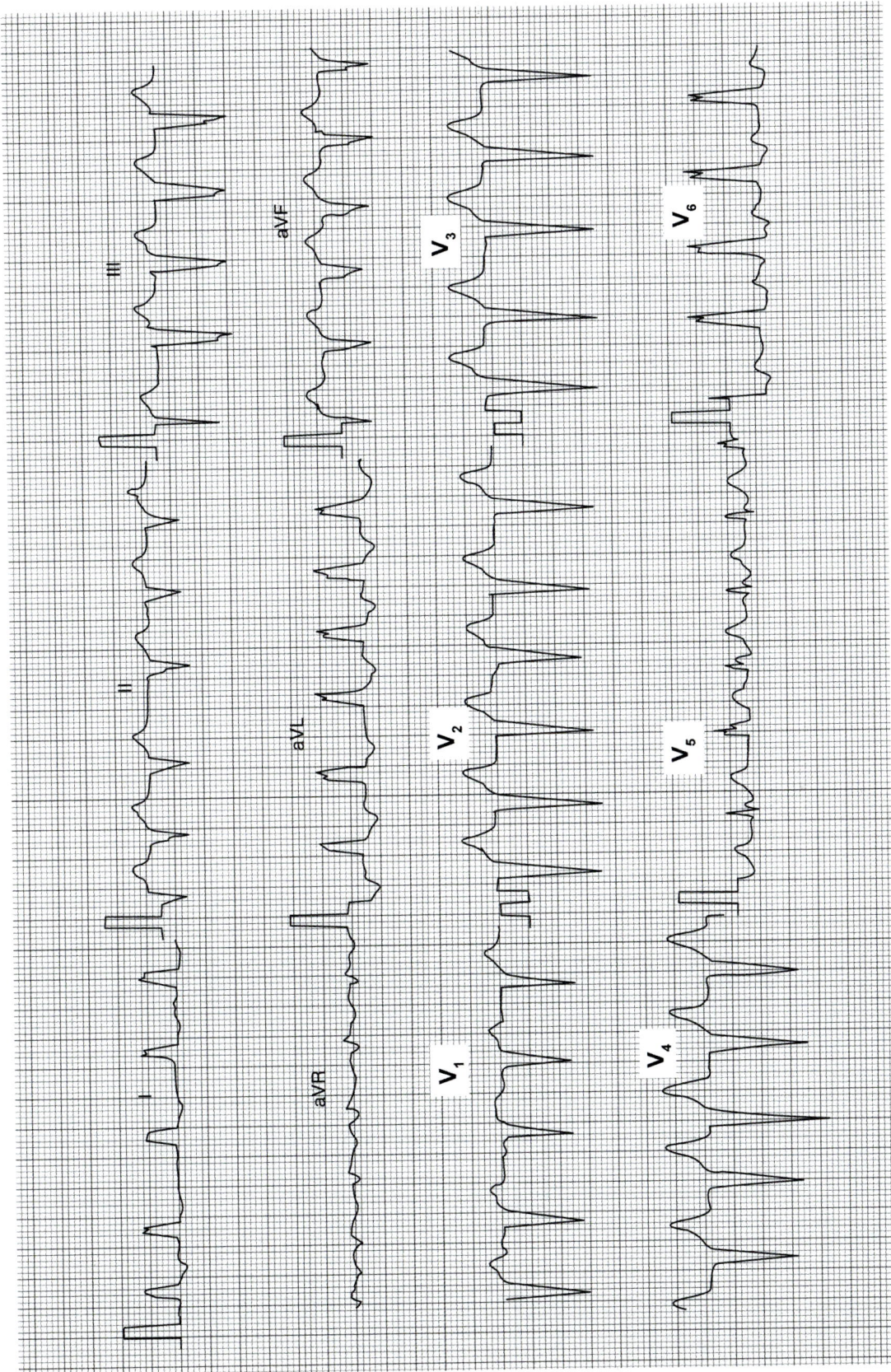

ECG NO. 34

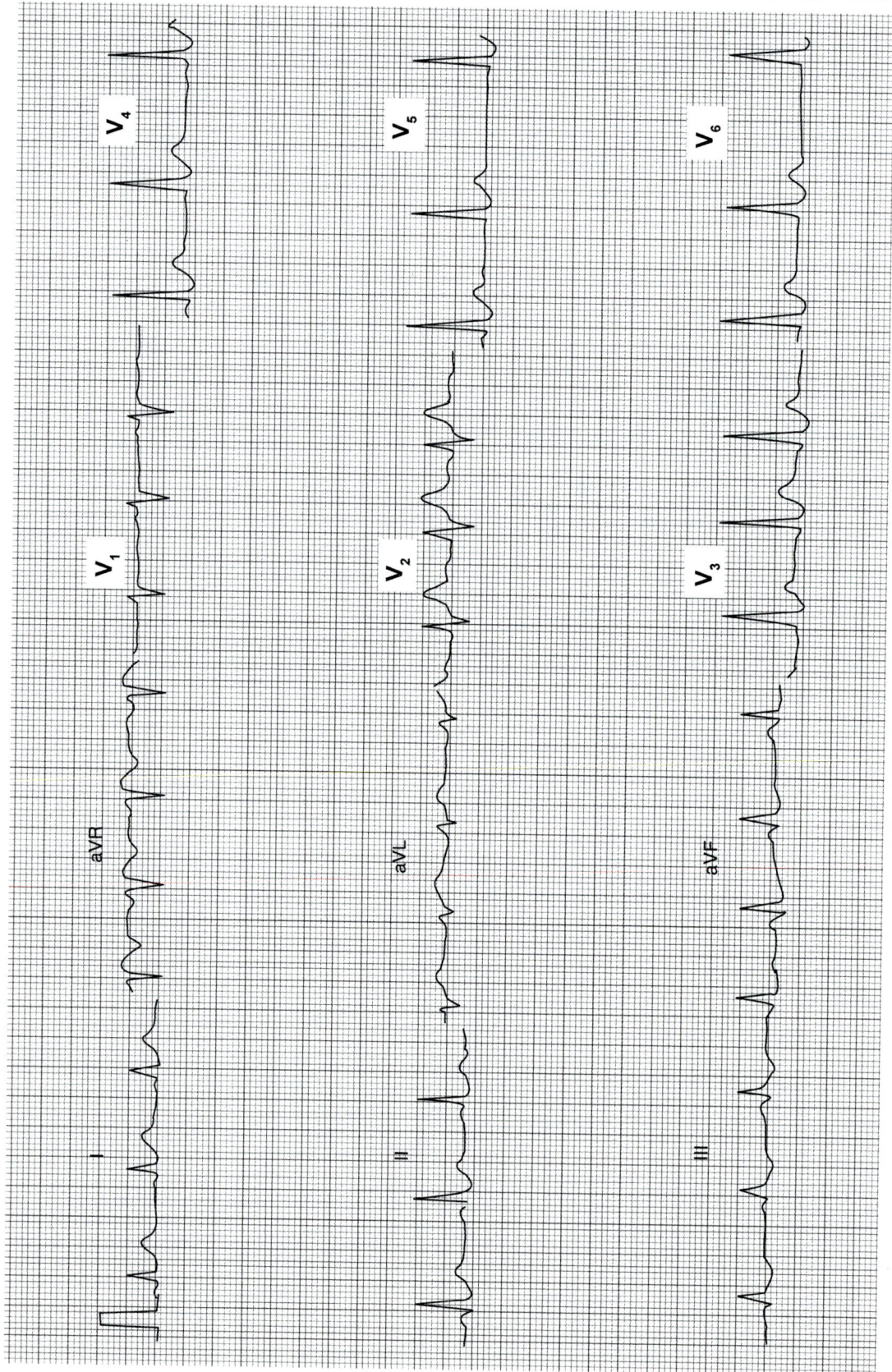

ECG NO. 35

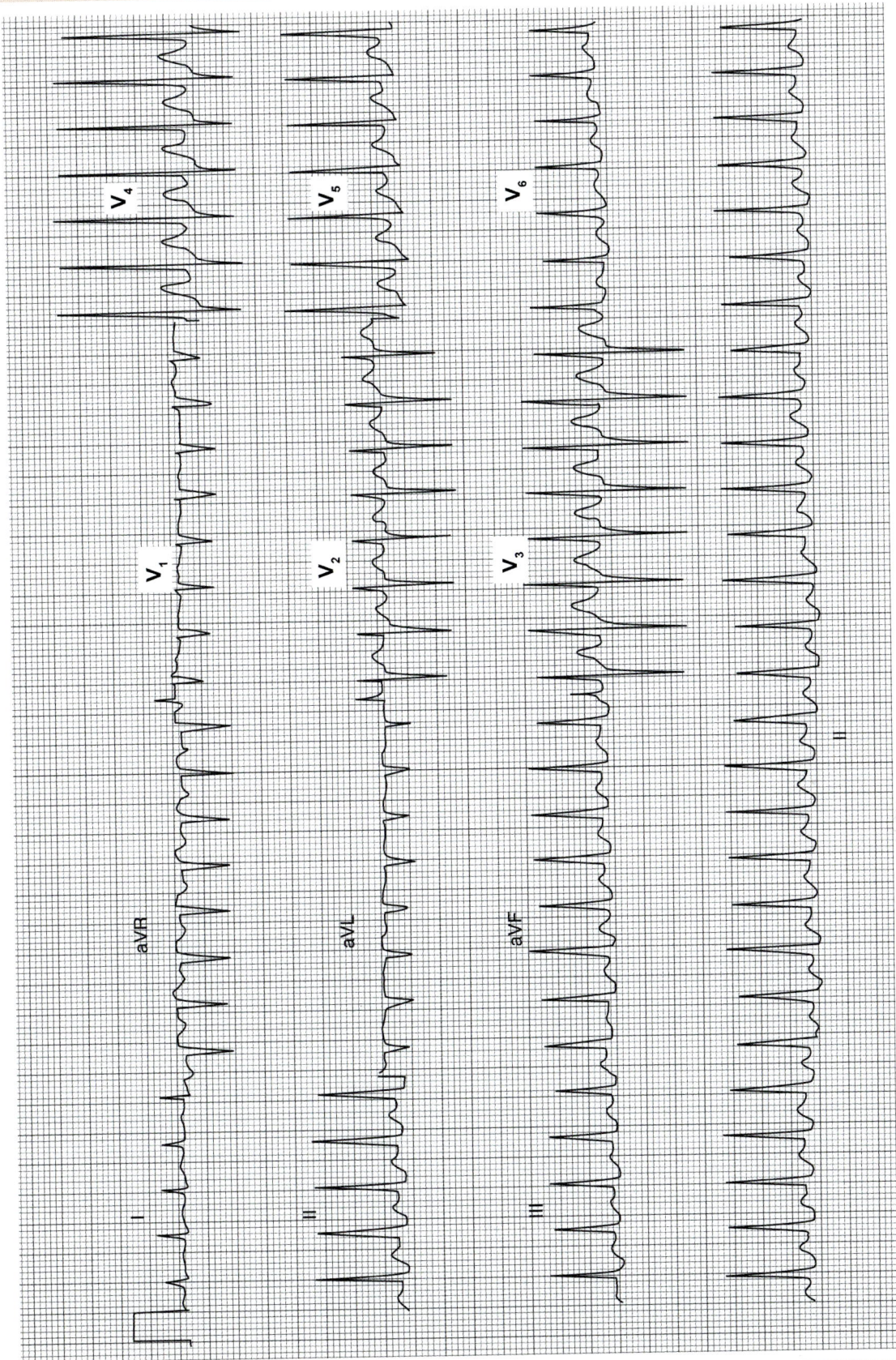

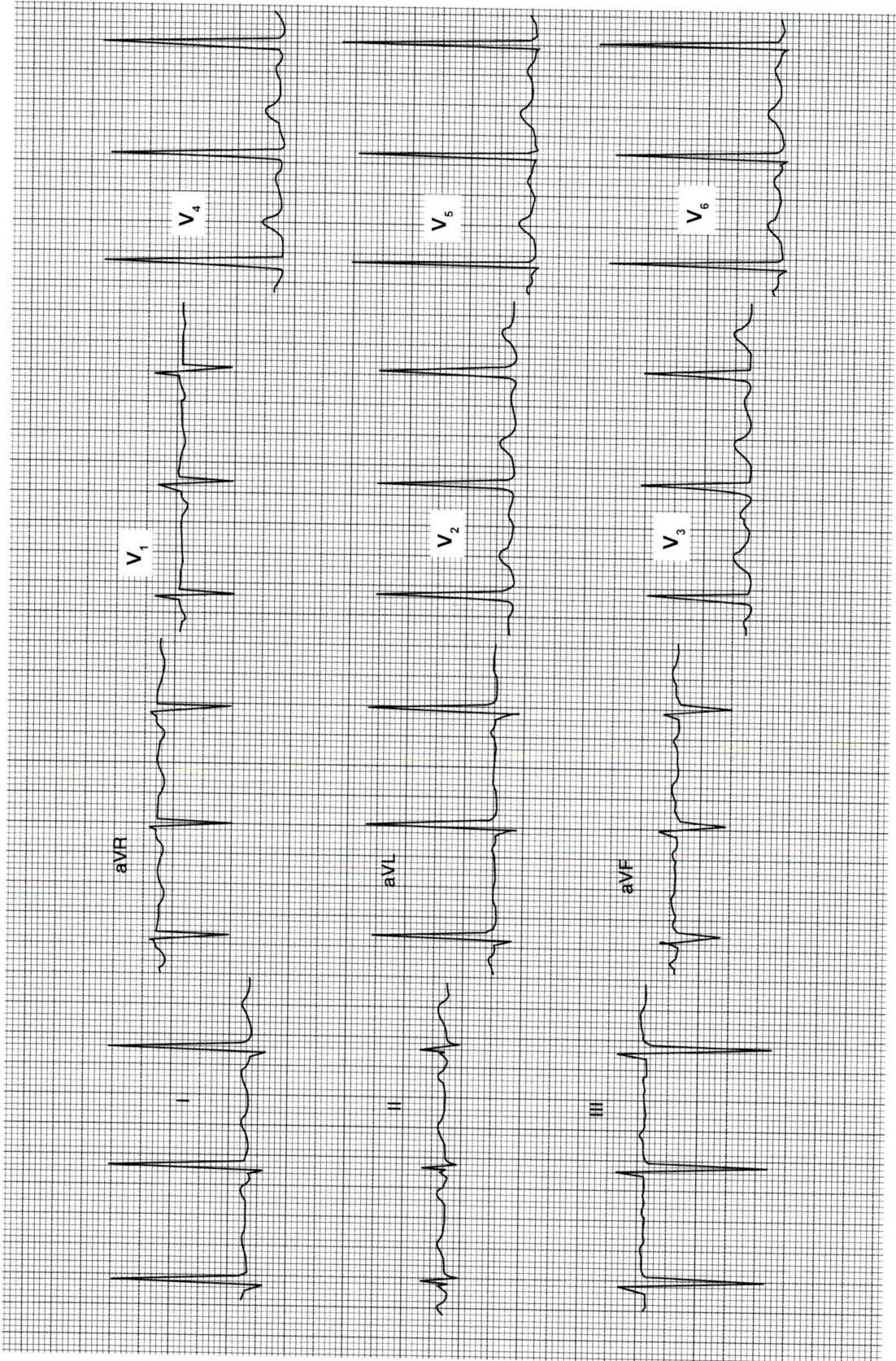

ECG NO. 37

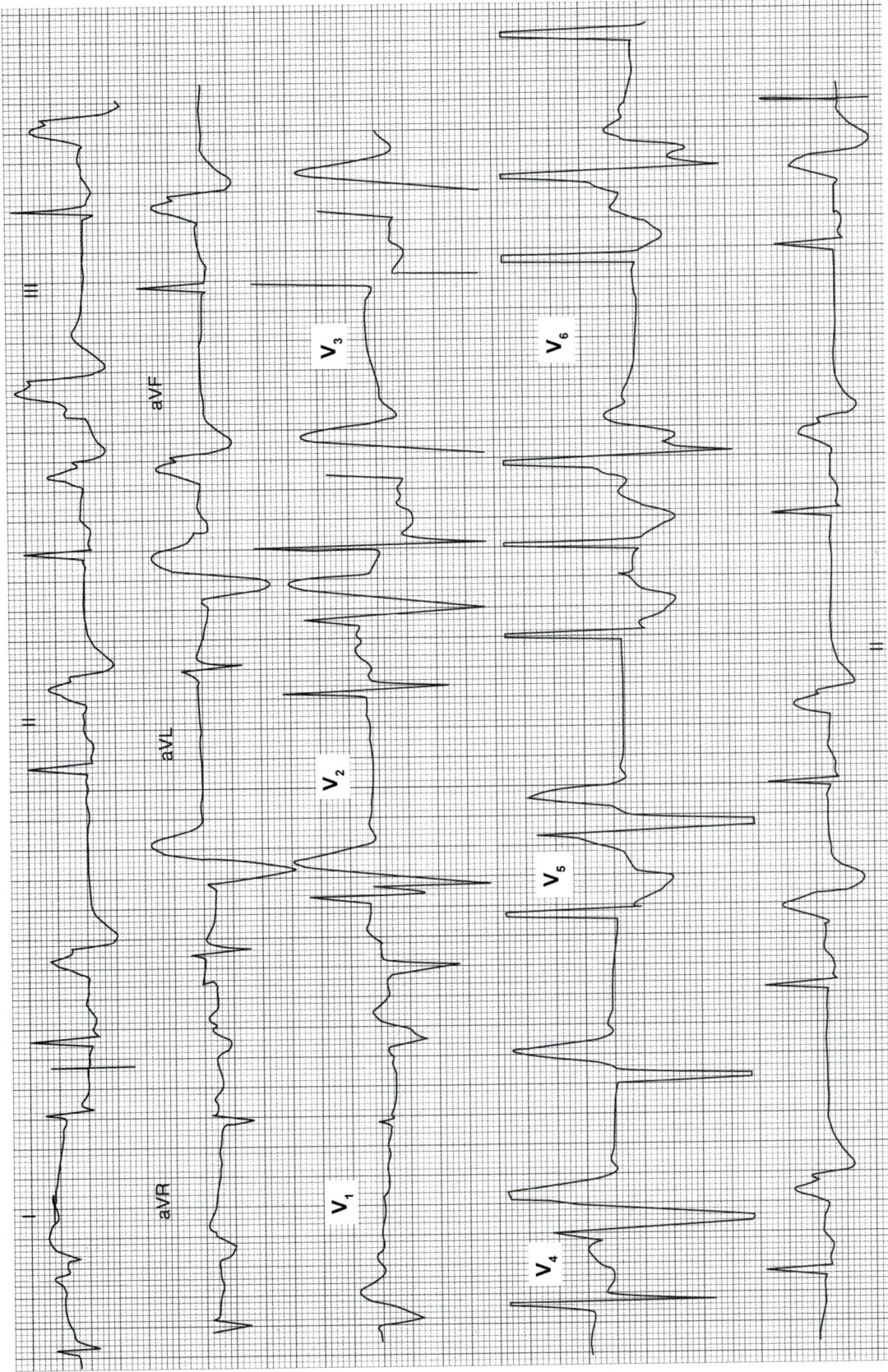

ECG NO. 38

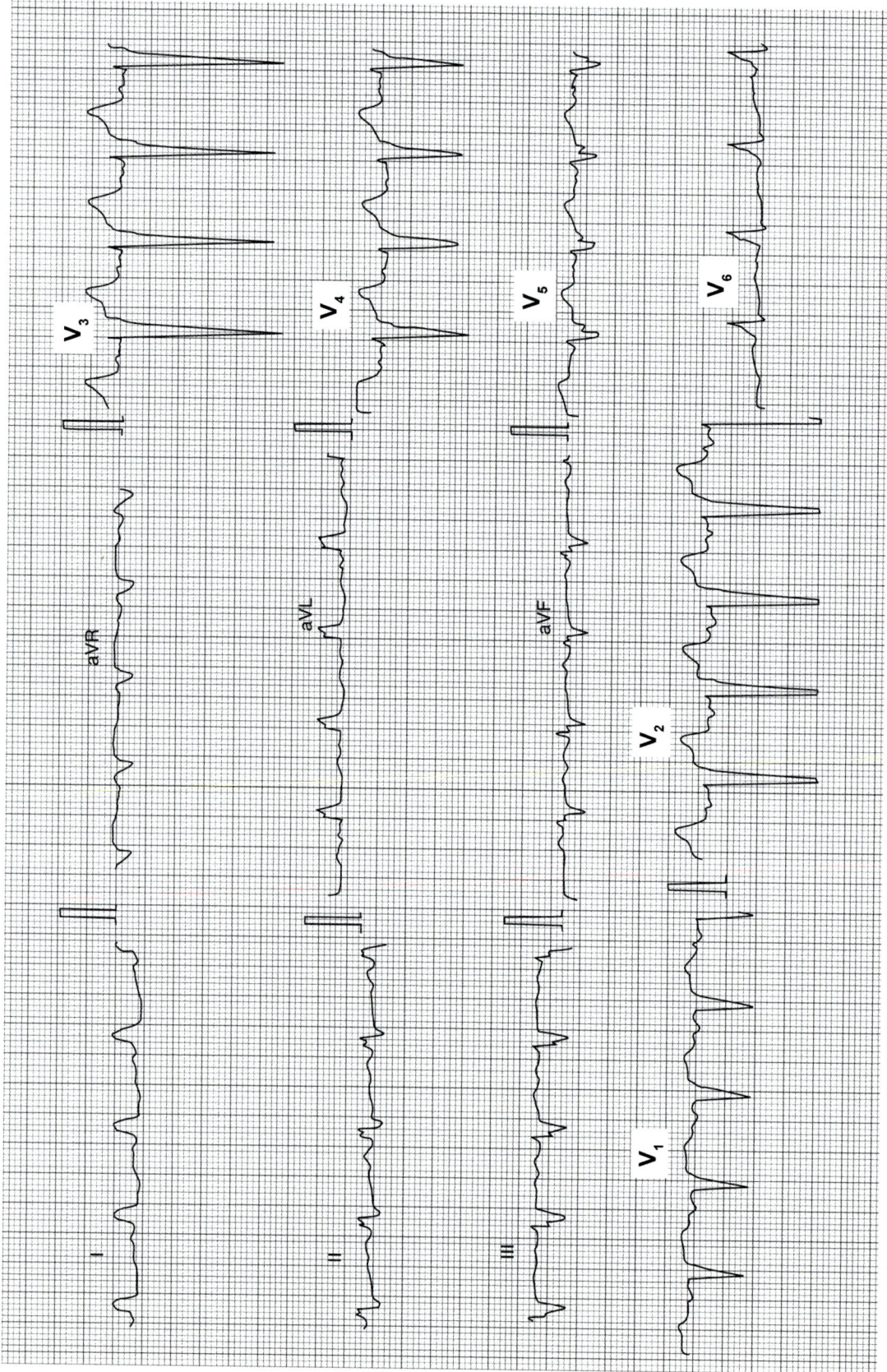

ECG NO. 39

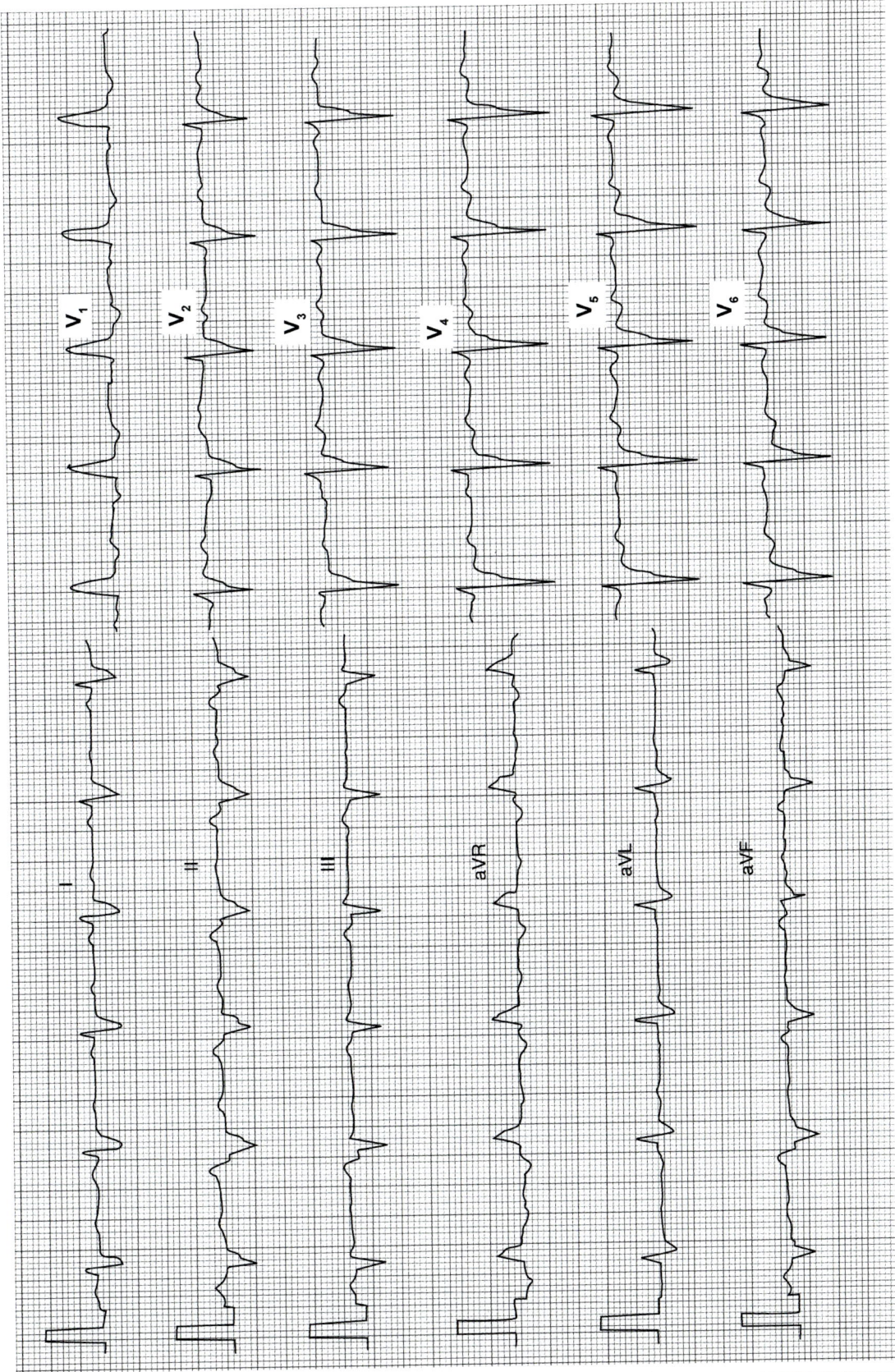

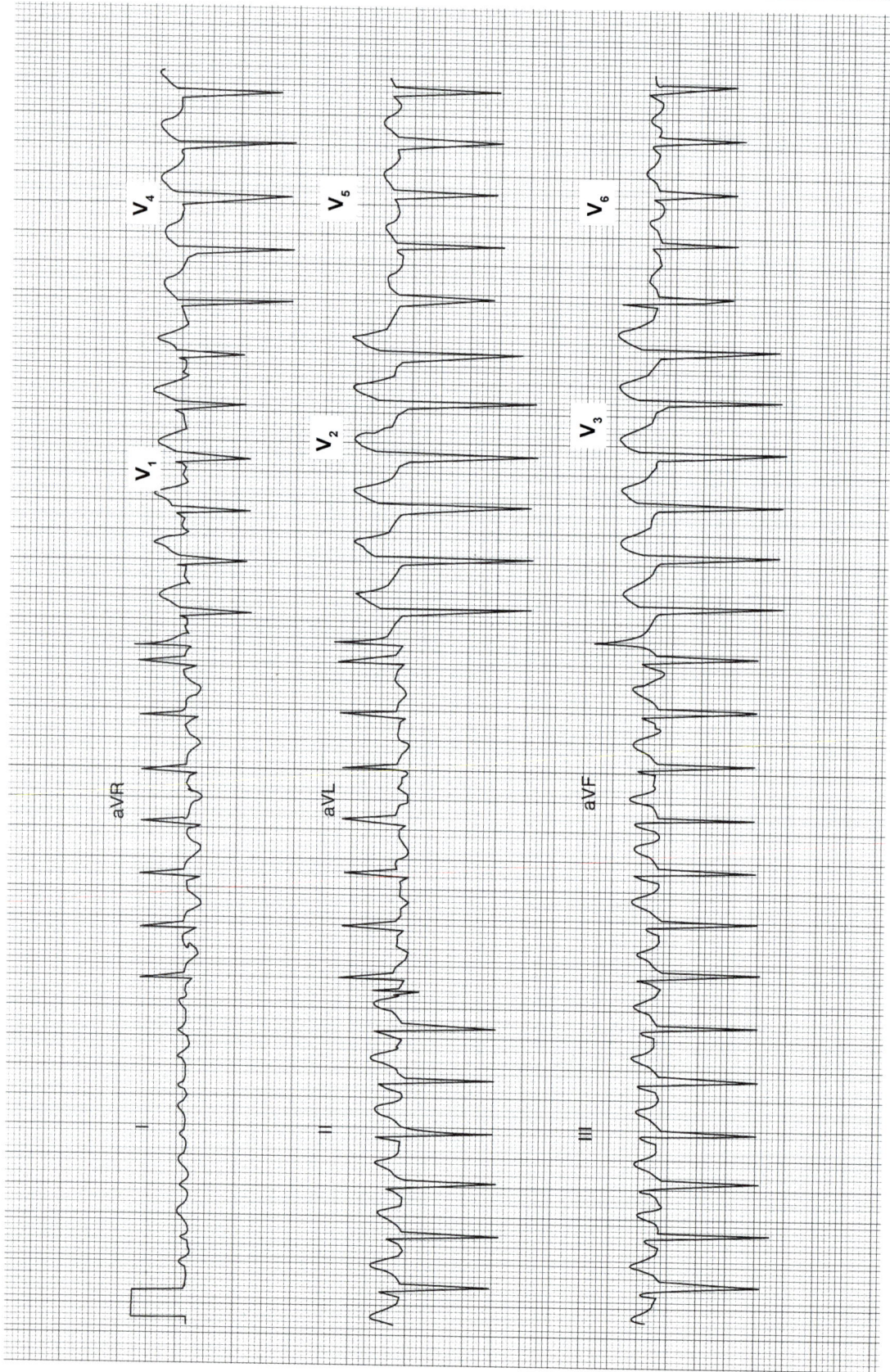

ECG NO. 40

ECG NO. 41

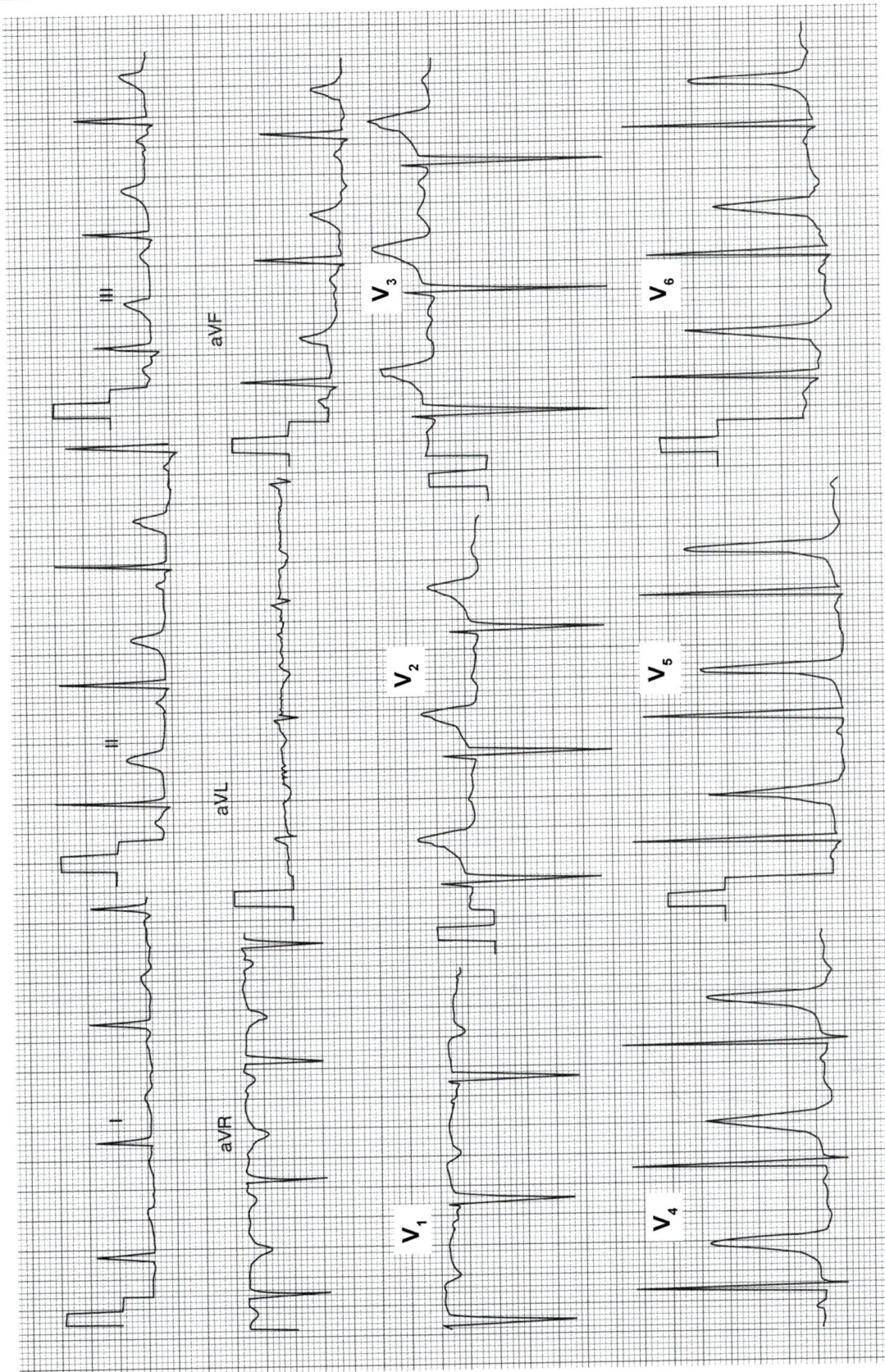

ECG NO. 42

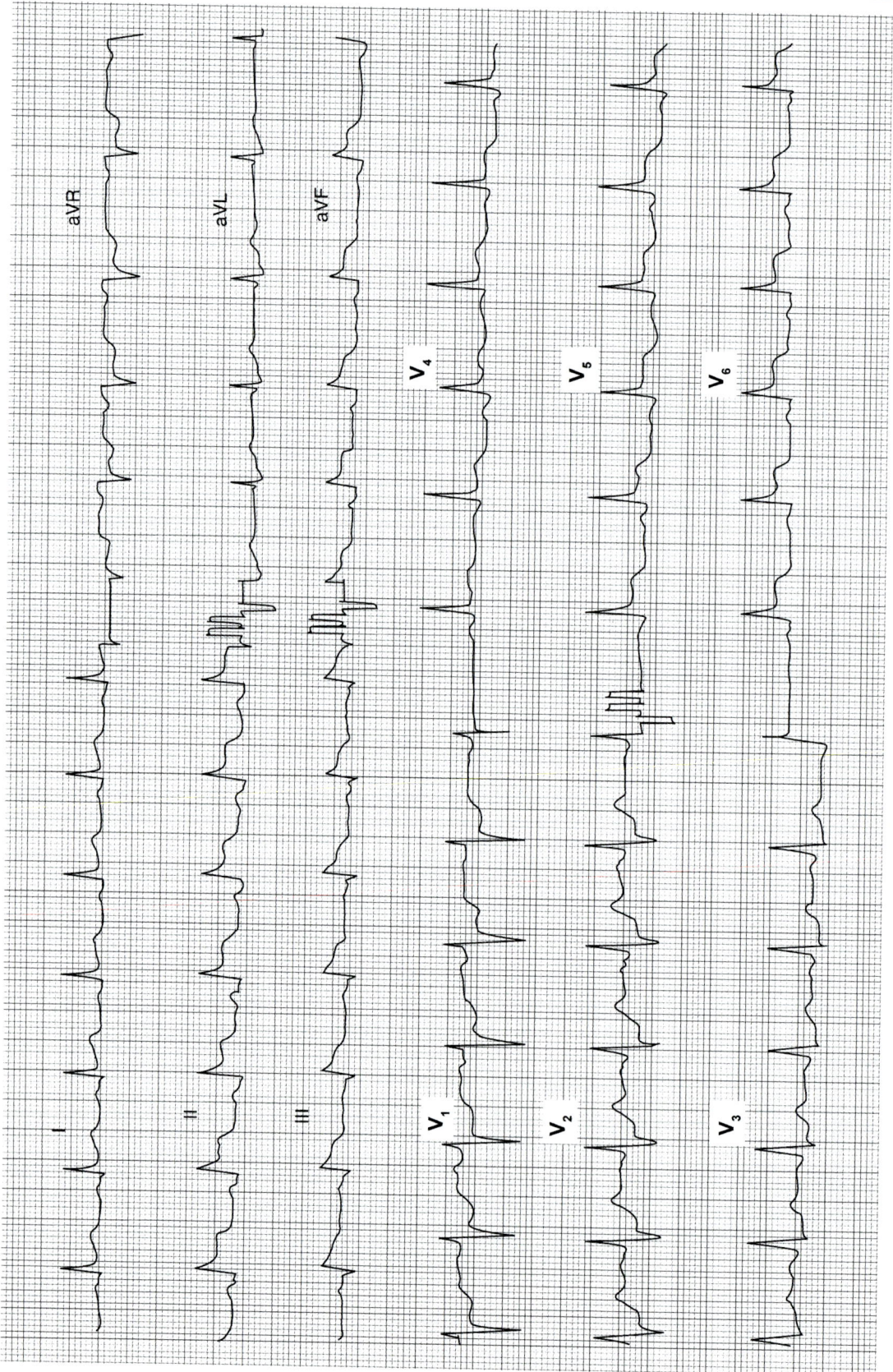

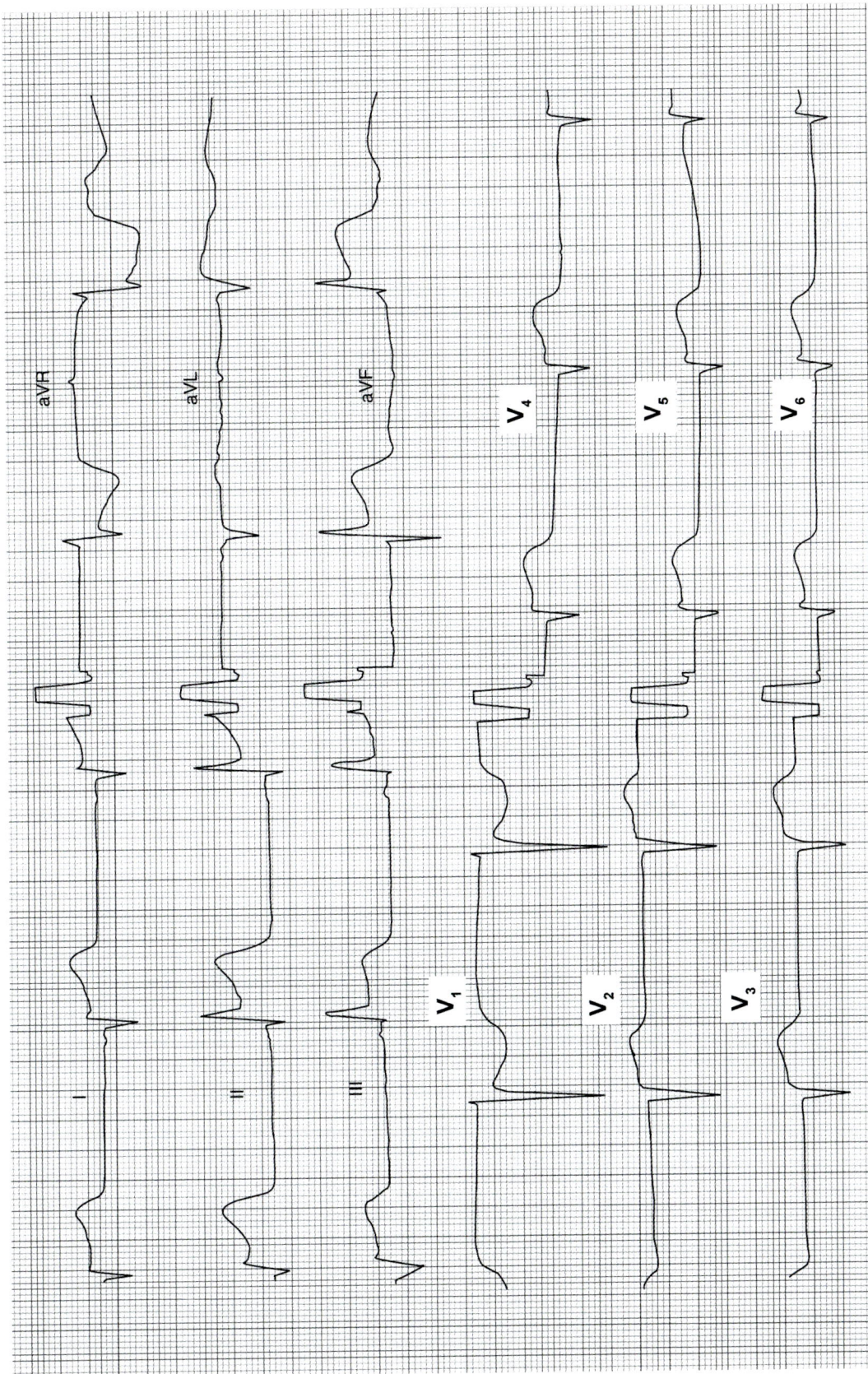

ECG NO. 43

aVR

aVL

aVF

V₄

V₅

V₆

I

II

III

V₁

V₂

V₃

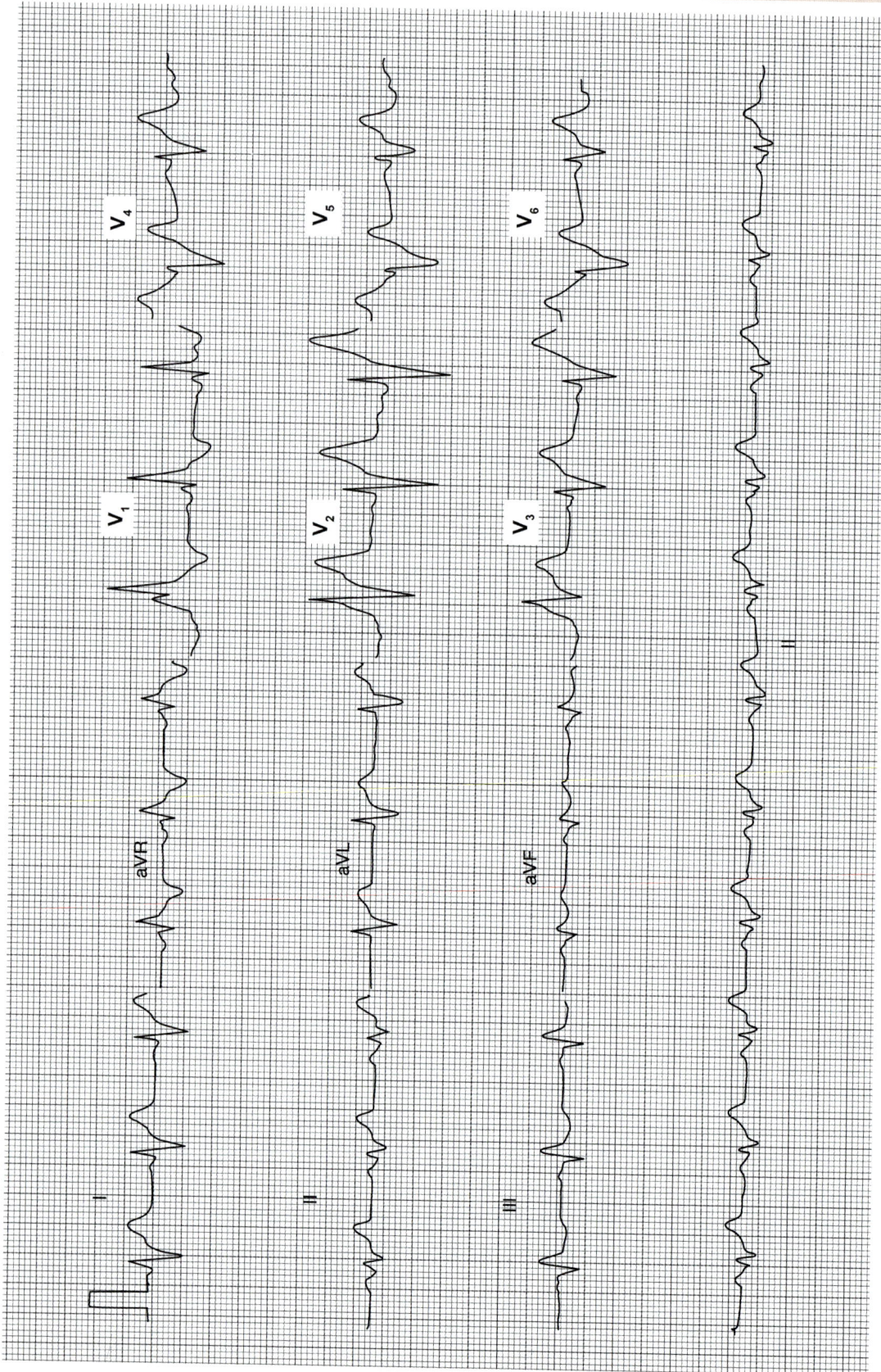

ECG NO. 45

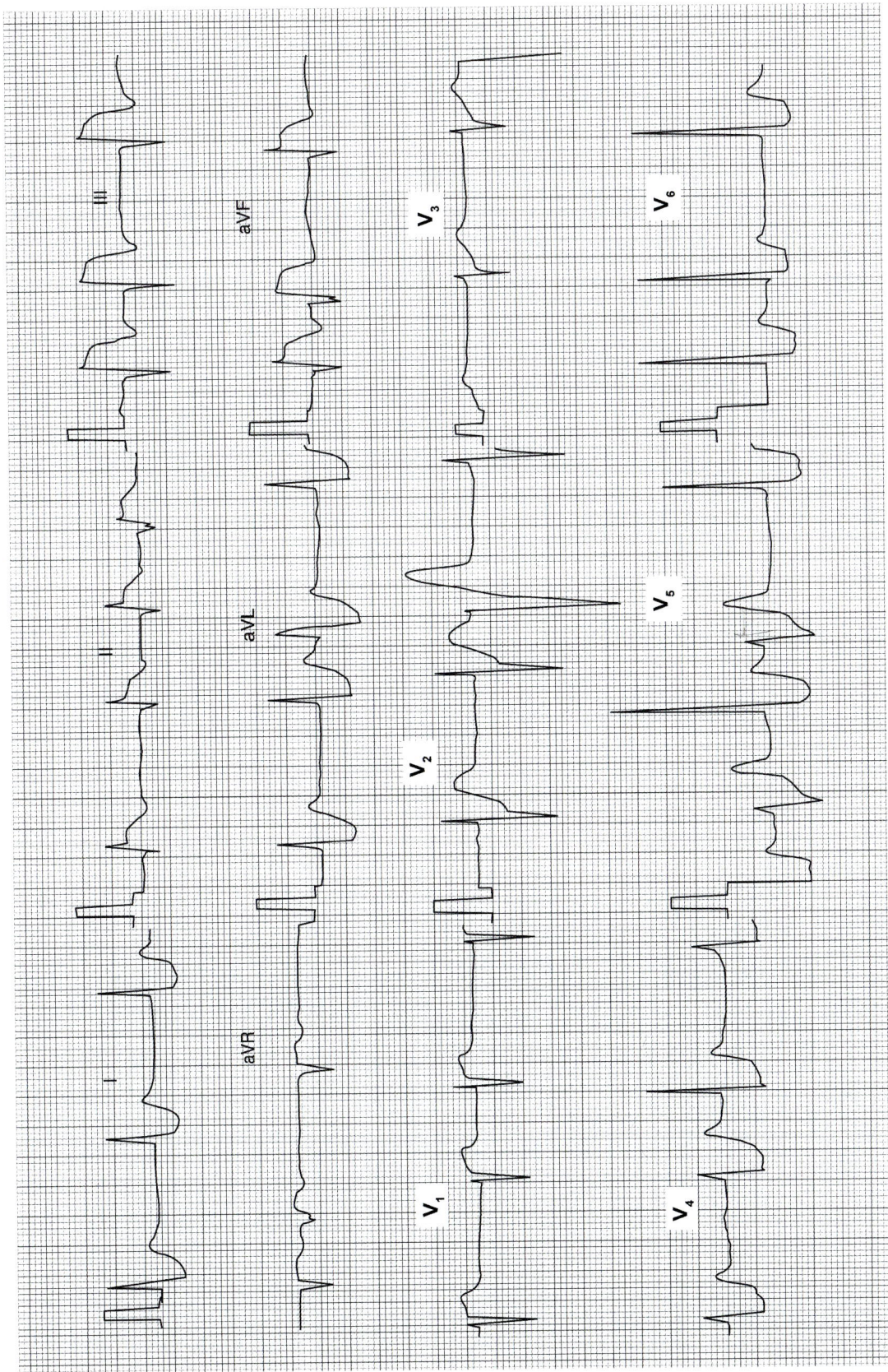

I
II
III
aVR
aVL
aVF
V₁
V₂
V₃
V₄
V₅
V₆

ECG NO. 46

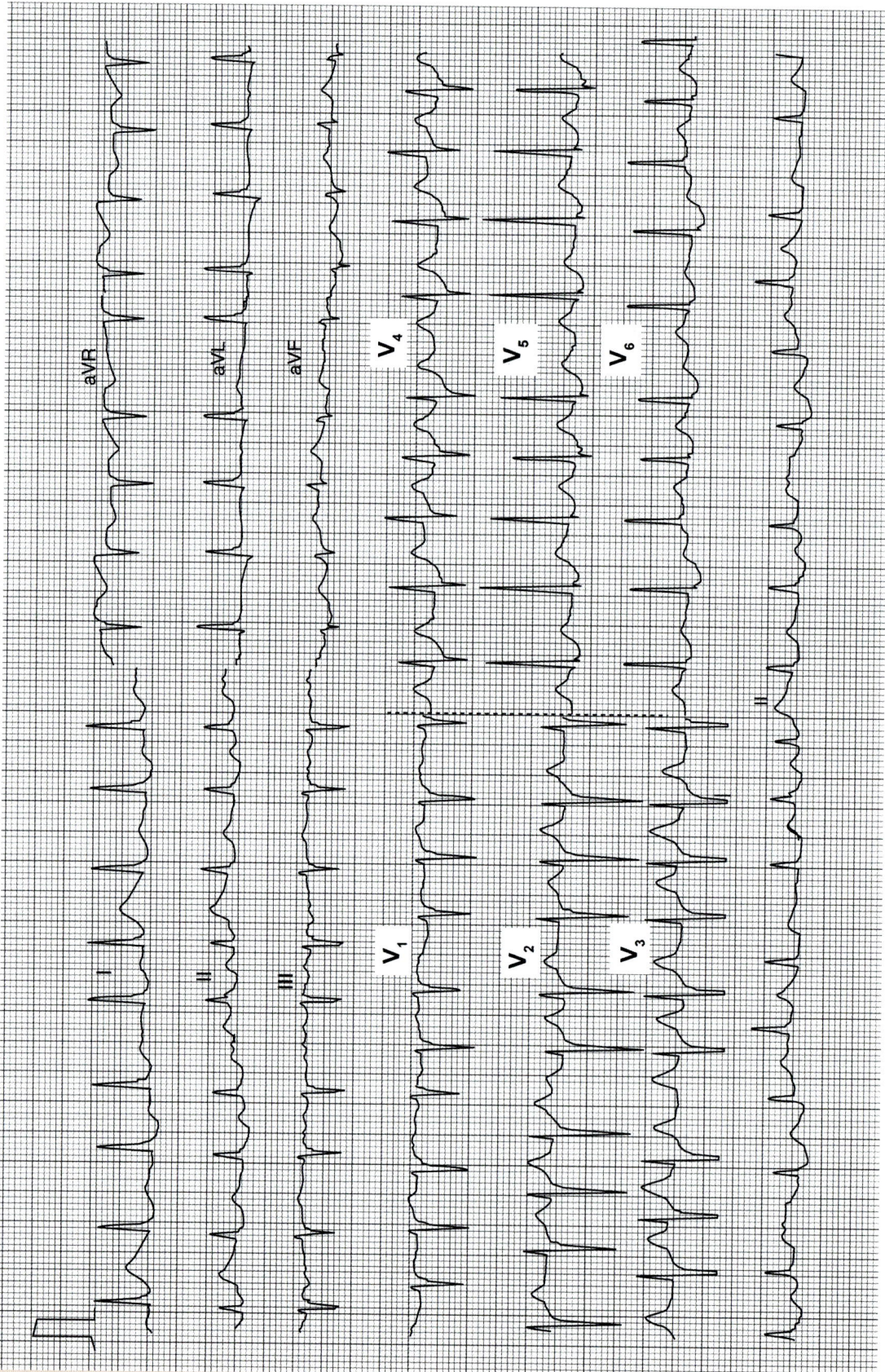

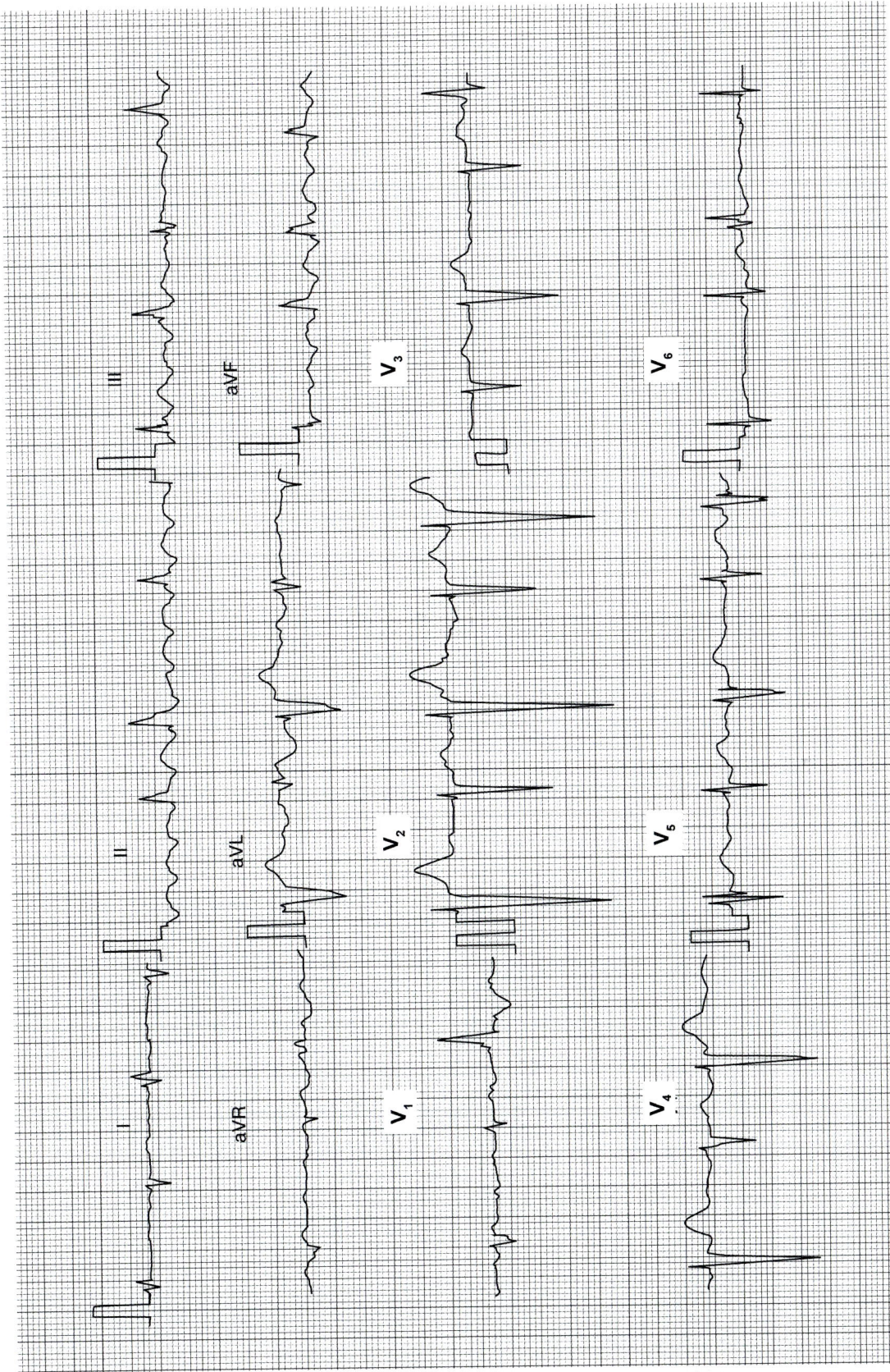

ECG NO. 47

I

II

III

aVR

aVL

aVF

V1

V2

V3

V4

V5

V6

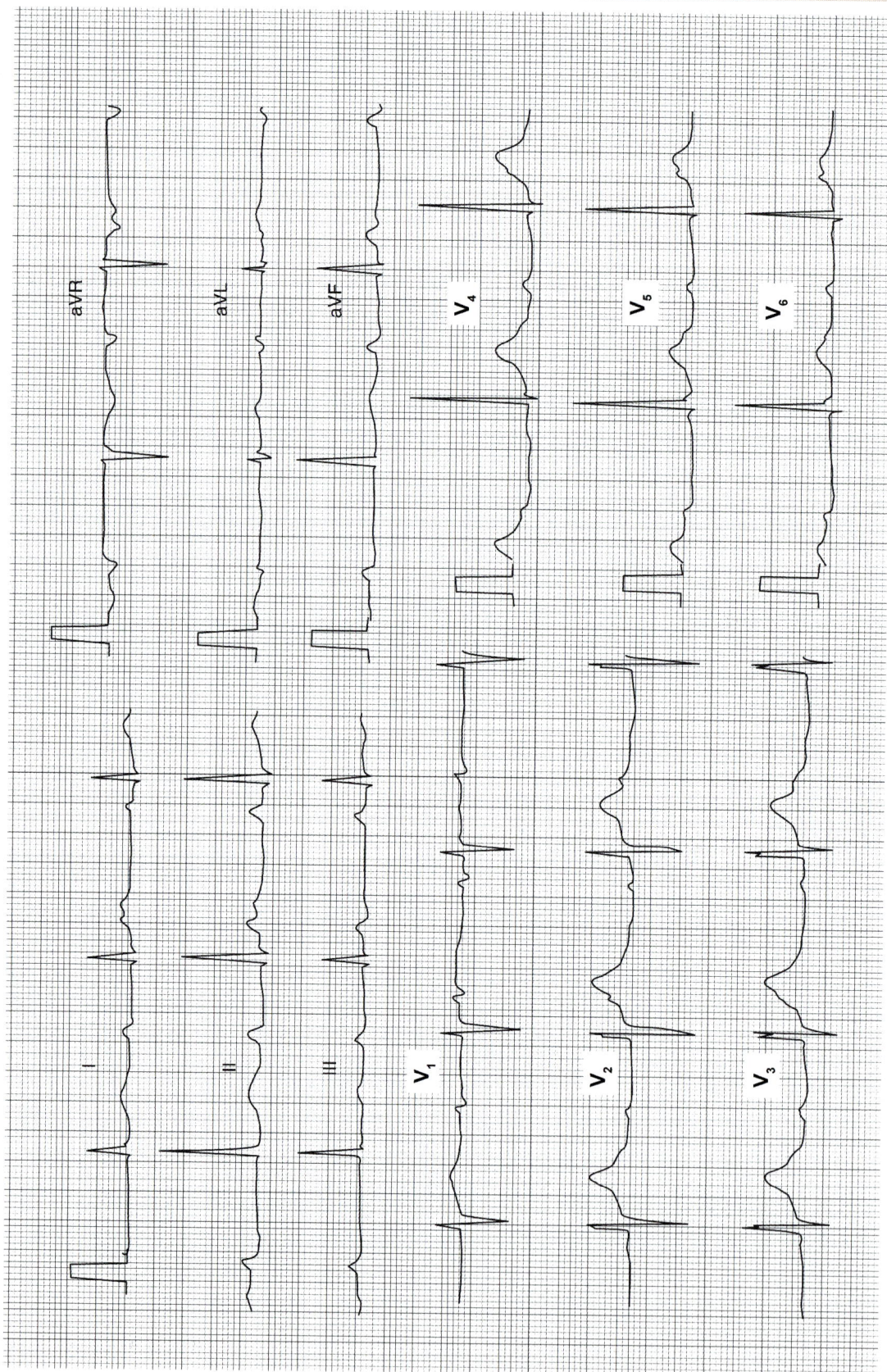

ECG NO. 49

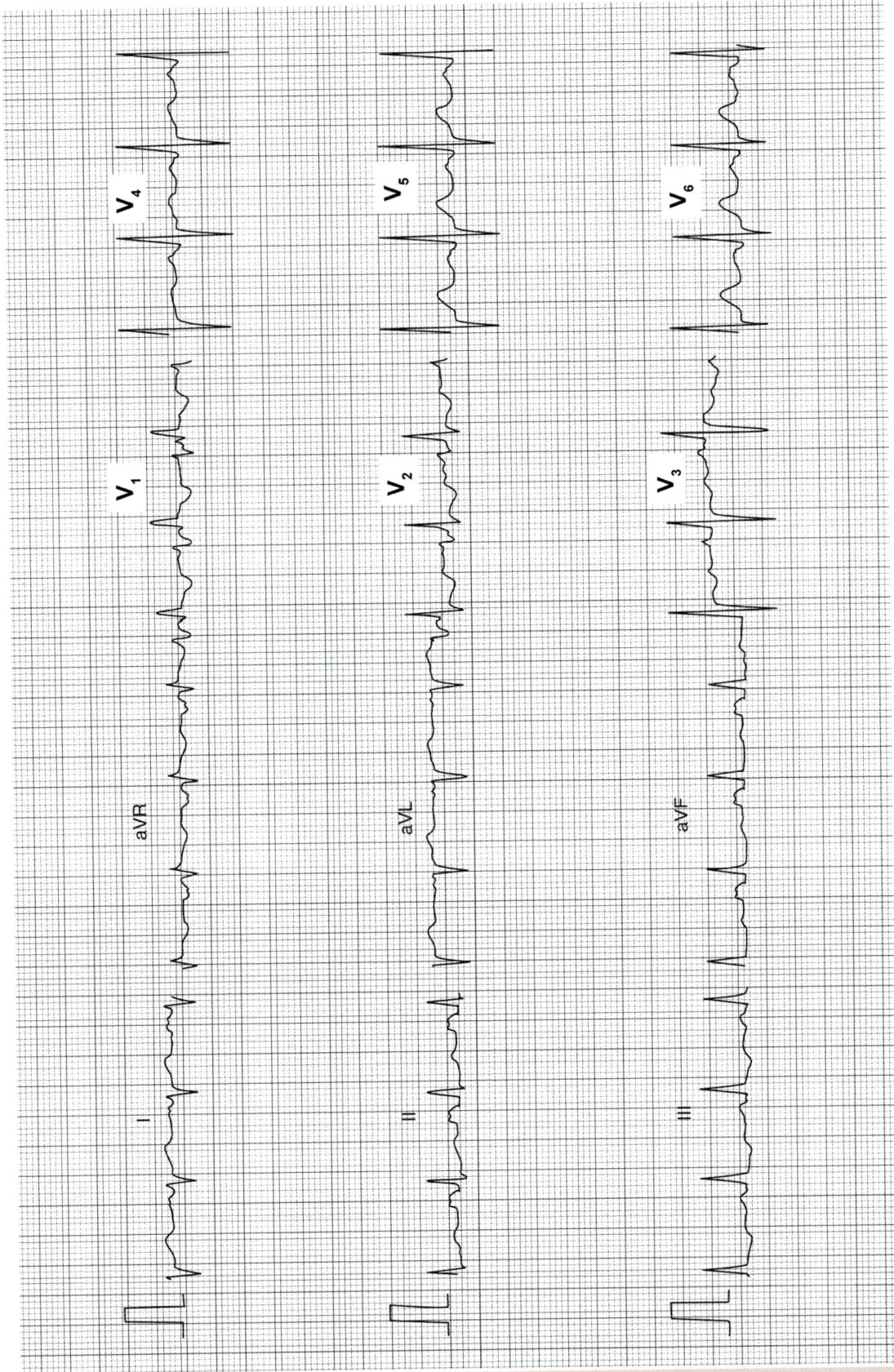

I

aVR

V₁

V₄

II

aVL

V₂

V₅

III

aVF

V₃

V₆

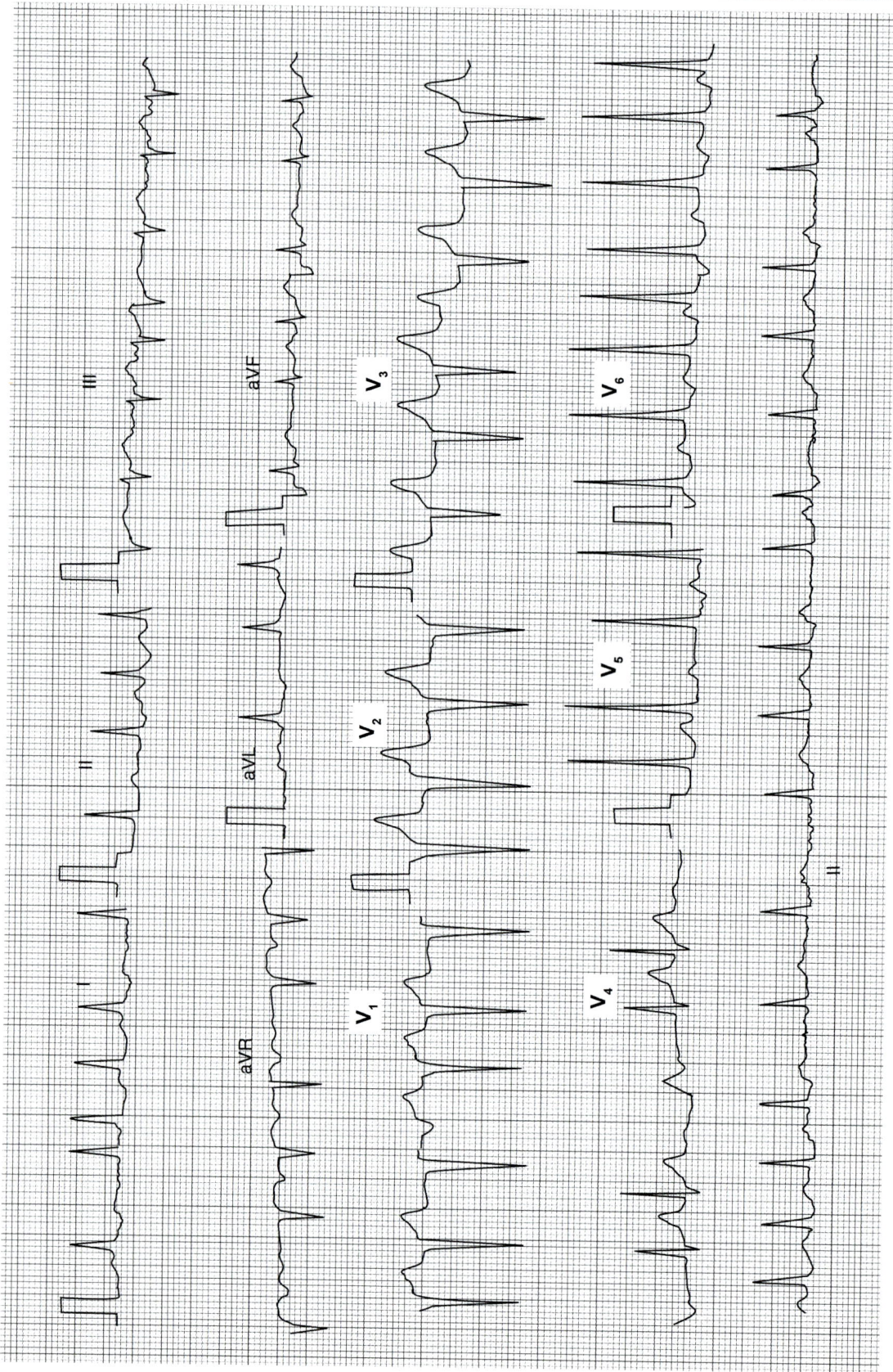

ECG NO. 50

ECG NO. 51

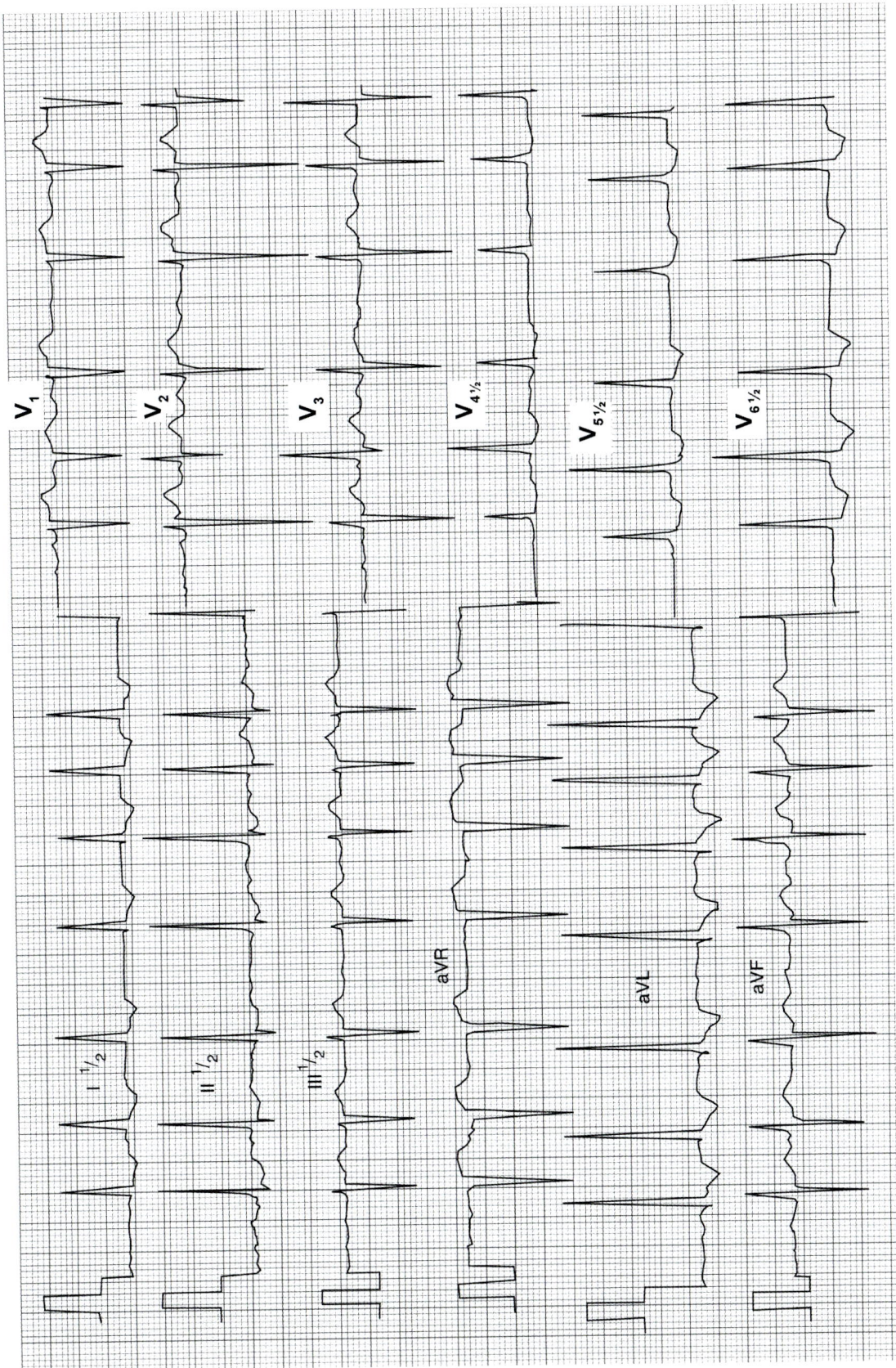

V_1 V_2 V_3 $V_{4½}$ $V_{5½}$ $V_{6½}$

$I_{½}$ $II_{½}$ $III_{½}$ aVR aVL aVF

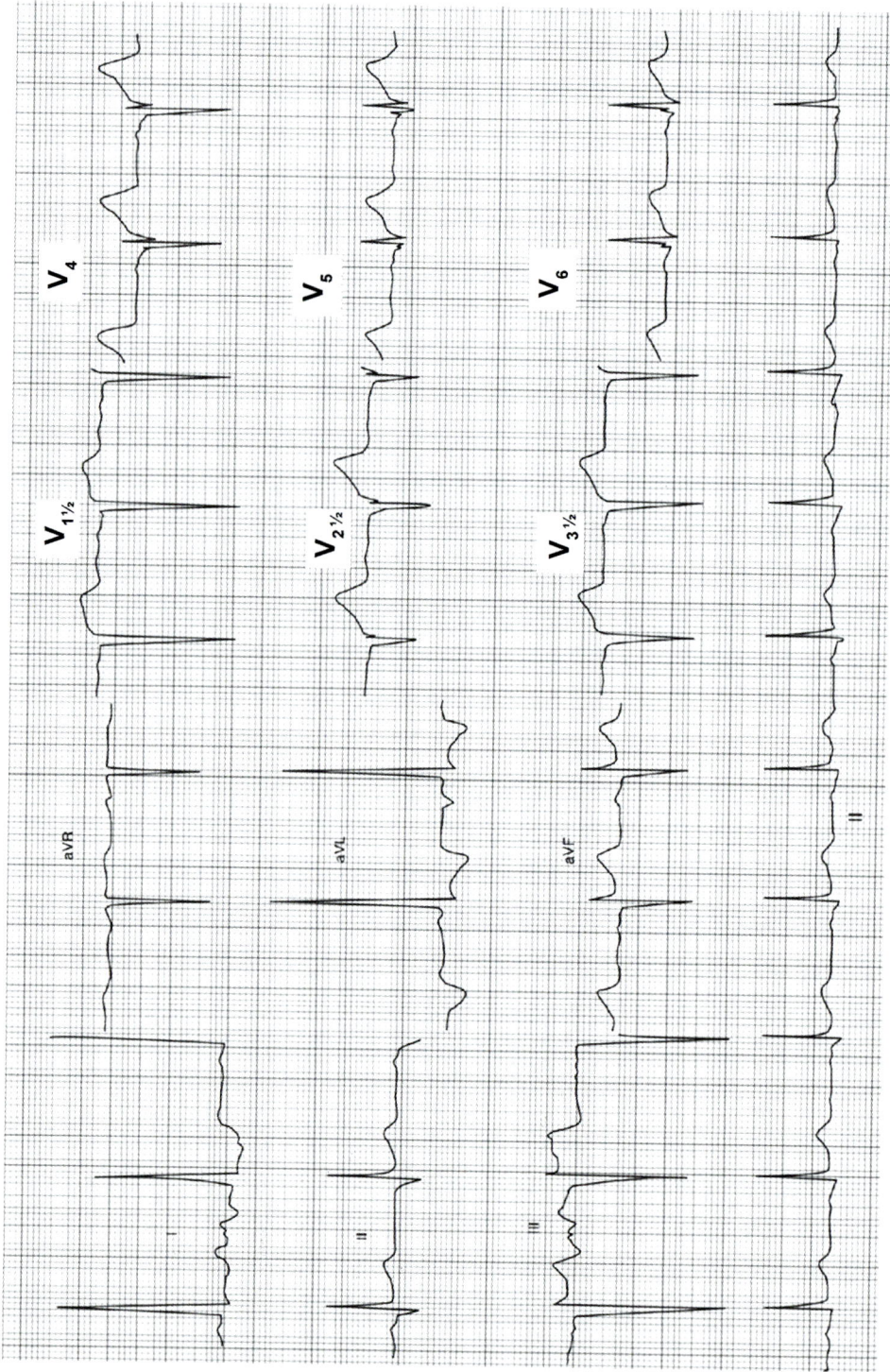

ECG NO. 53

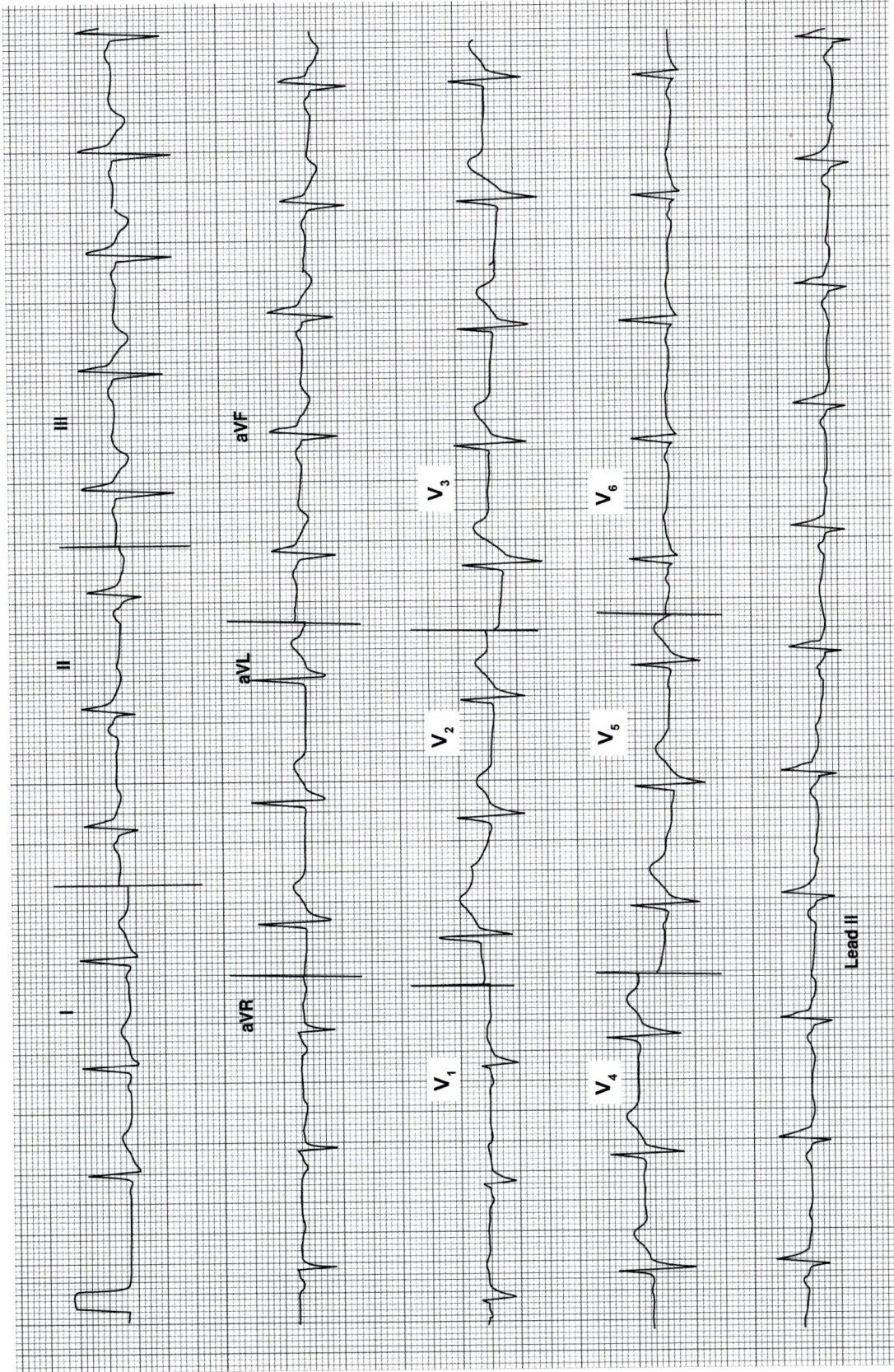

I   aVR   V1   V4

II   aVL   V2   V5

III   aVF   V3   V6

Lead II

ECG NO. 54

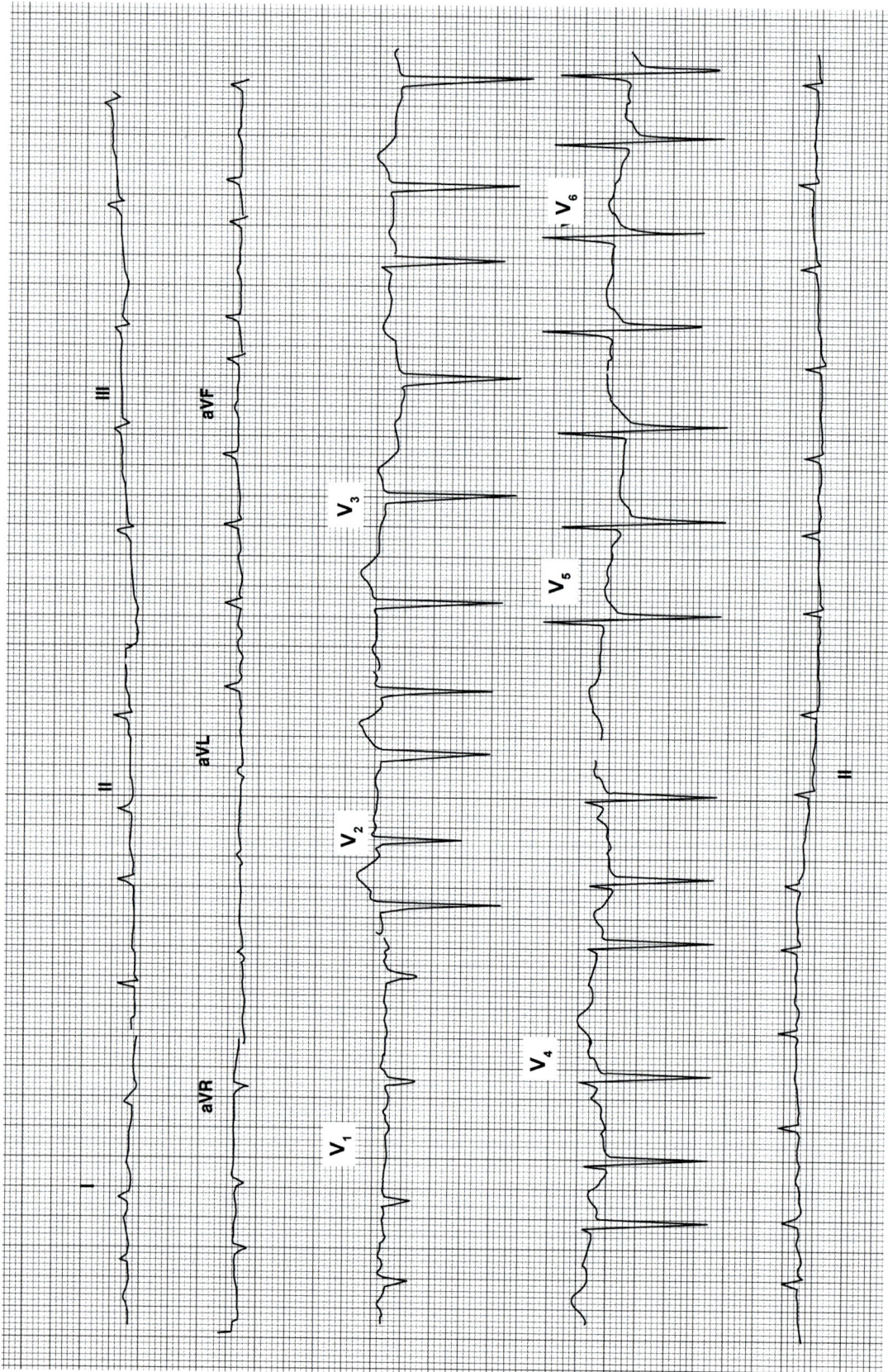

ECG NO. 55

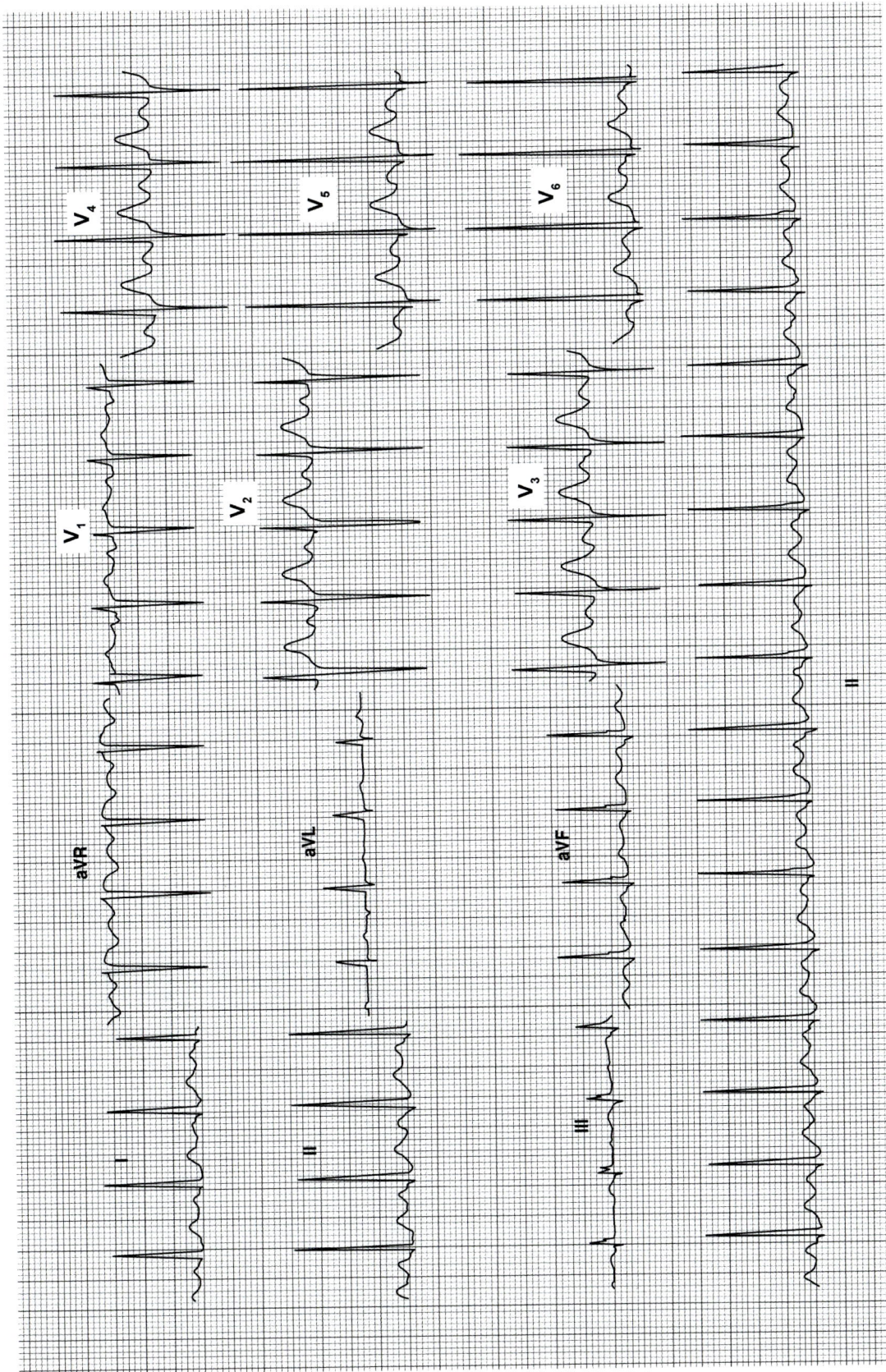

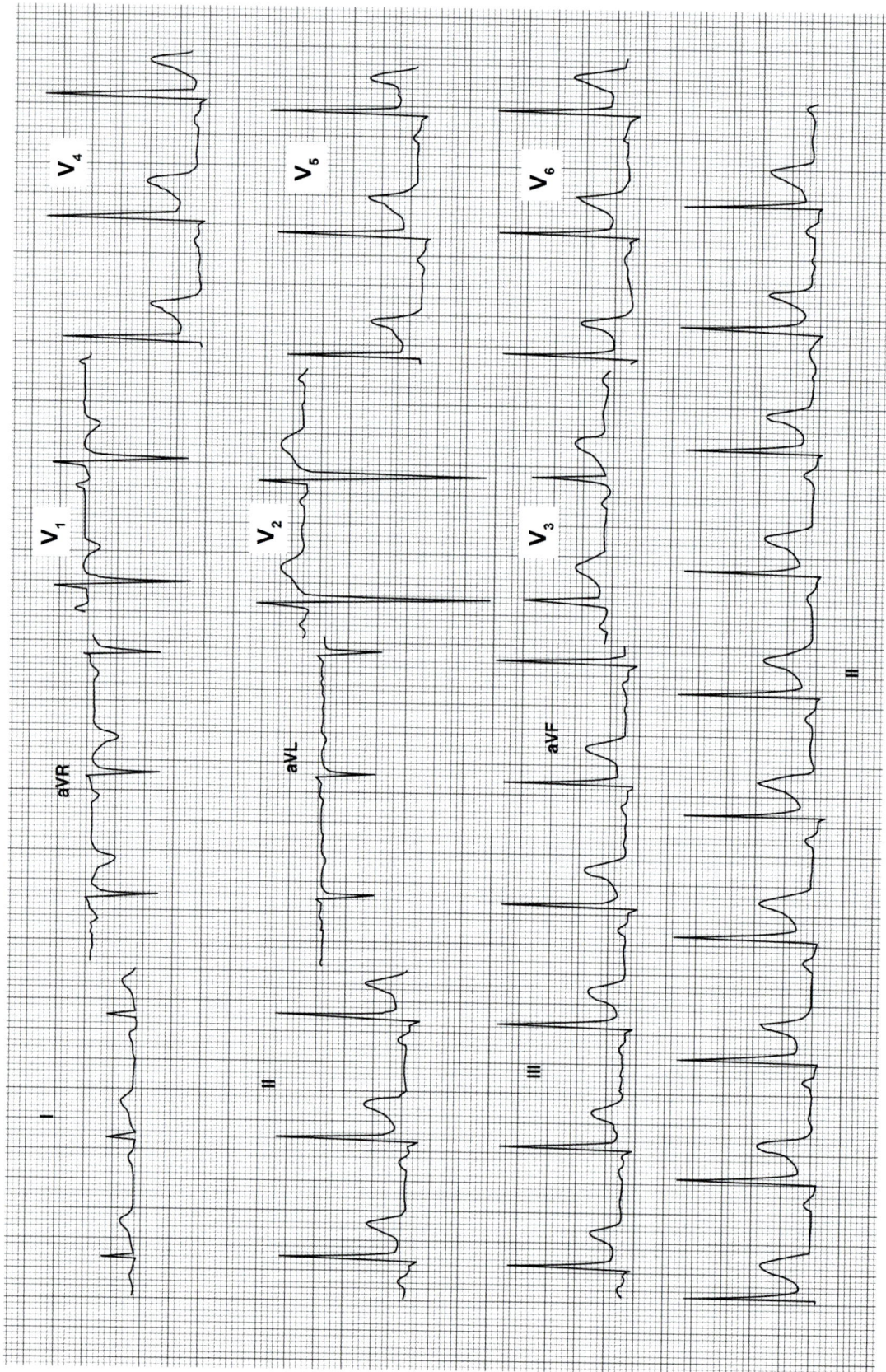

ECG NO. 56

ECG NO. 57

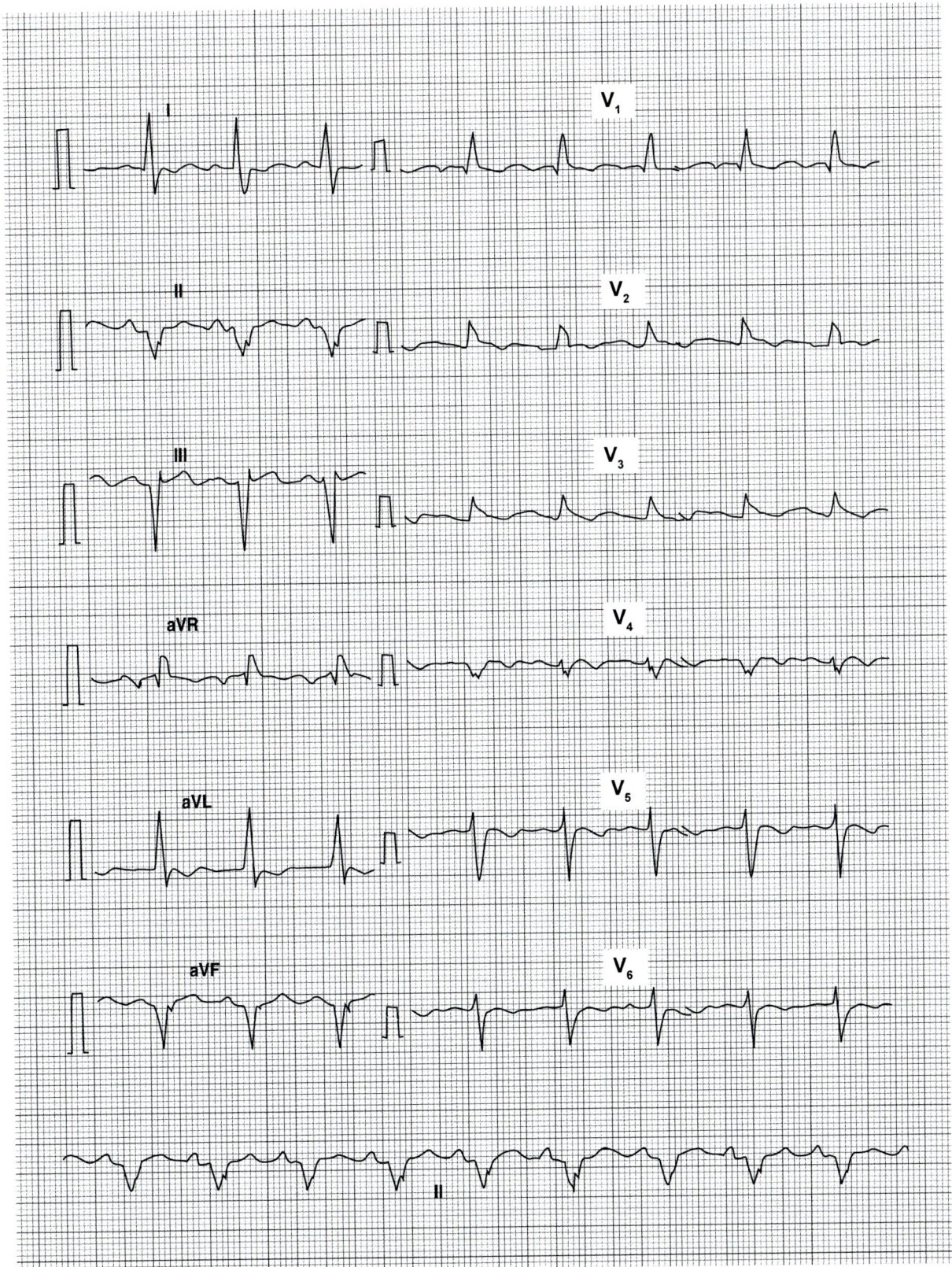

ECG NO. 58

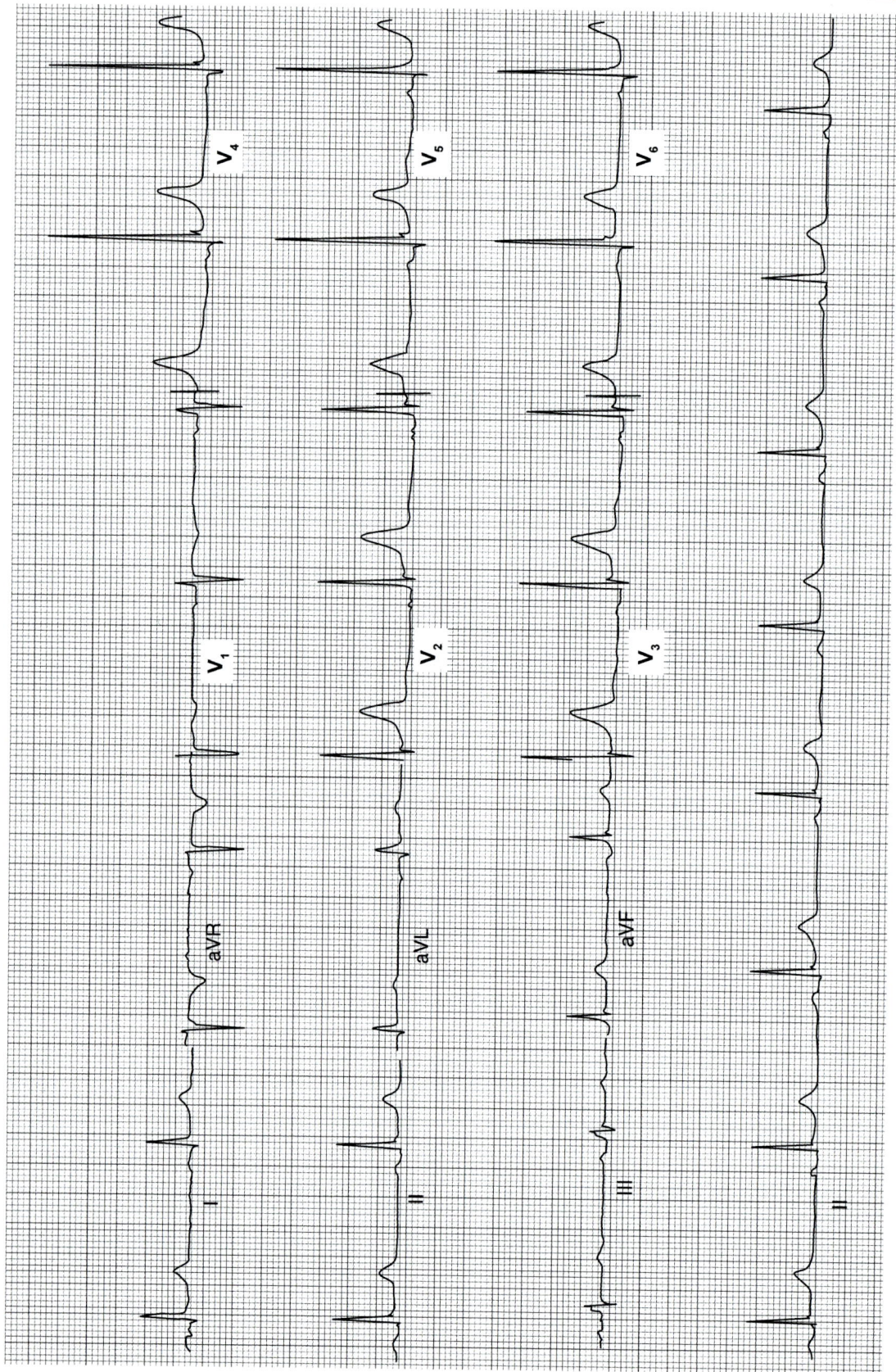

ECG NO. 59

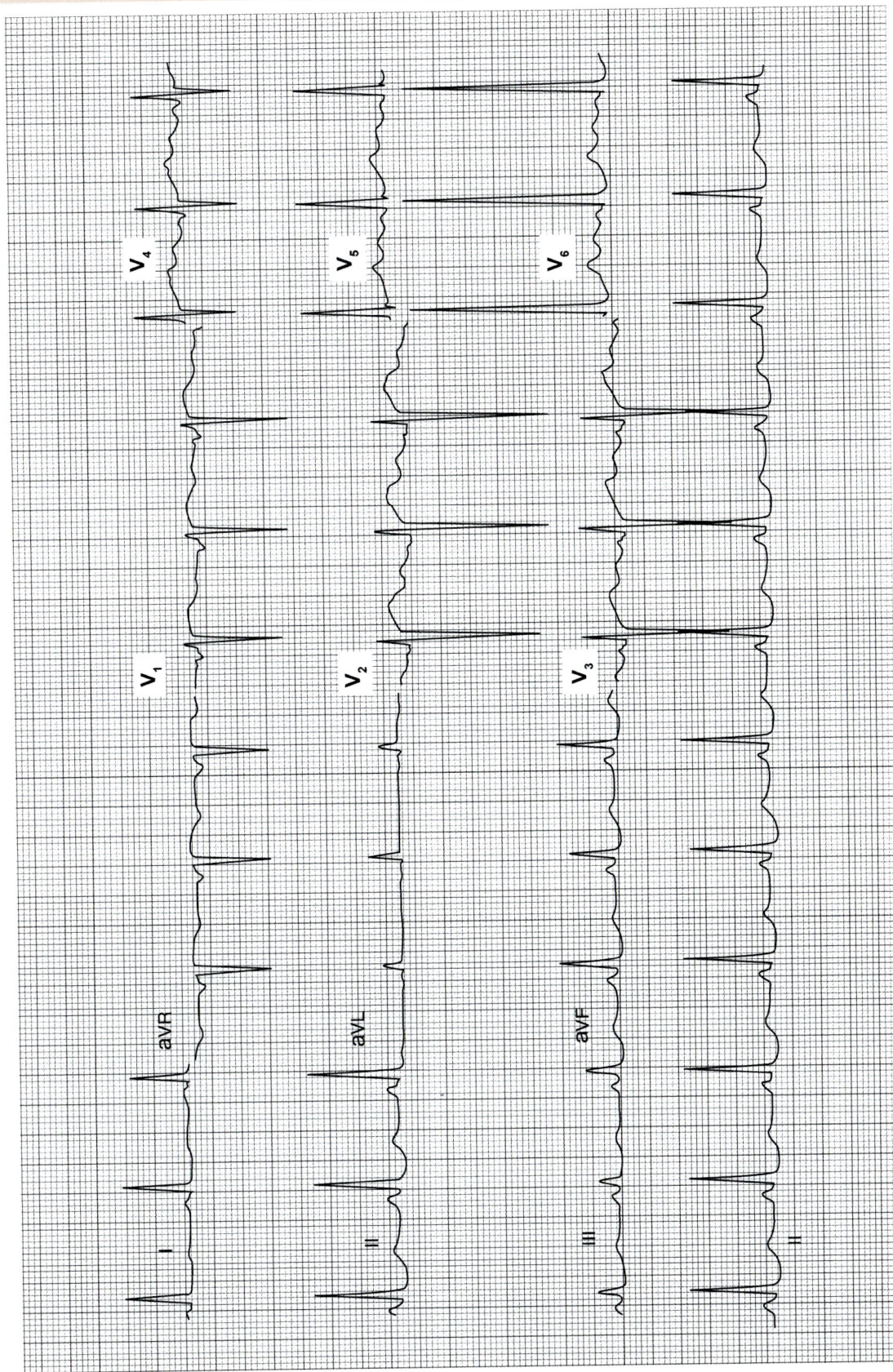

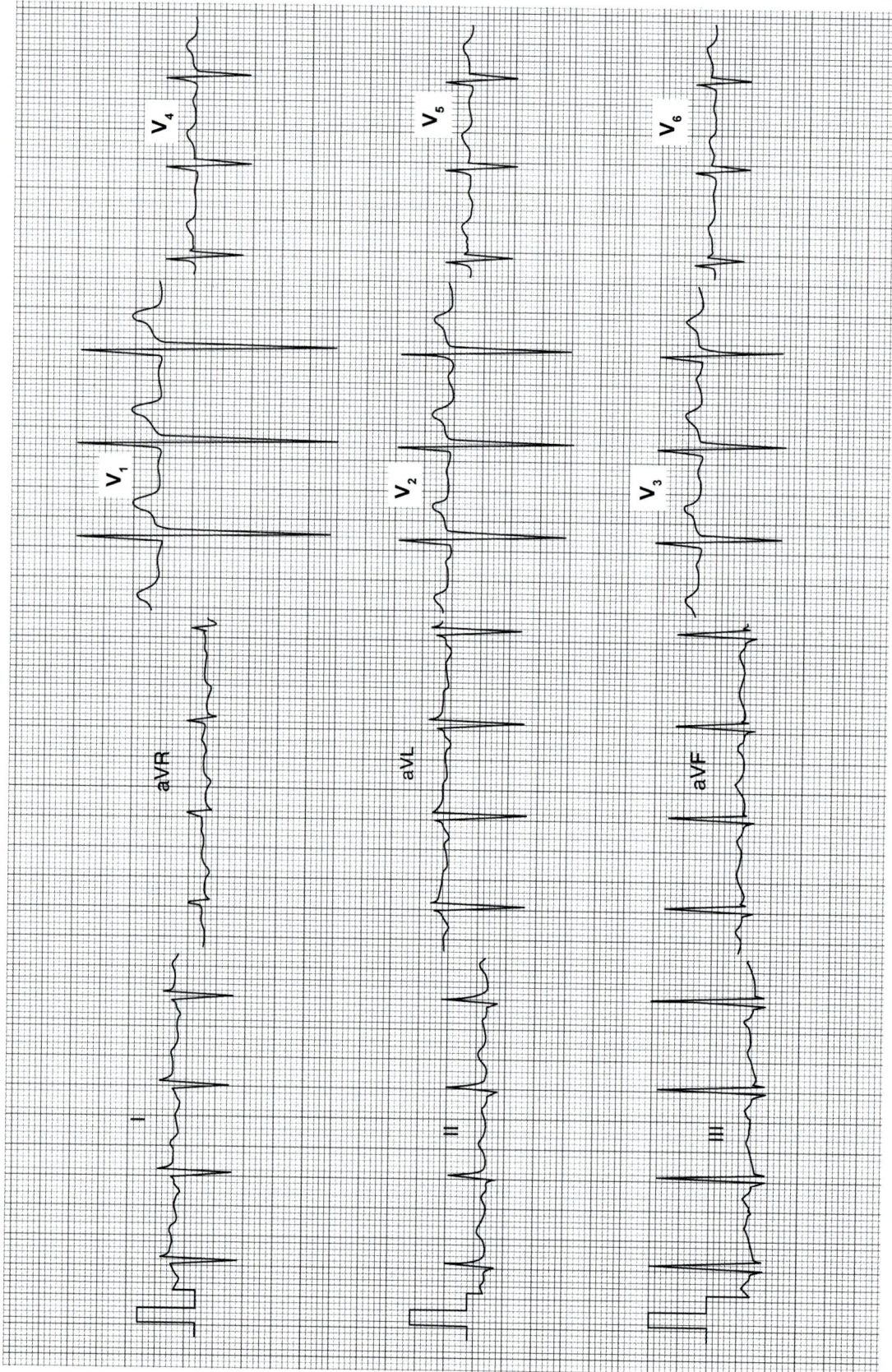

ECG NO. 60

ECG NO. 61

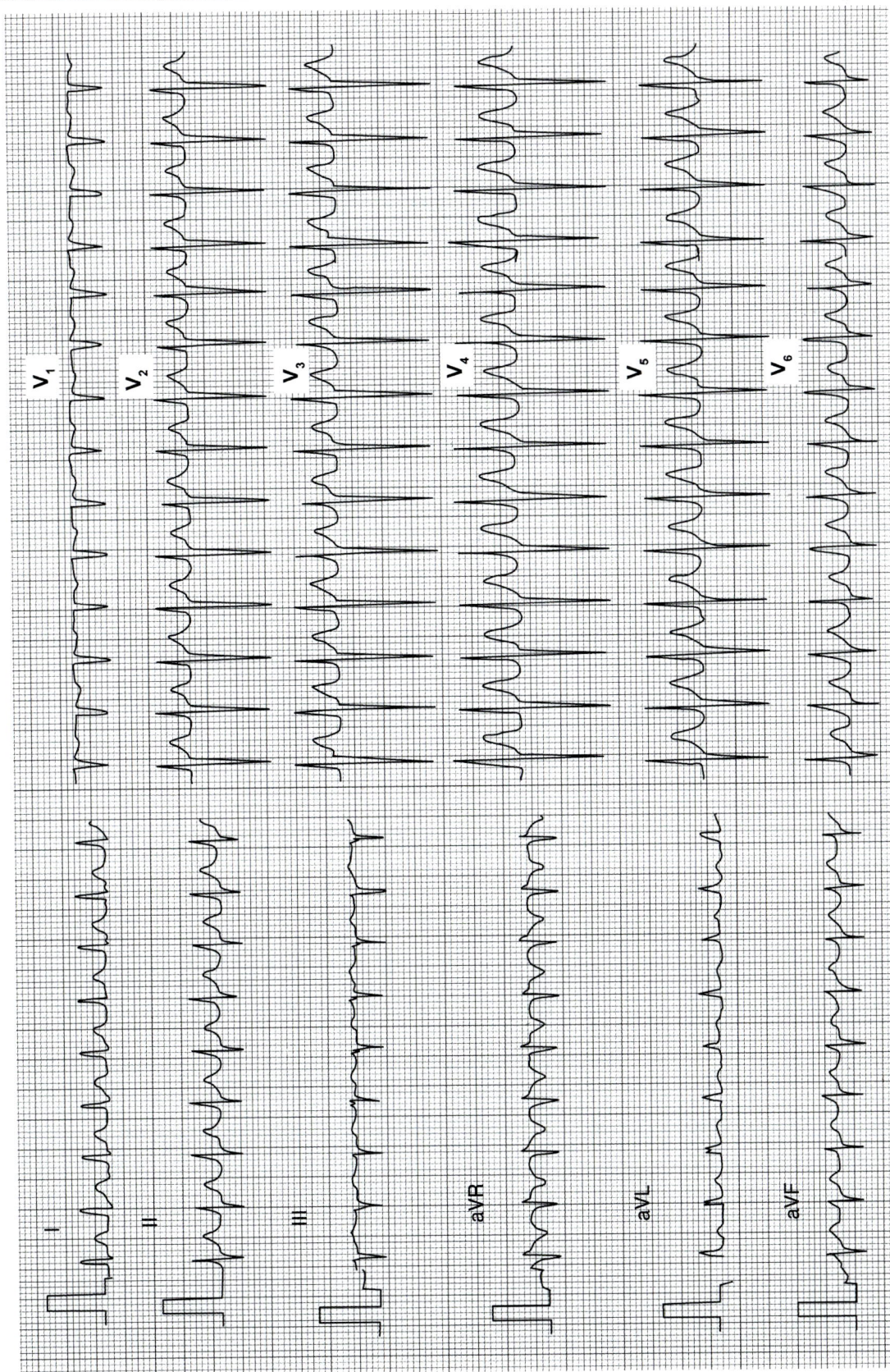

I

II

III

aVR

aVL

aVF

V₁

V₂

V₃

V₄

V₅

V₆

ECG NO. 62

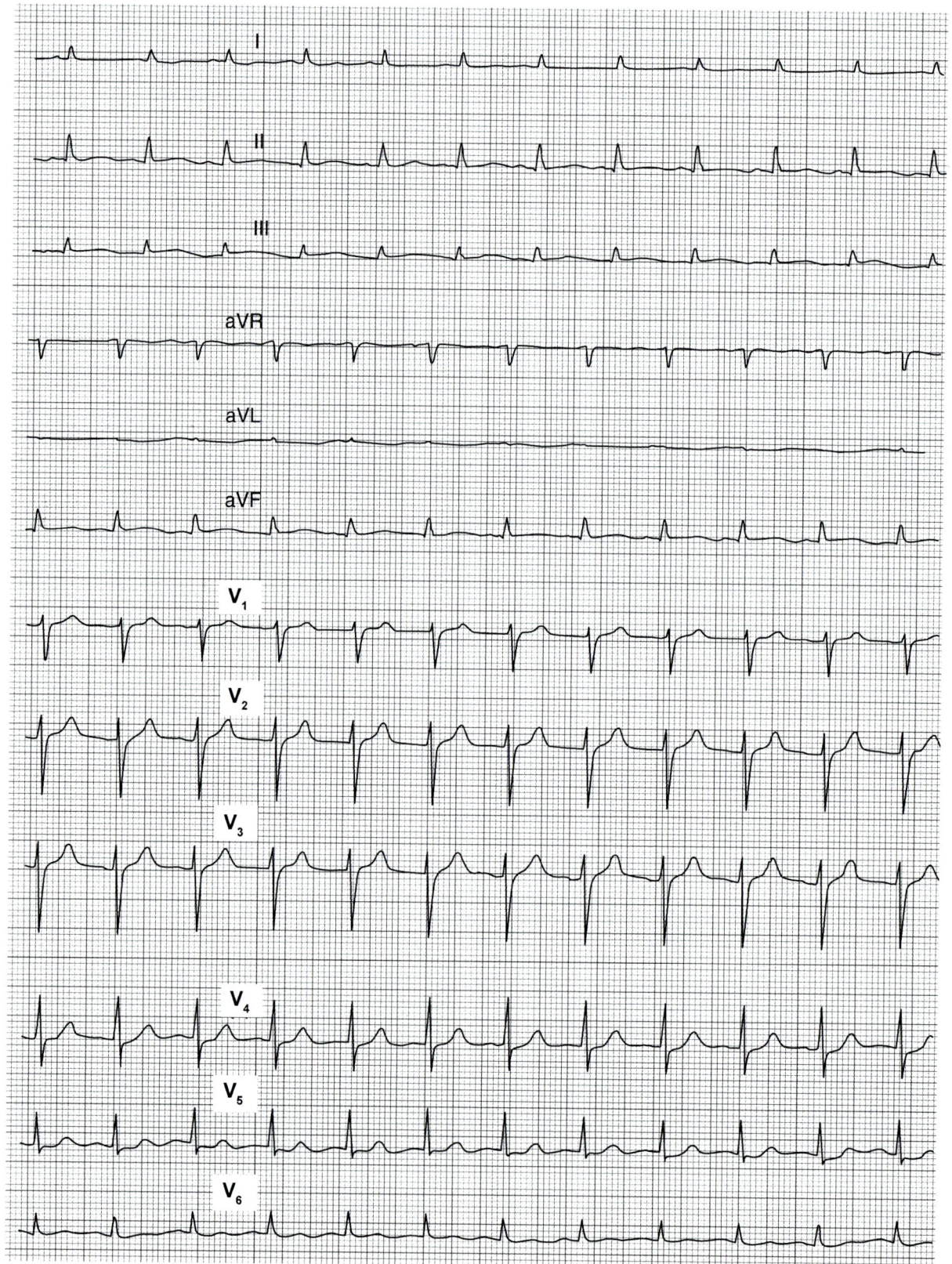

ECG NO. 63

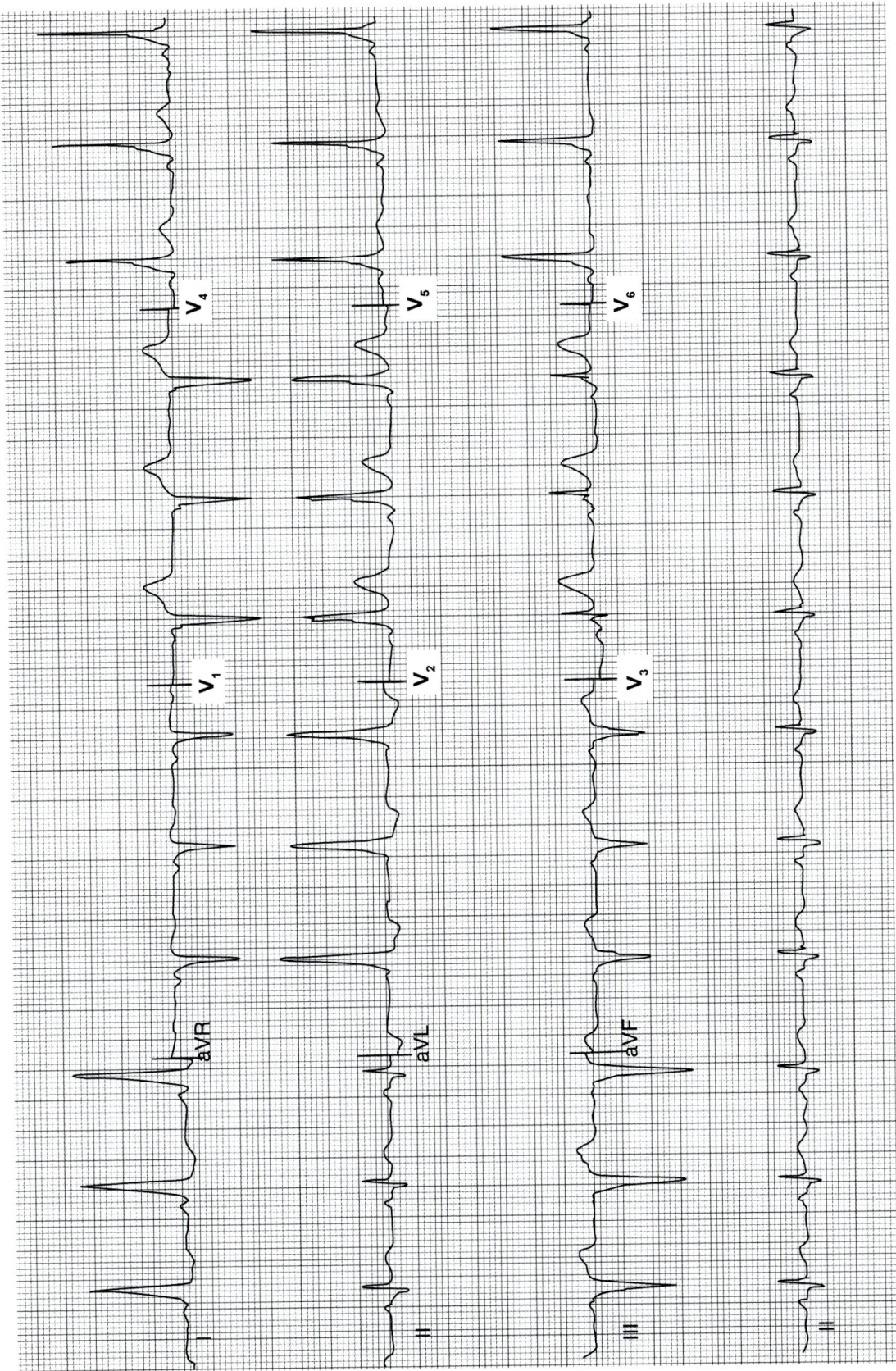

aVR

aVL

aVF

V₁

V₂

V₃

V₄

V₅

V₆

I

II

III

II

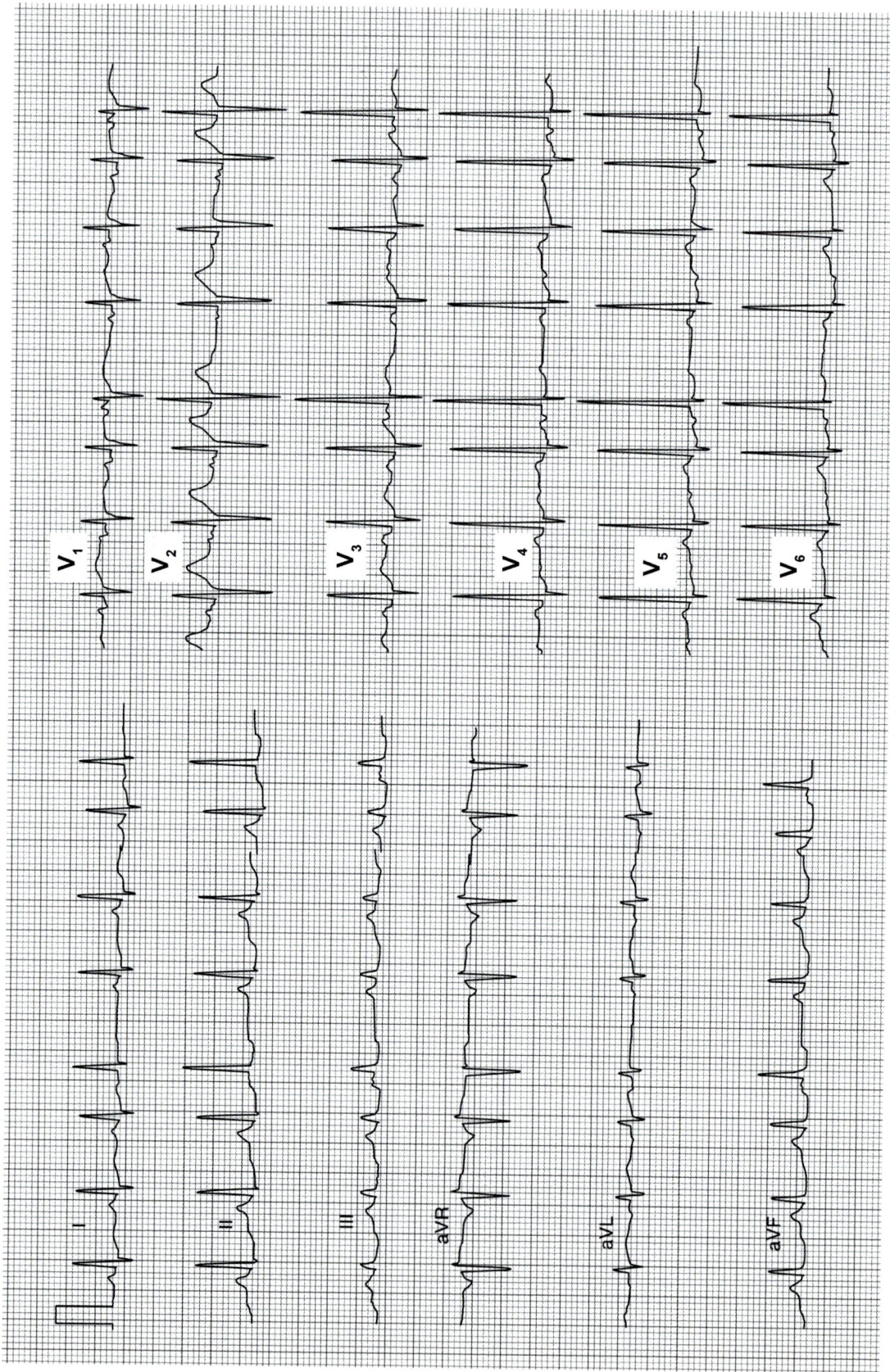

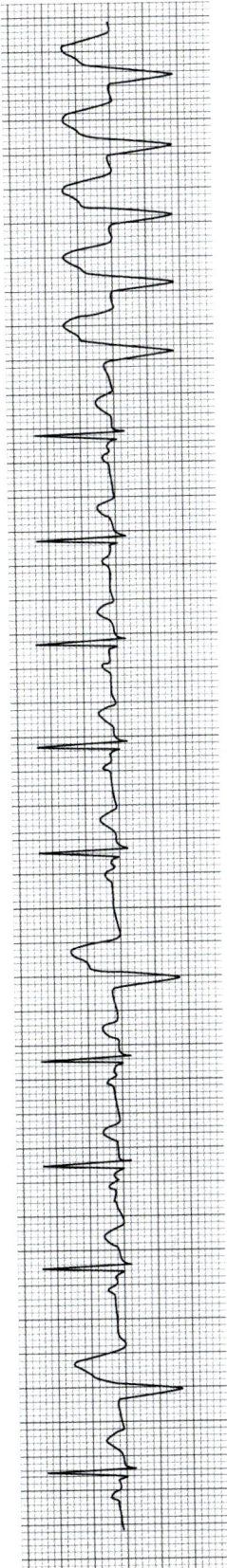

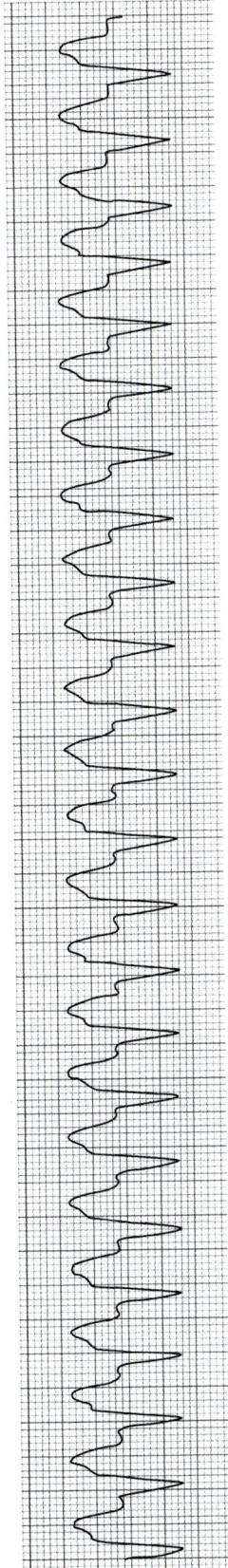

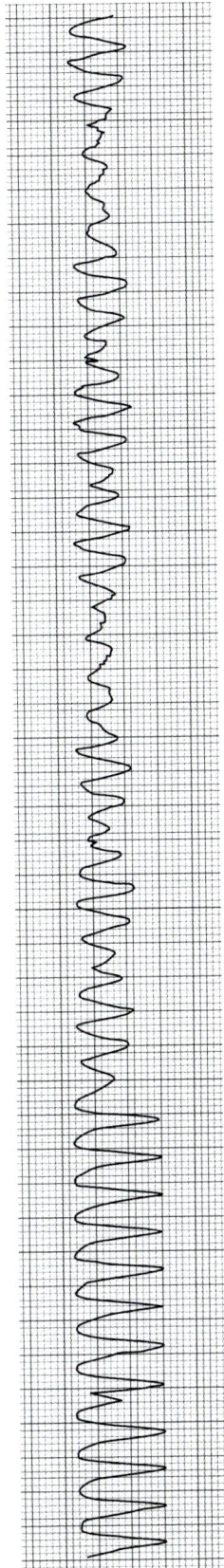

ECG NO. 65

ECG NO. 66

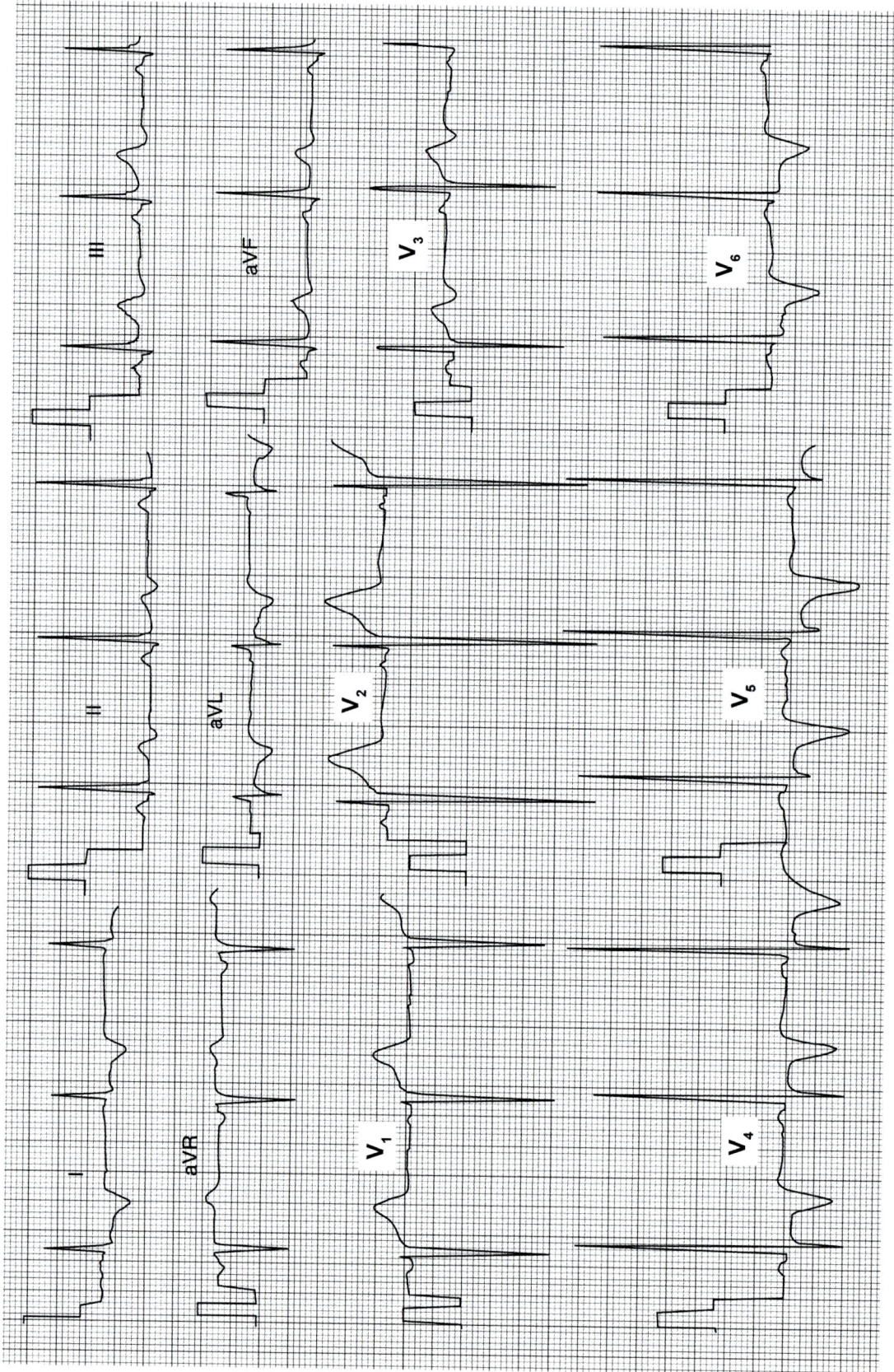

ECG NO. 67

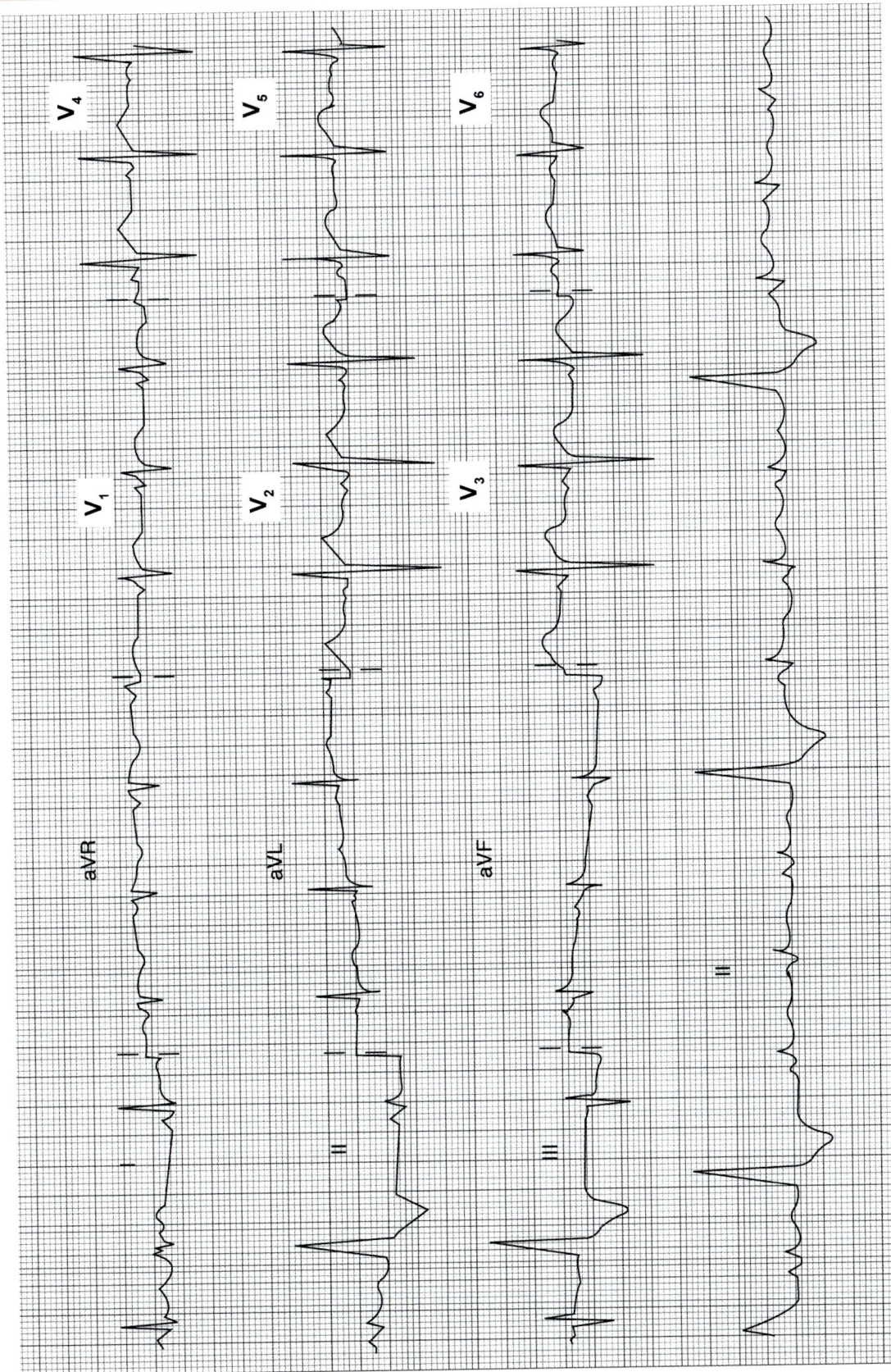

V₁

V₂

V₃

V₄

V₅

V₆

aVR

aVL

aVF

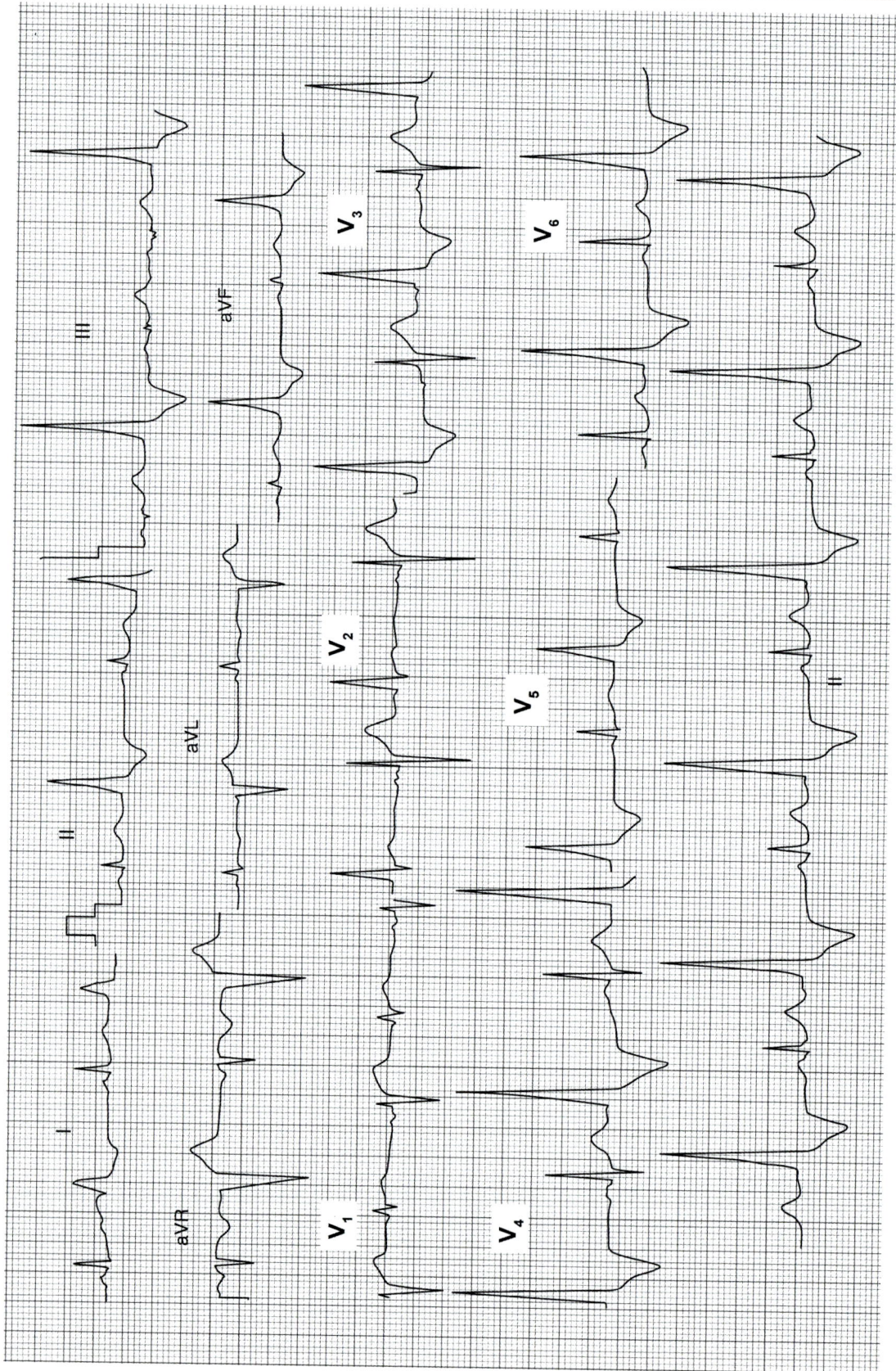

ECG NO. 68

ECG NO. 69

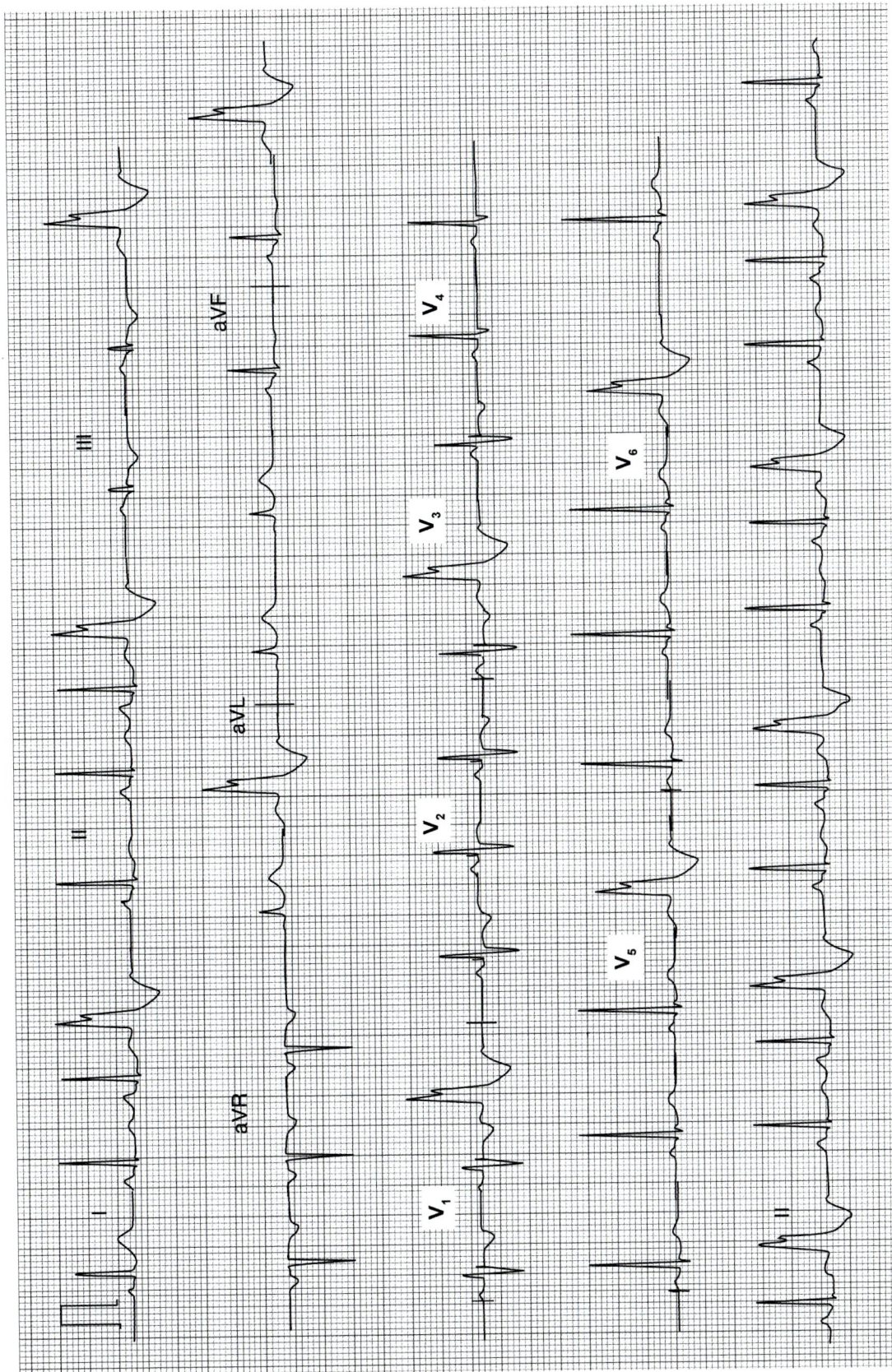

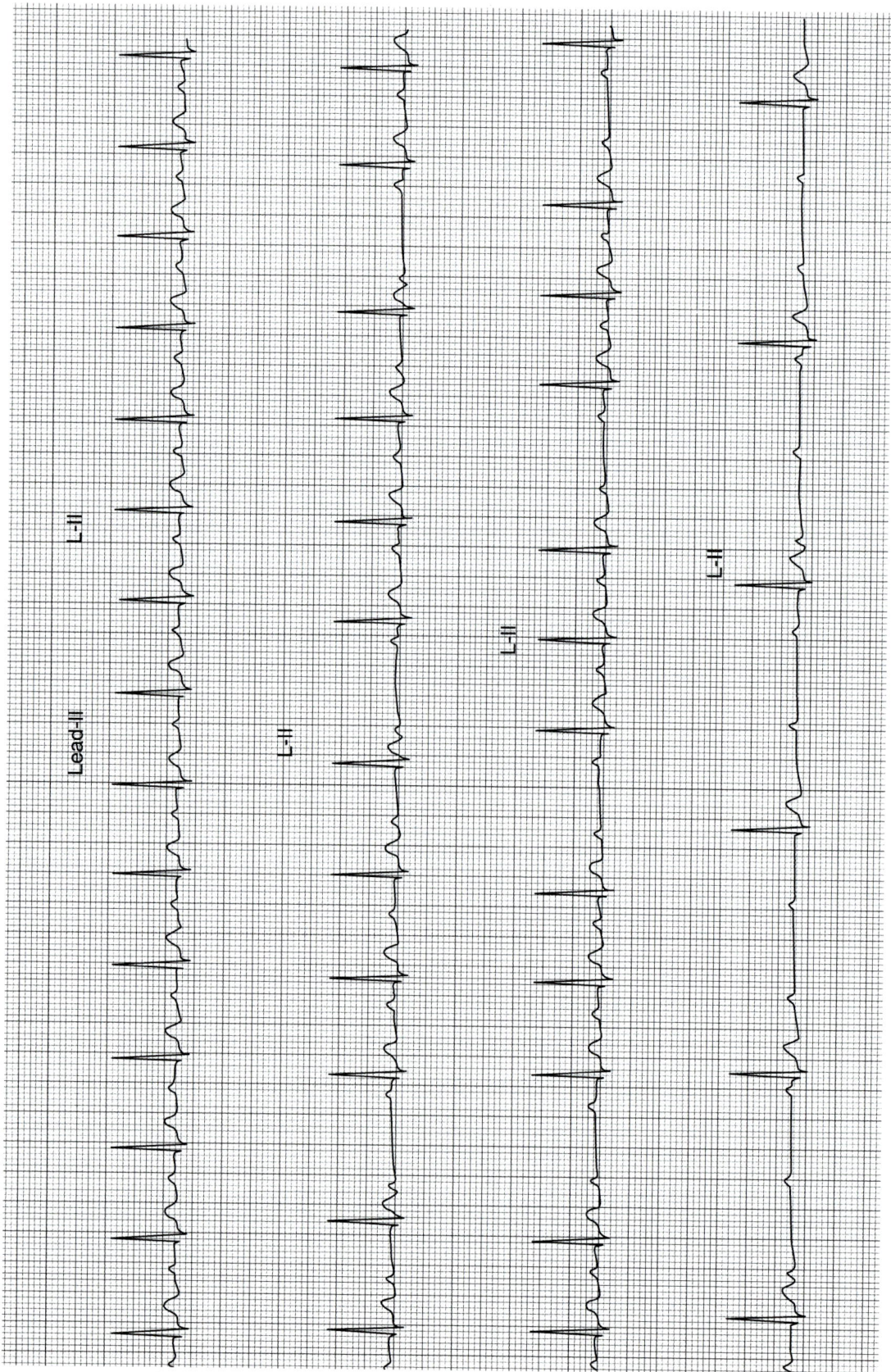

ECG NO. 70

Lead-II

L-II

L-II

L-II

L-II

ECG NO. 71

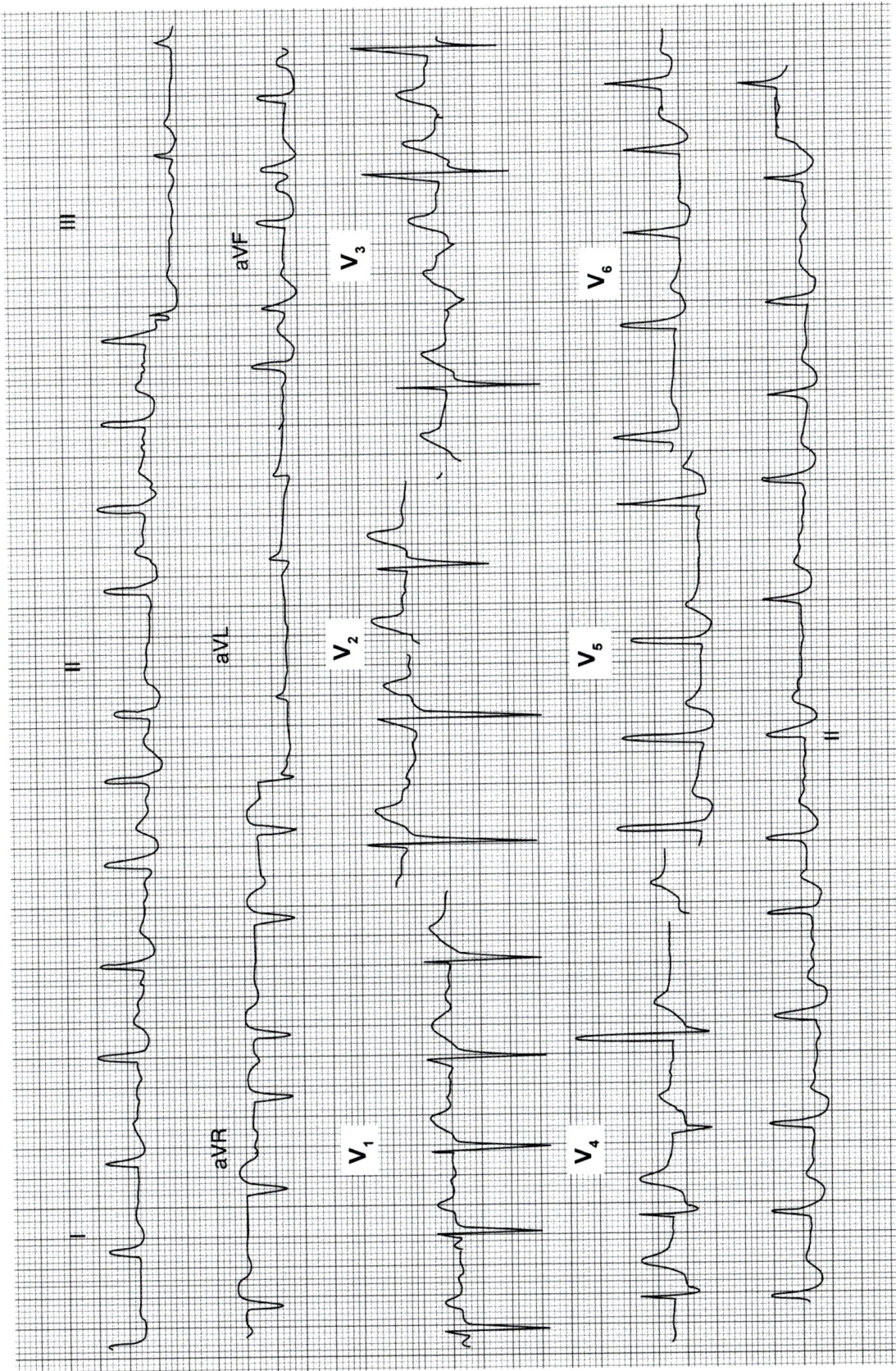

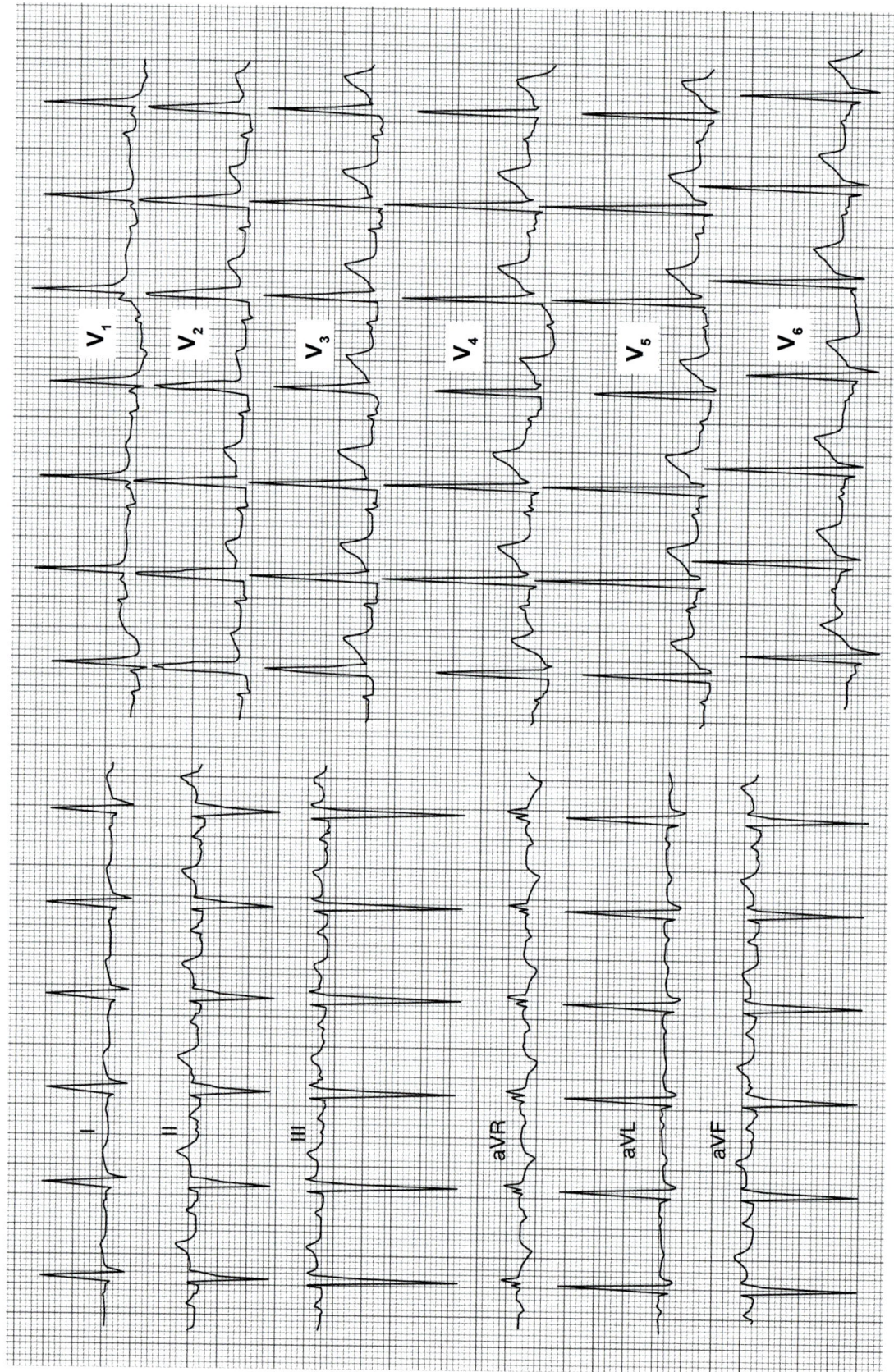

ECG NO. 72

I

II

III

aVR

aVL

aVF

V₁

V₂

V₃

V₄

V₅

V₆

ECG NO. 73

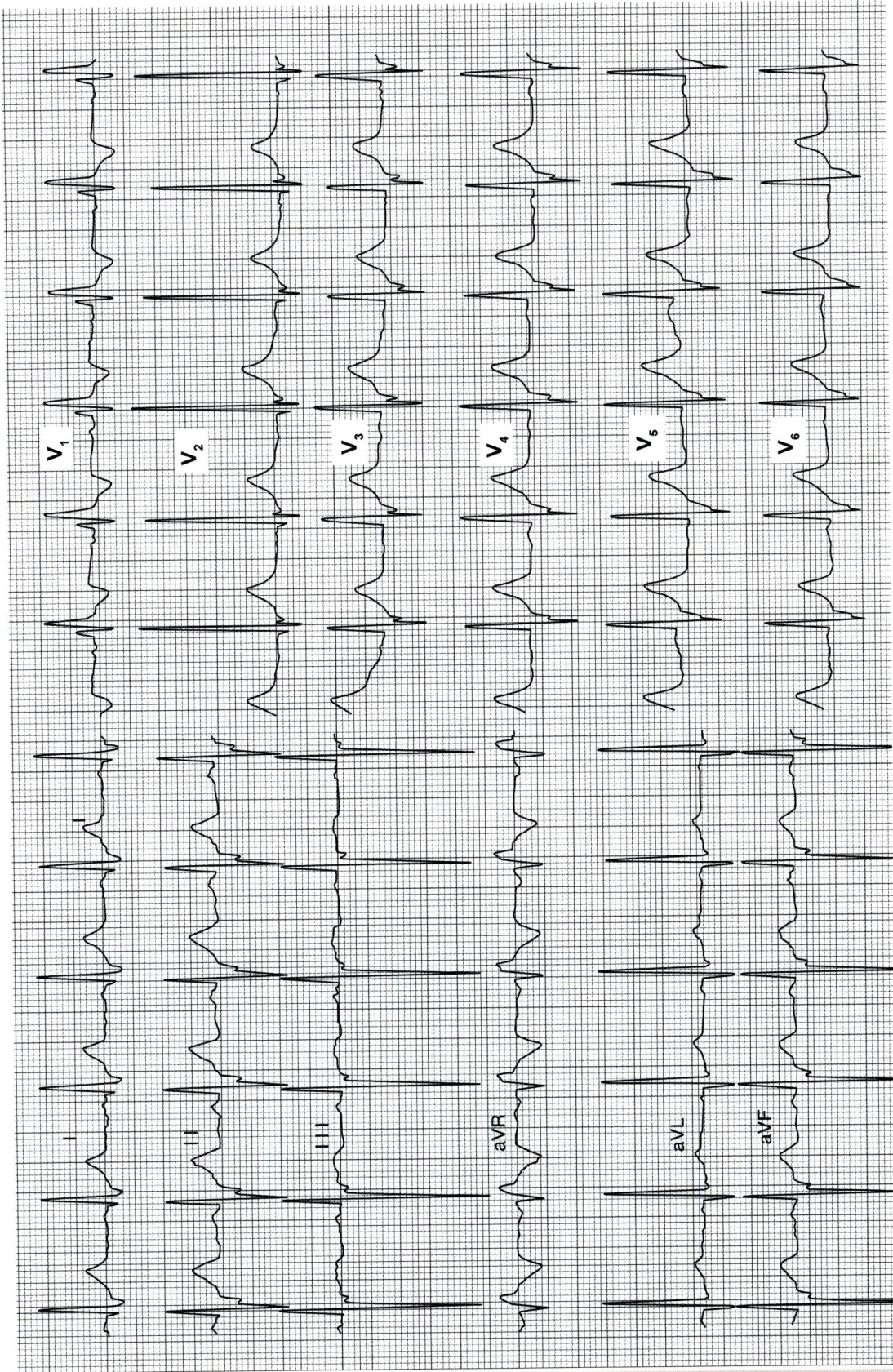

V₁

V₂

V₃

V₄

V₅

V₆

I

II

III

aVR

aVL

aVF

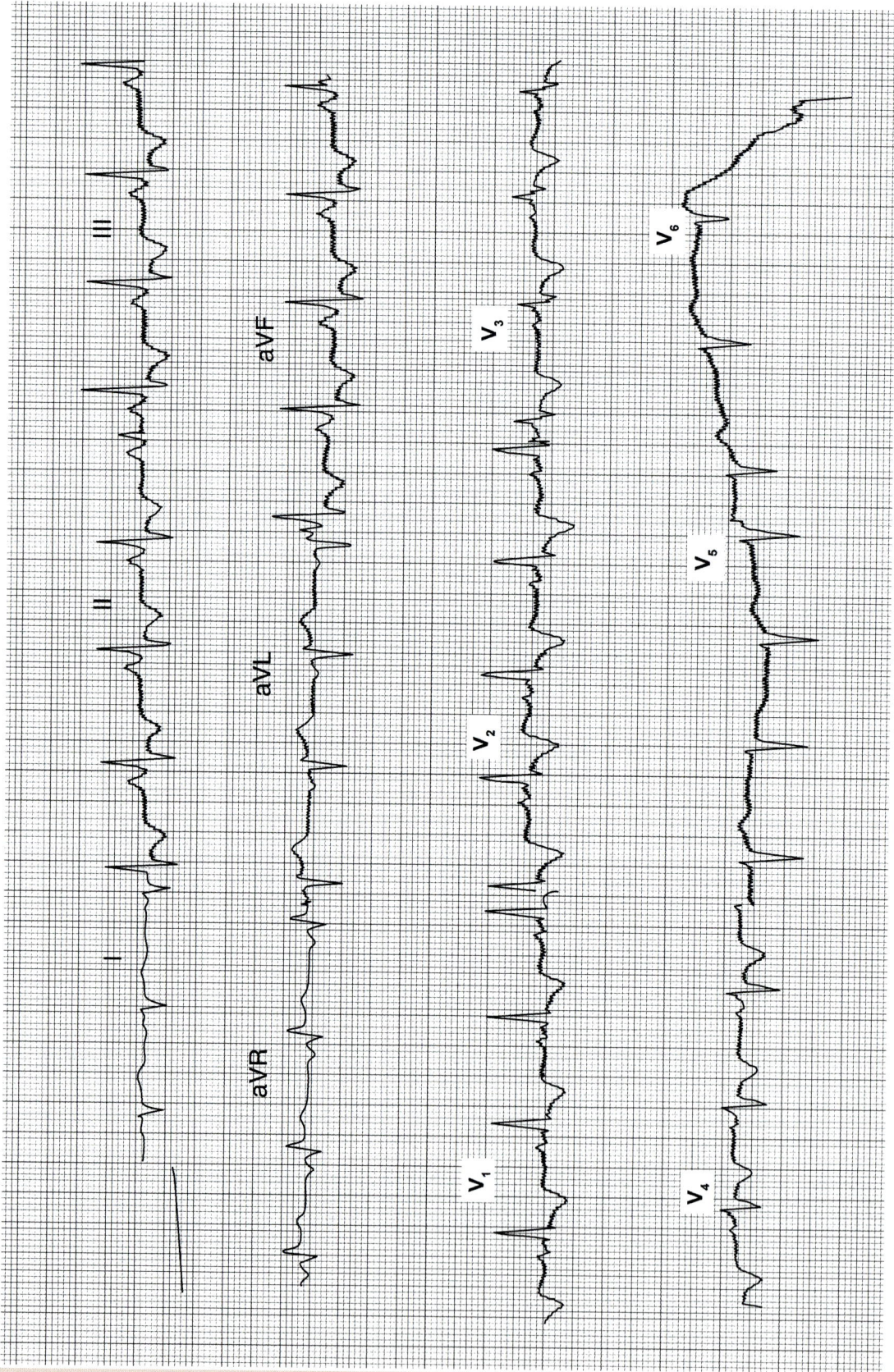

ECG NO. 74

I

II

III

aVR

aVL

aVF

V₁

V₂

V₃

V₄

V₅

V₆

ECG NO. 75

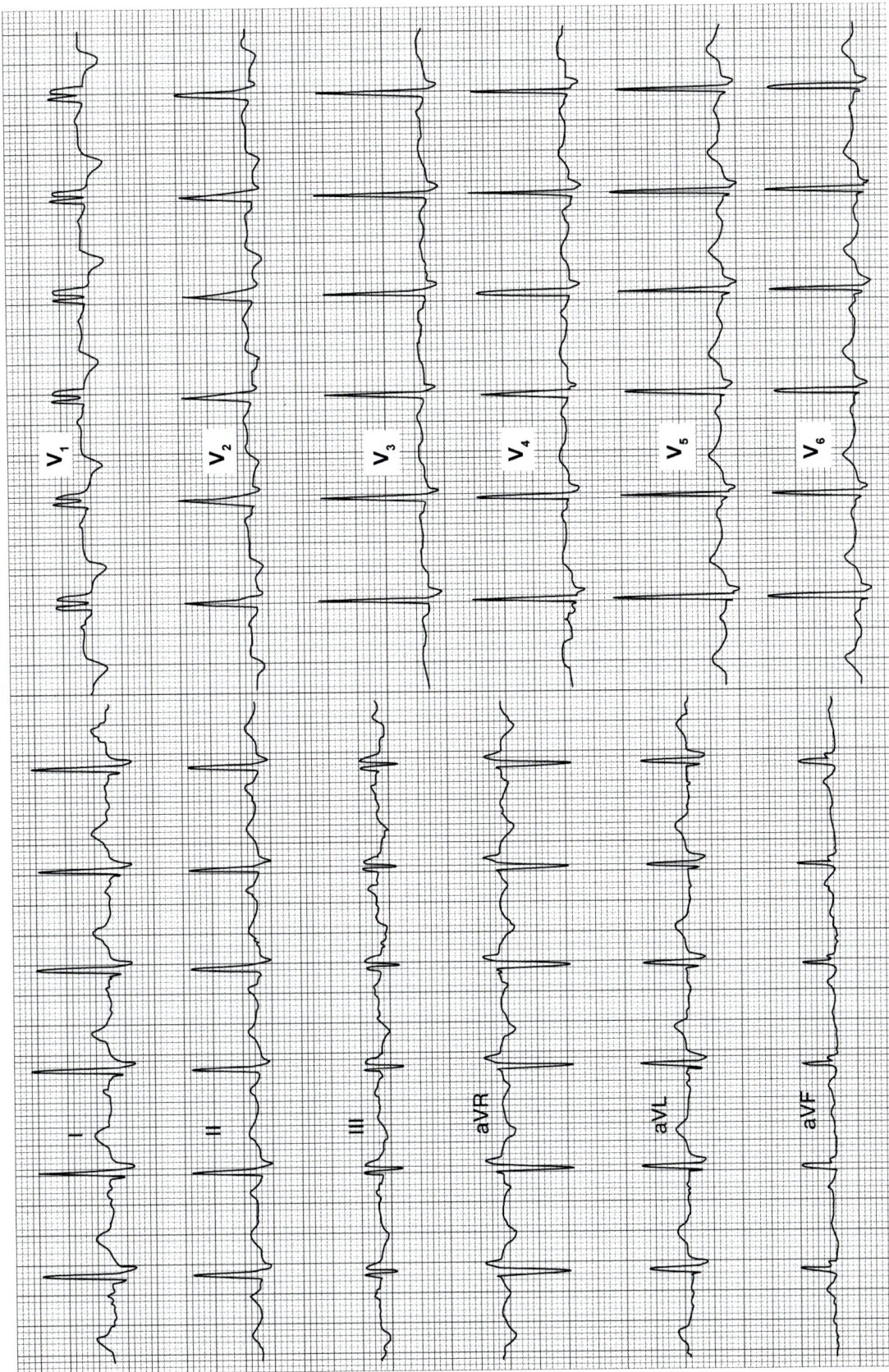

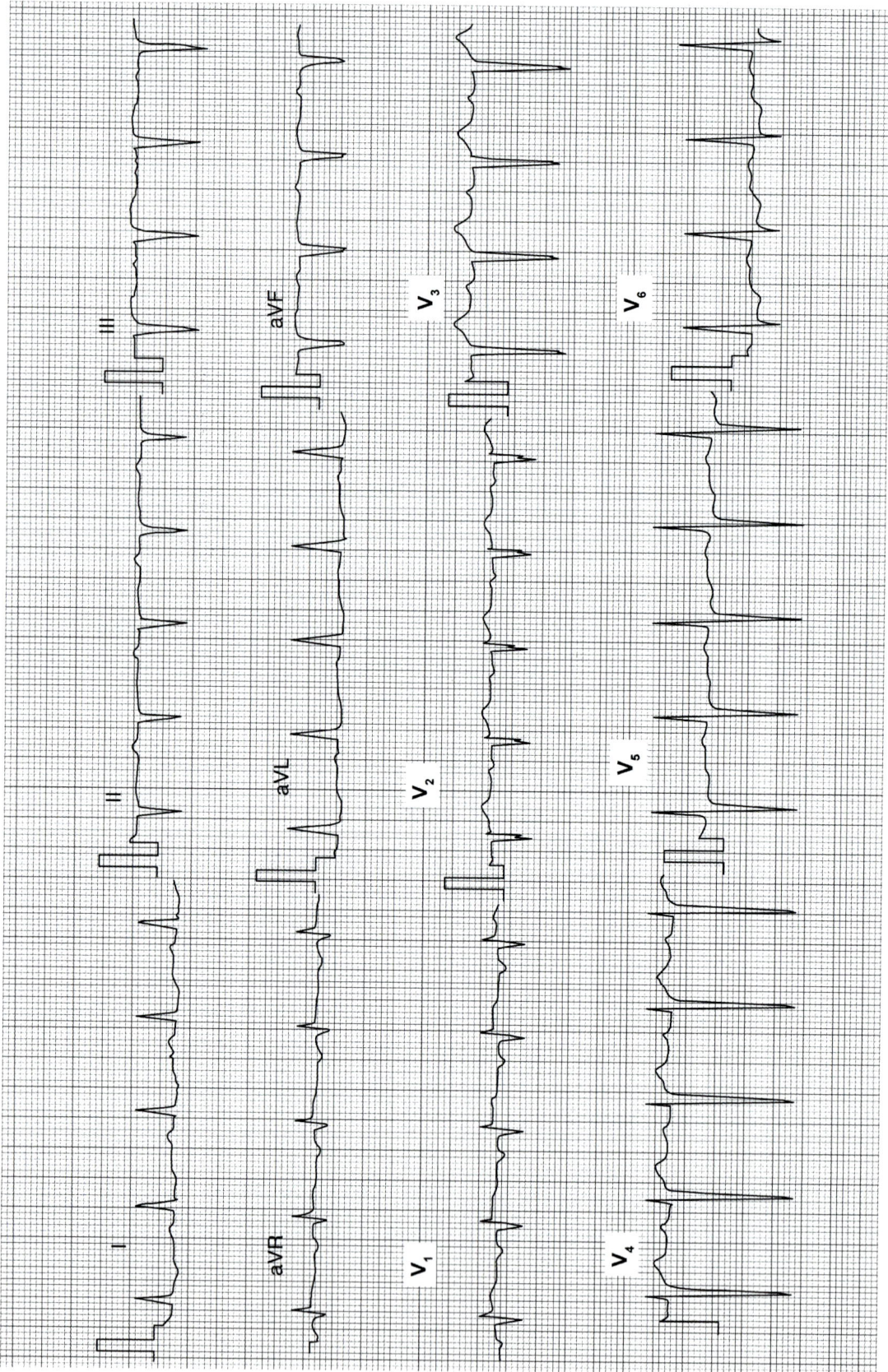

ECG NO. 76

ECG NO. 77

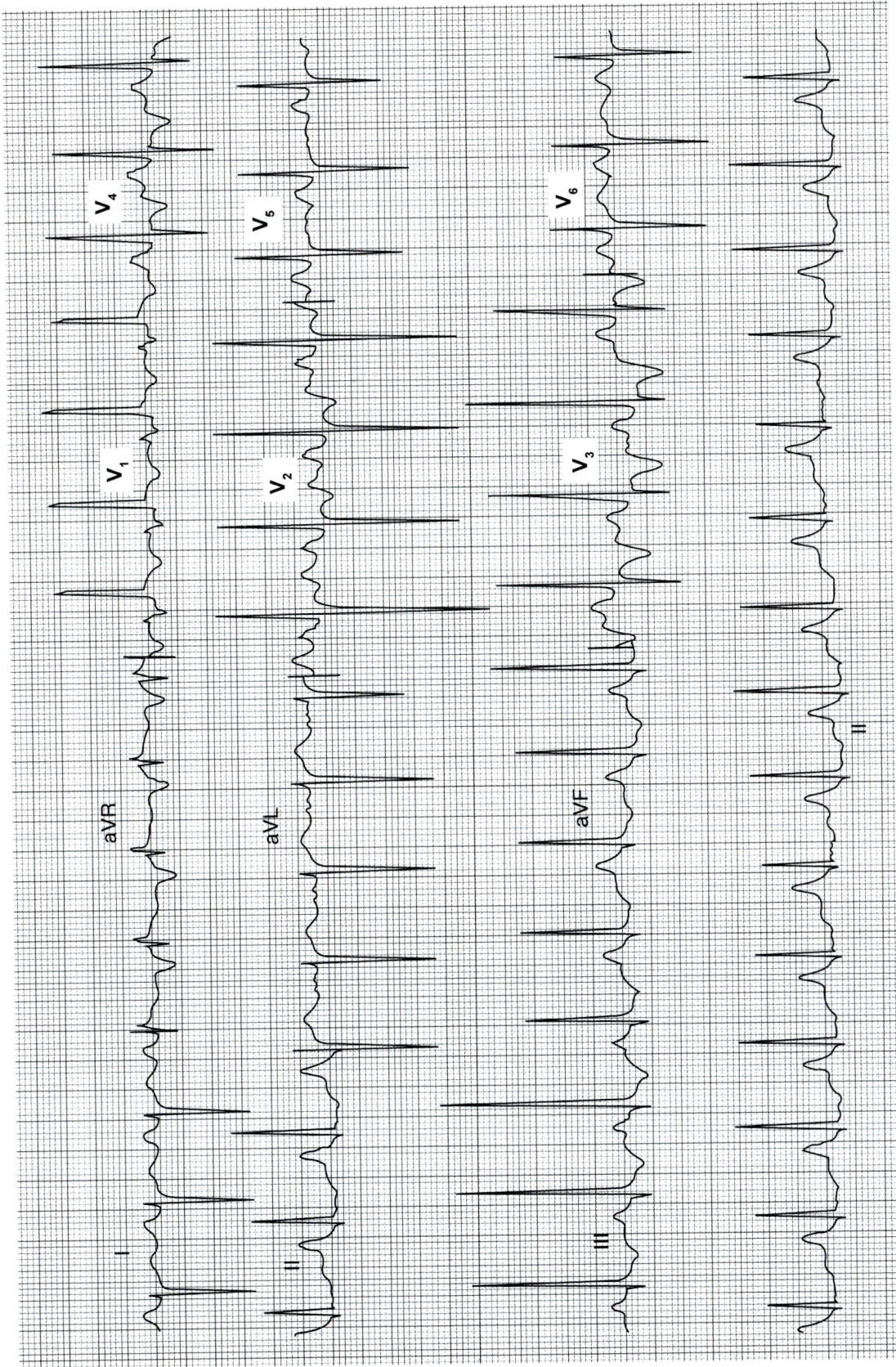

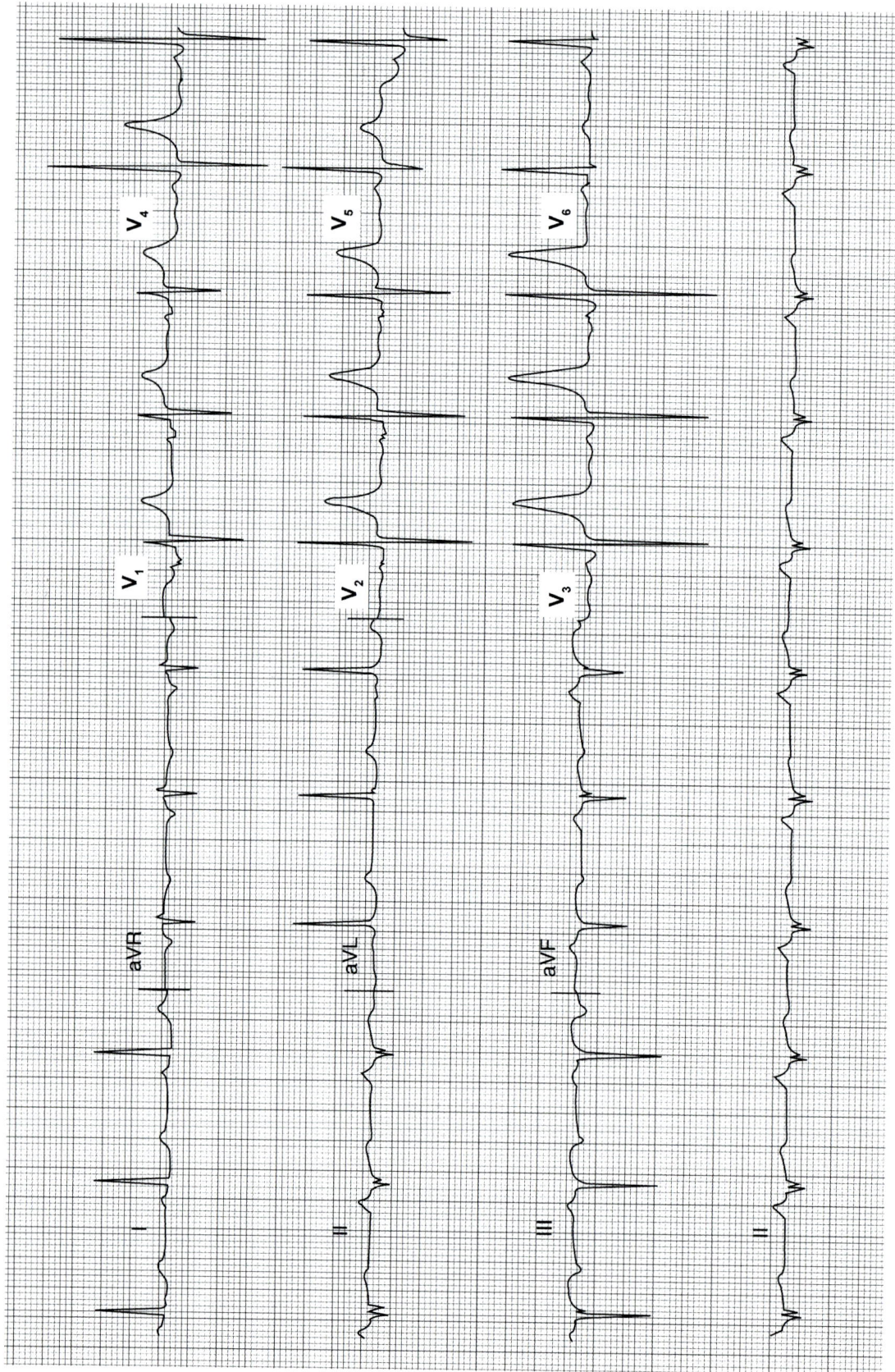

ECG NO. 79

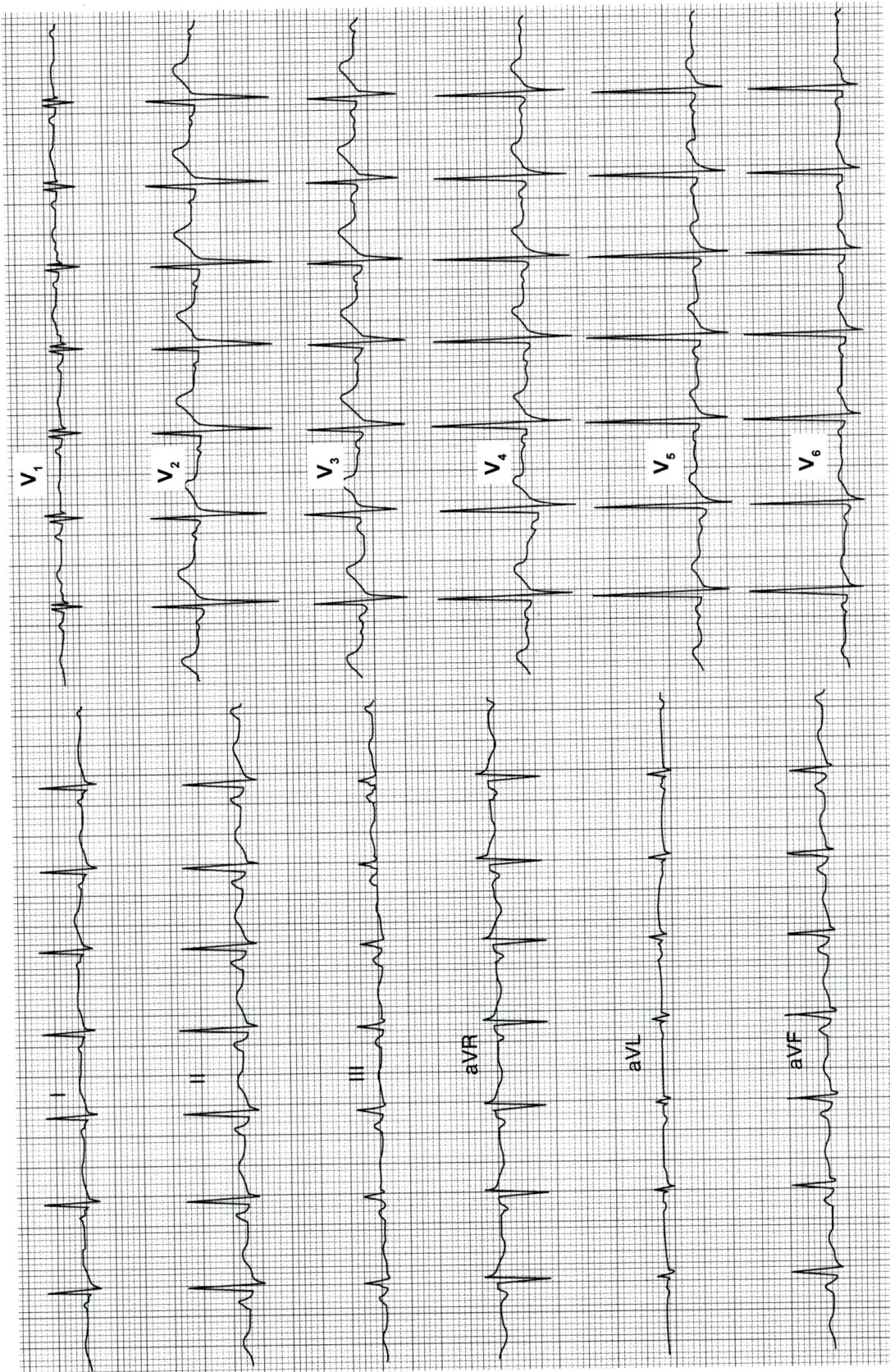

V₁ V₂ V₃ V₄ V₅ V₆ I II III aVR aVL aVF

ECG NO. 80

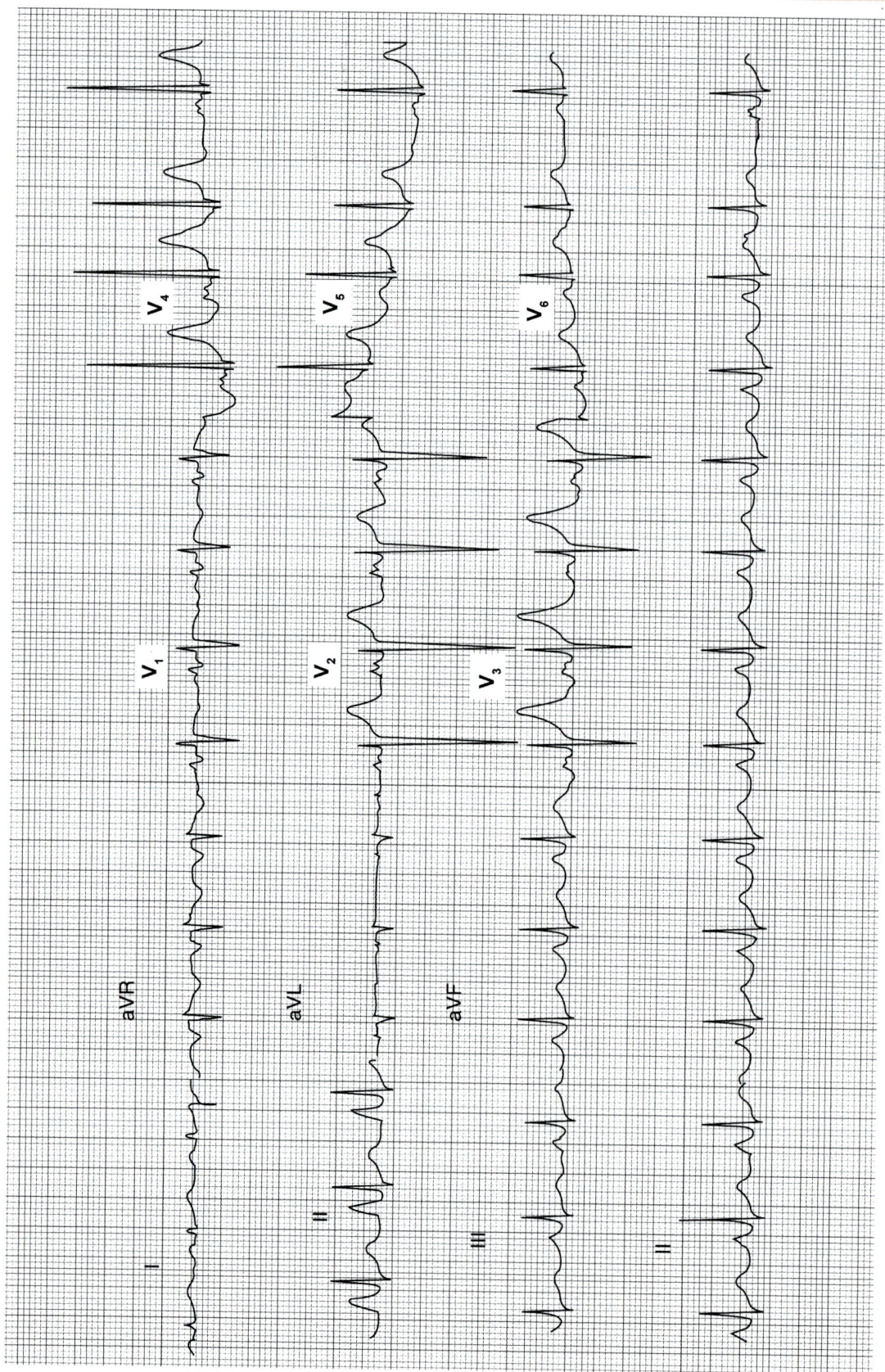

ECG NO. 81

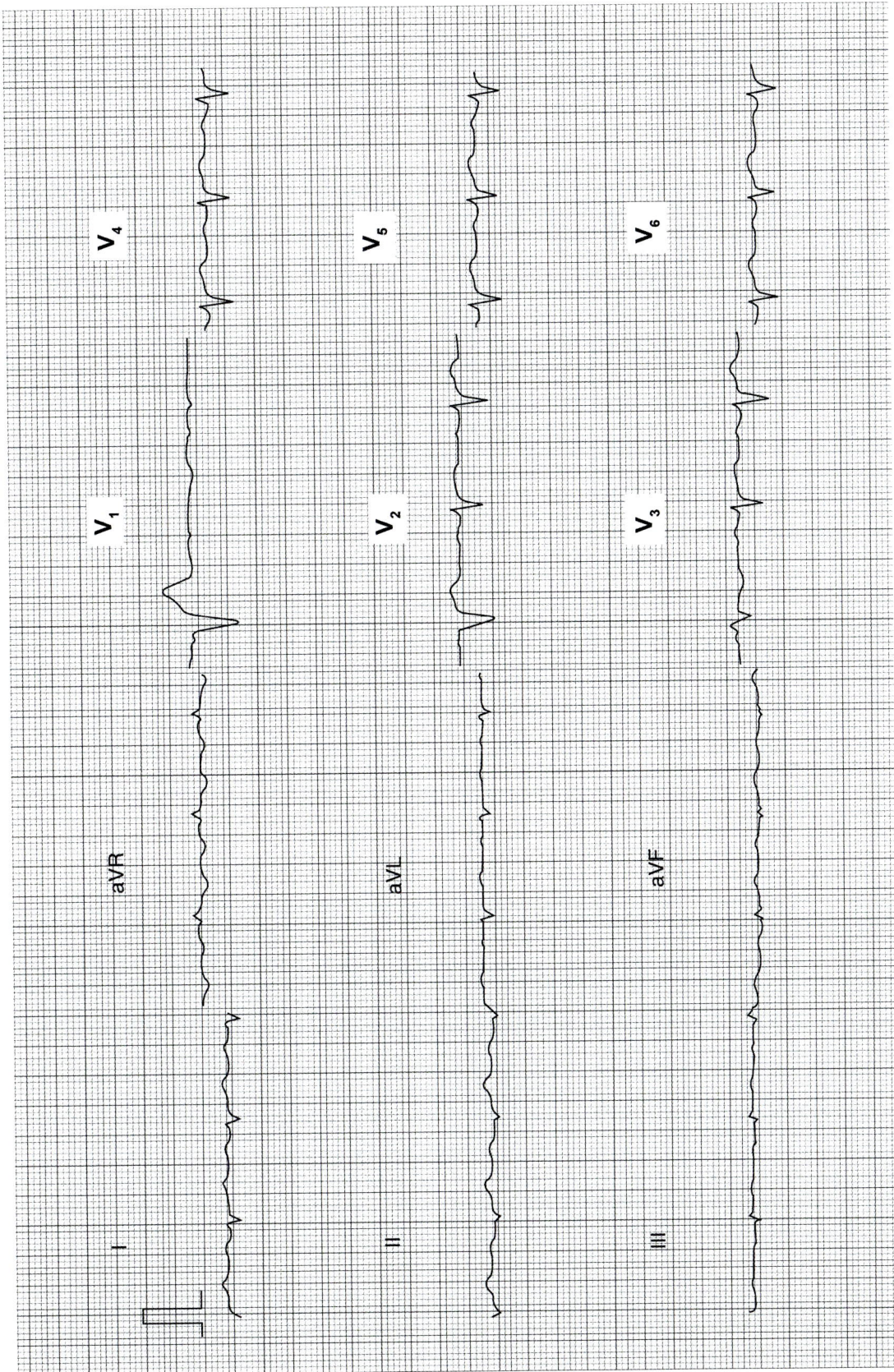

ECG NO. 82

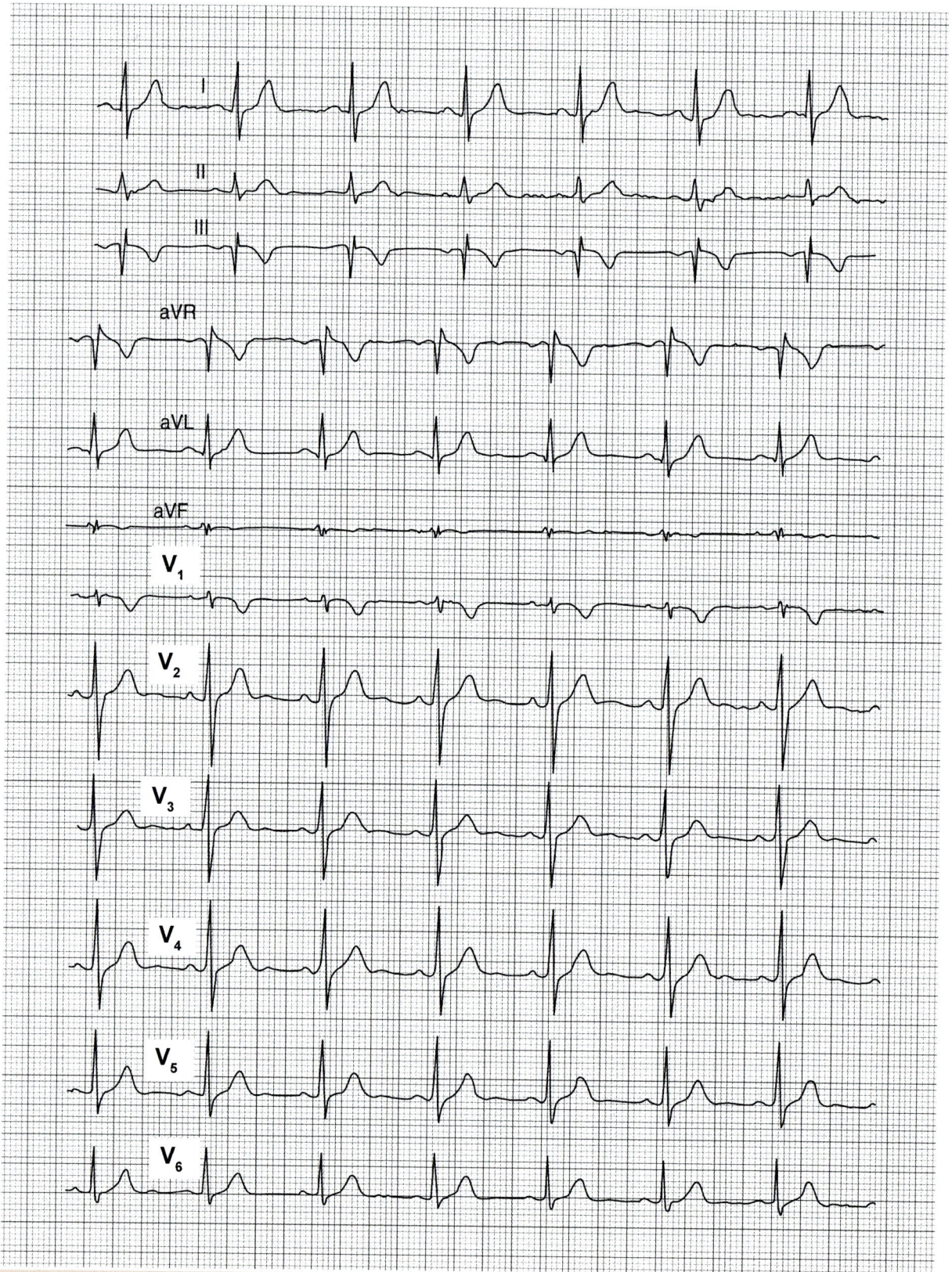

ECG NO. 83

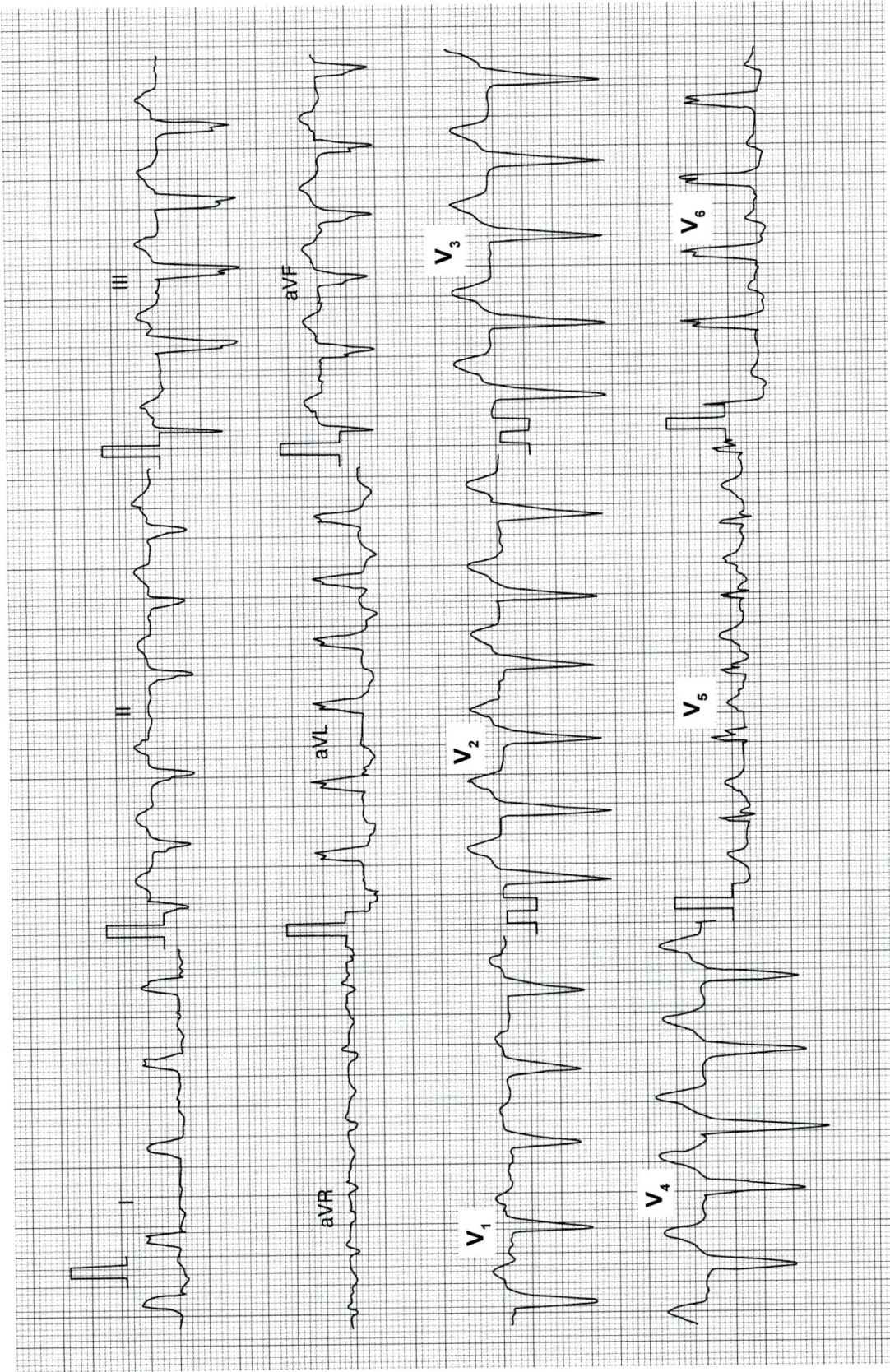

ECG NO. 84

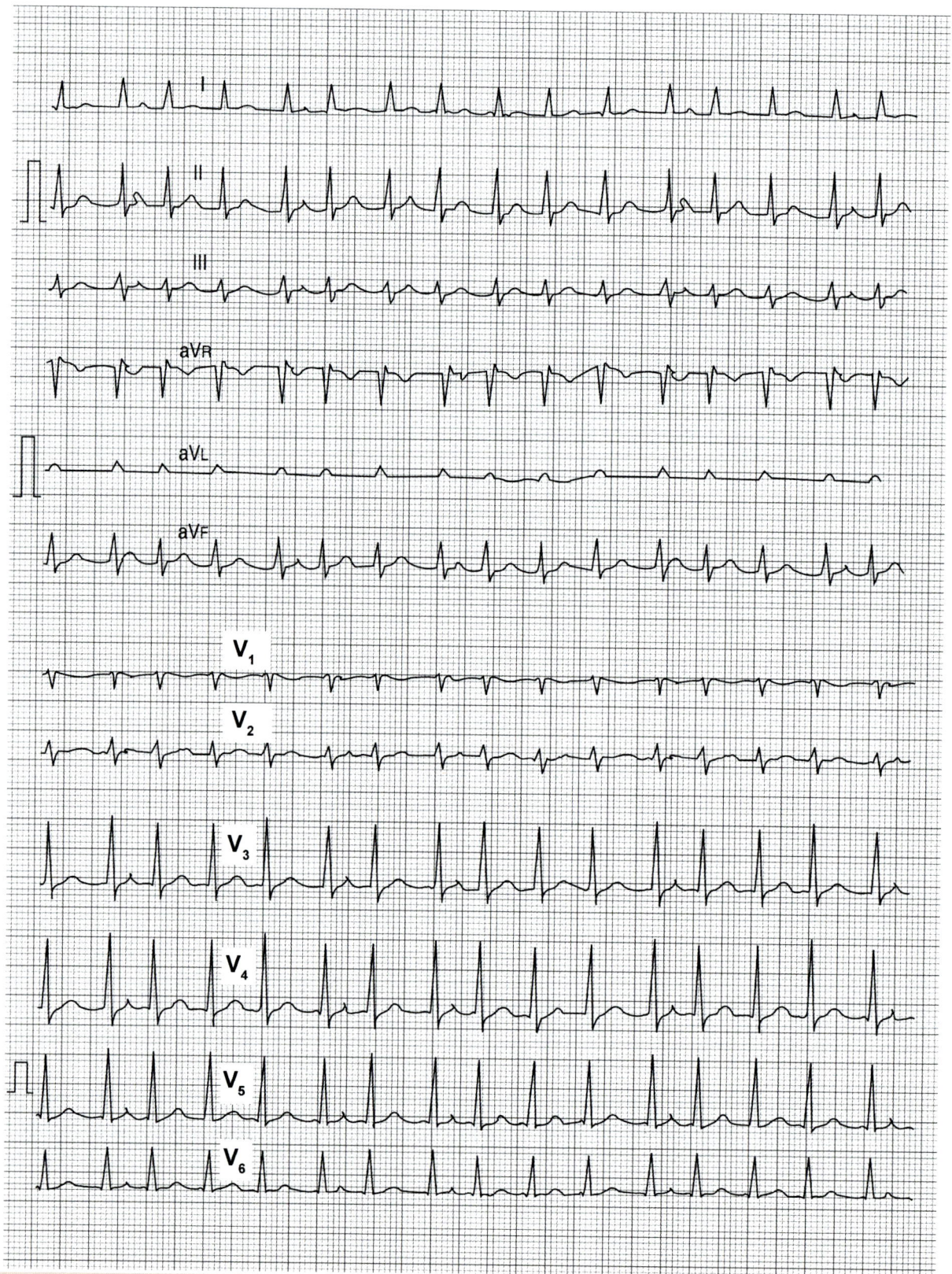

ECG NO. 85

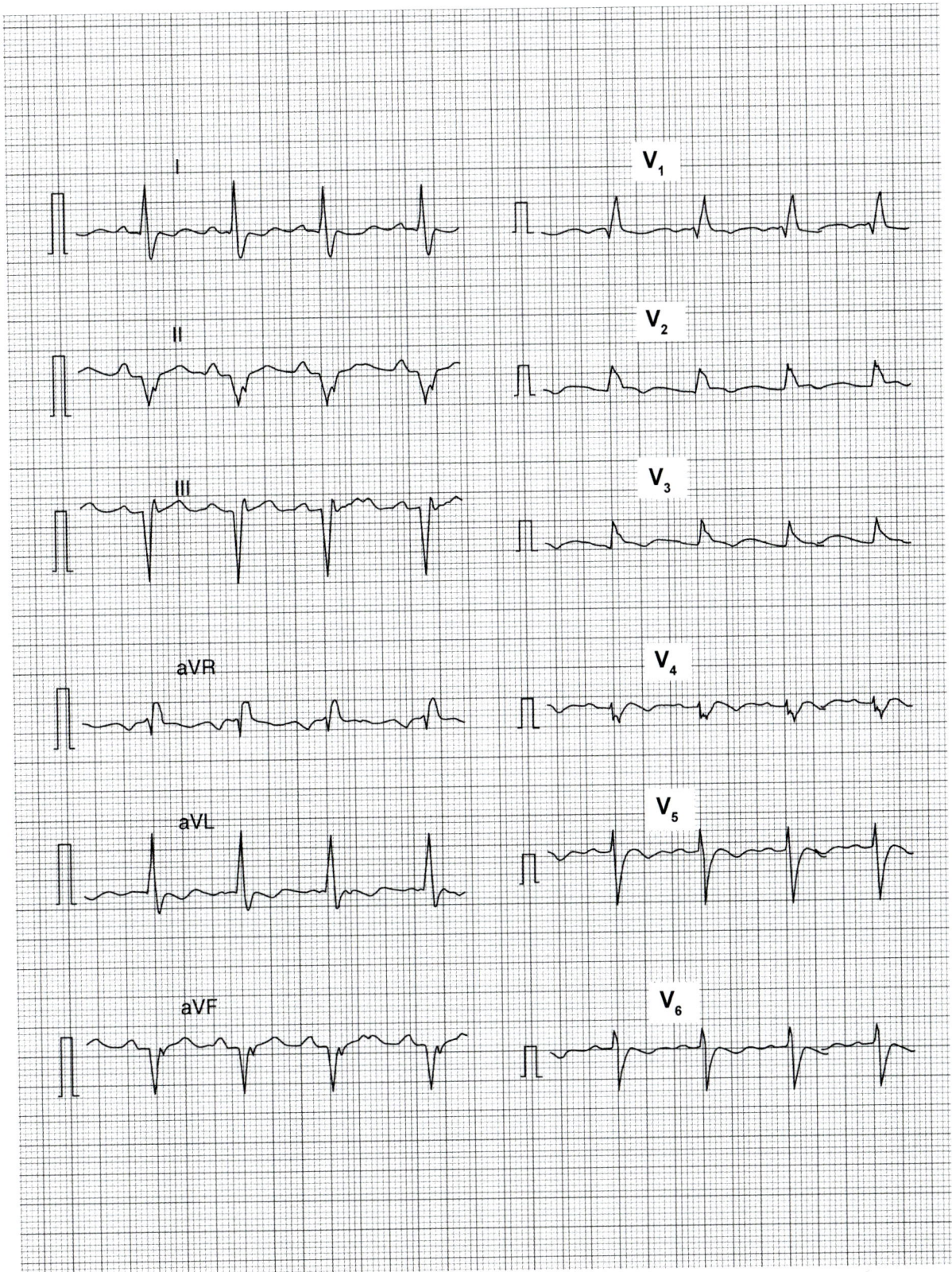

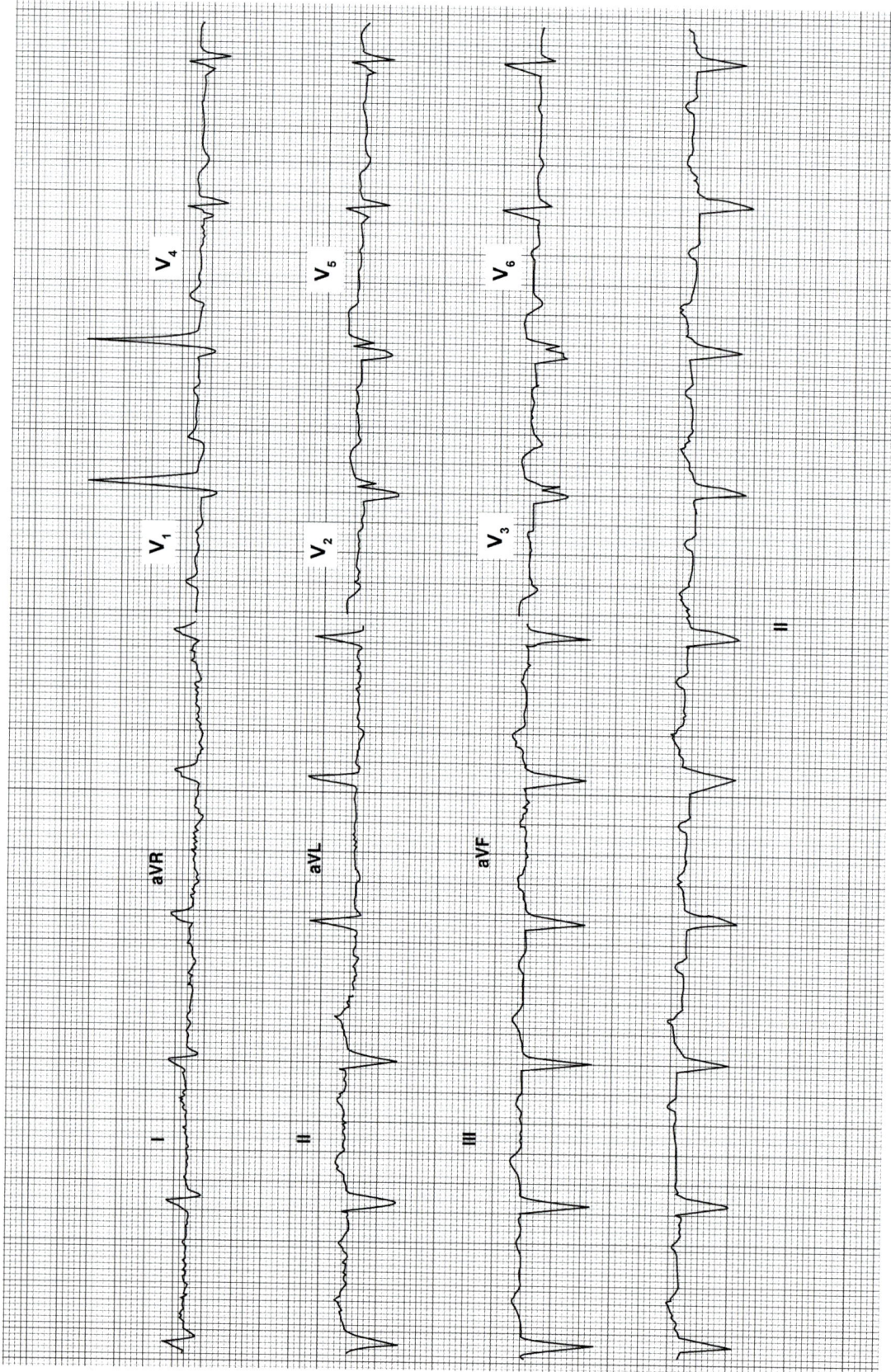

ECG NO. 87

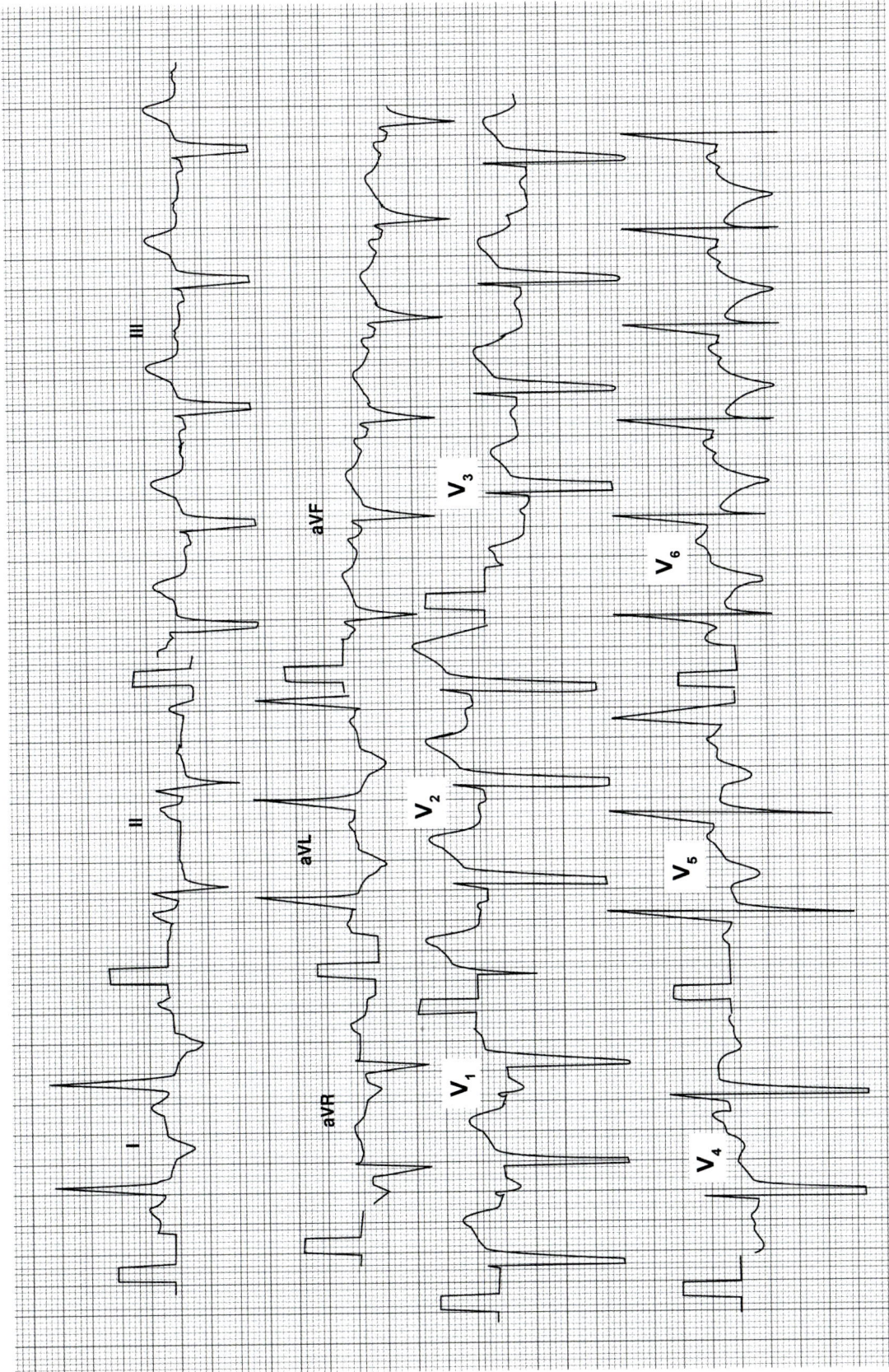

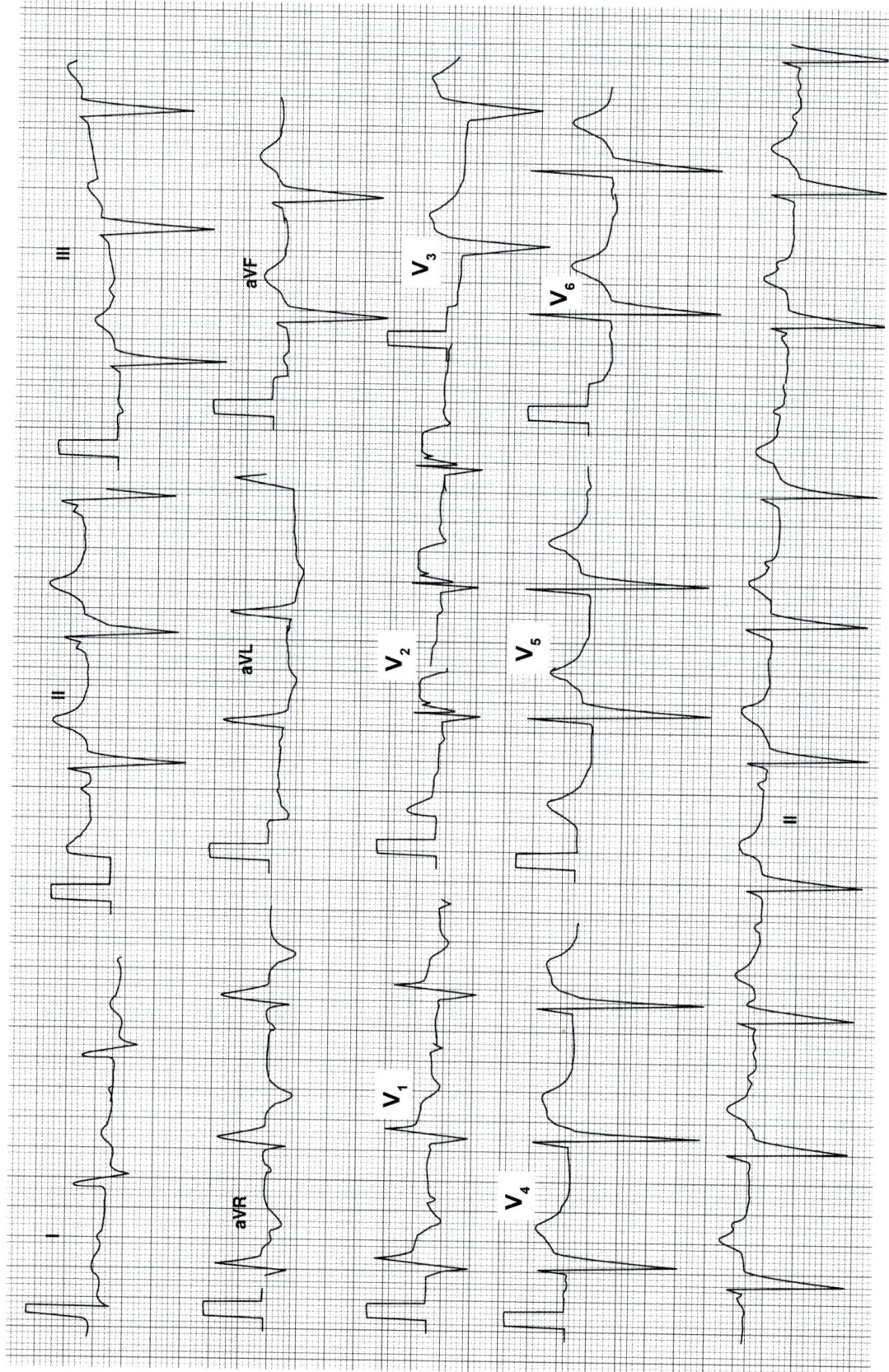

ECG NO. 89

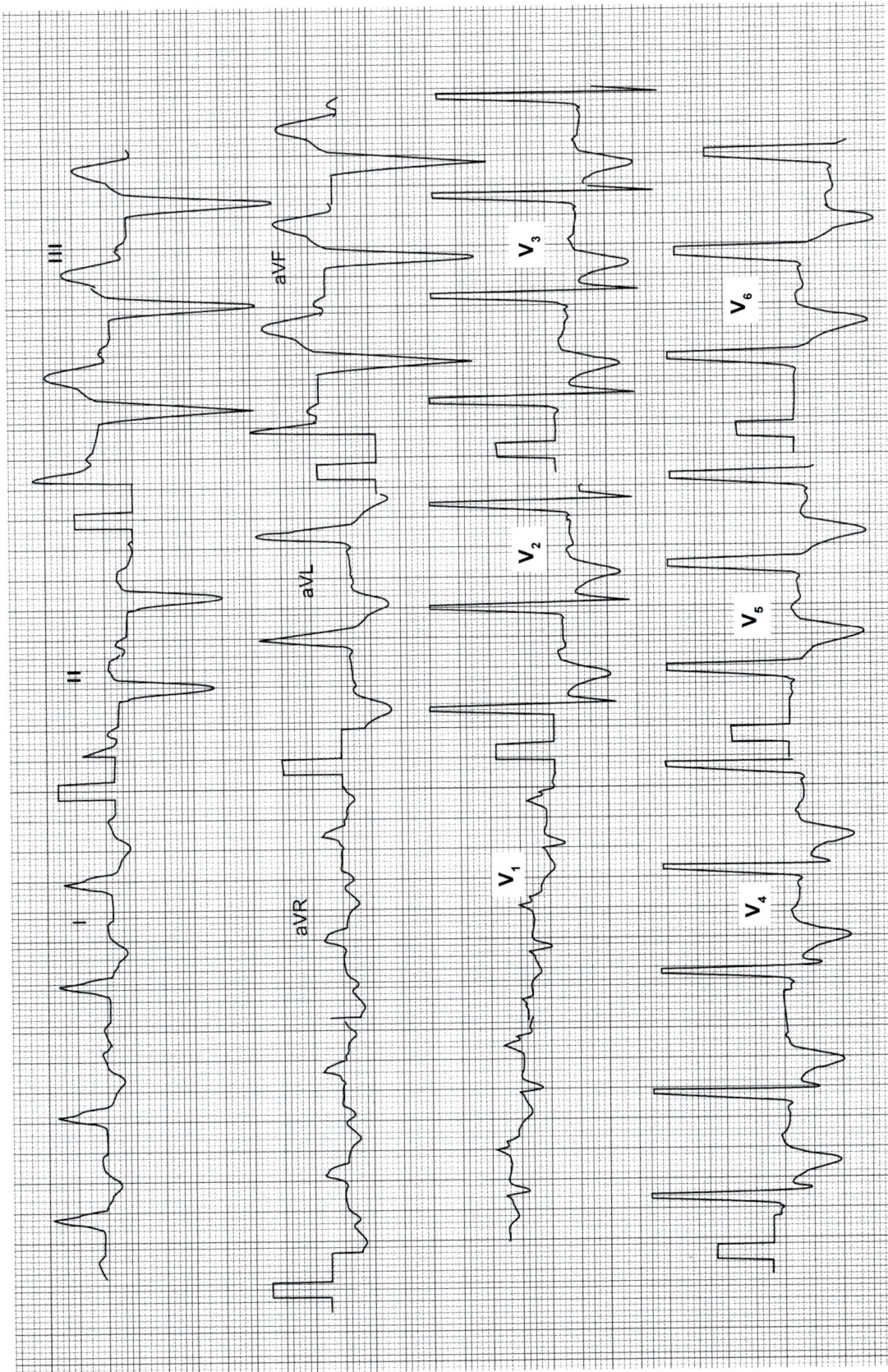

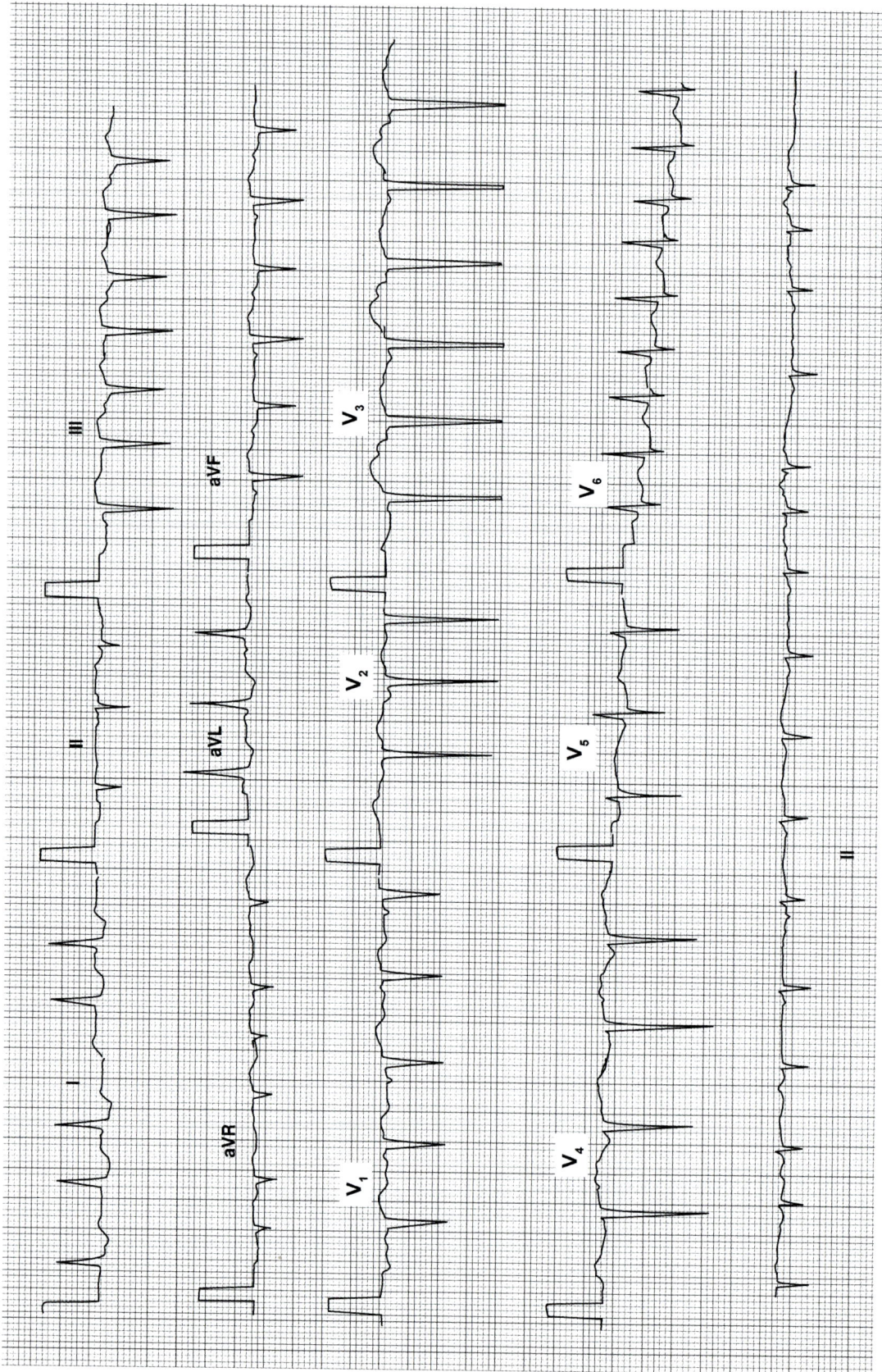

ECG NO. 90

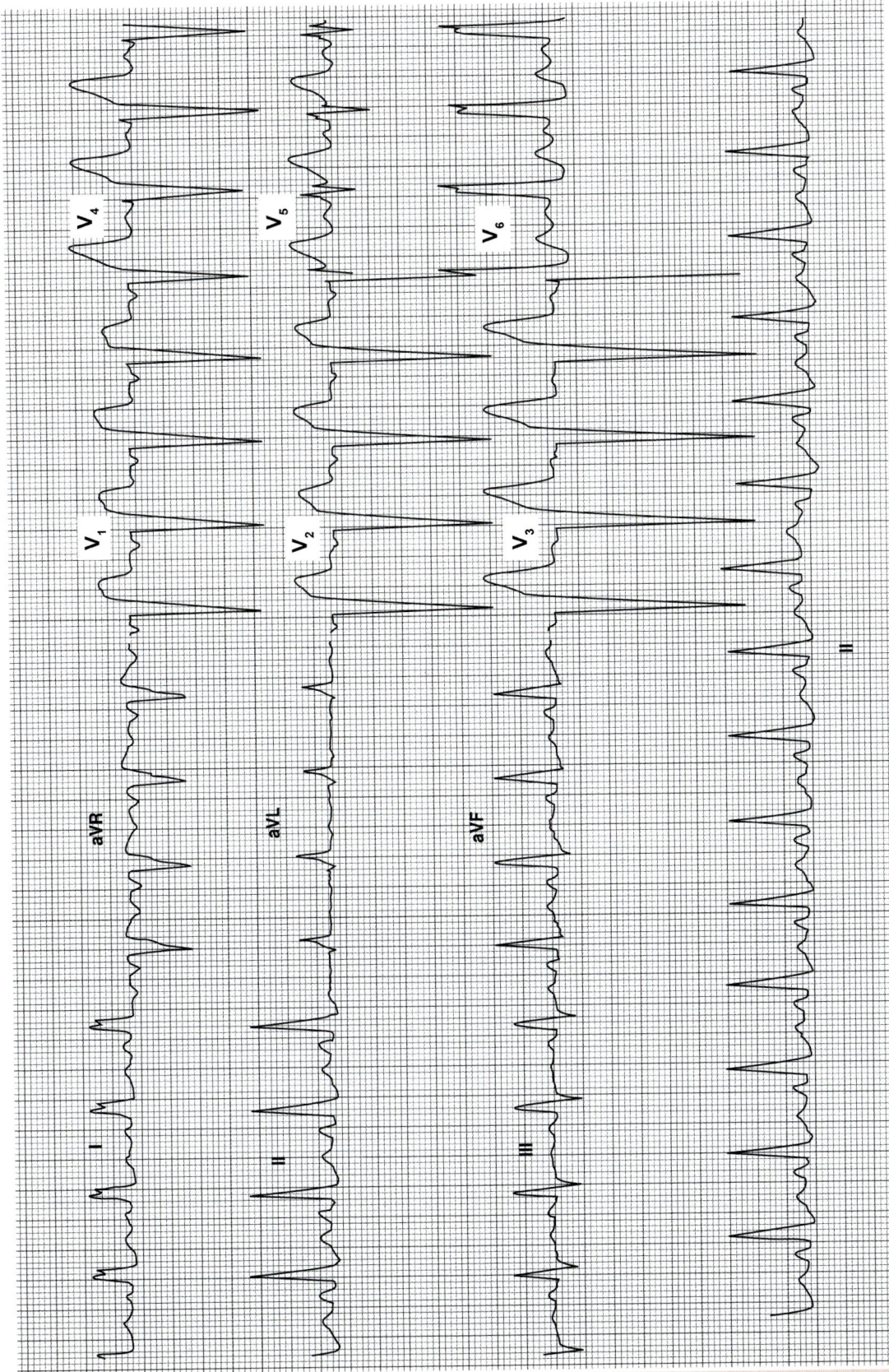

ECG NO. 91

aVR

aVL

aVF

I

II

III

V₁

V₂

V₃

V₄

V₅

V₆

II

ECG NO. 92

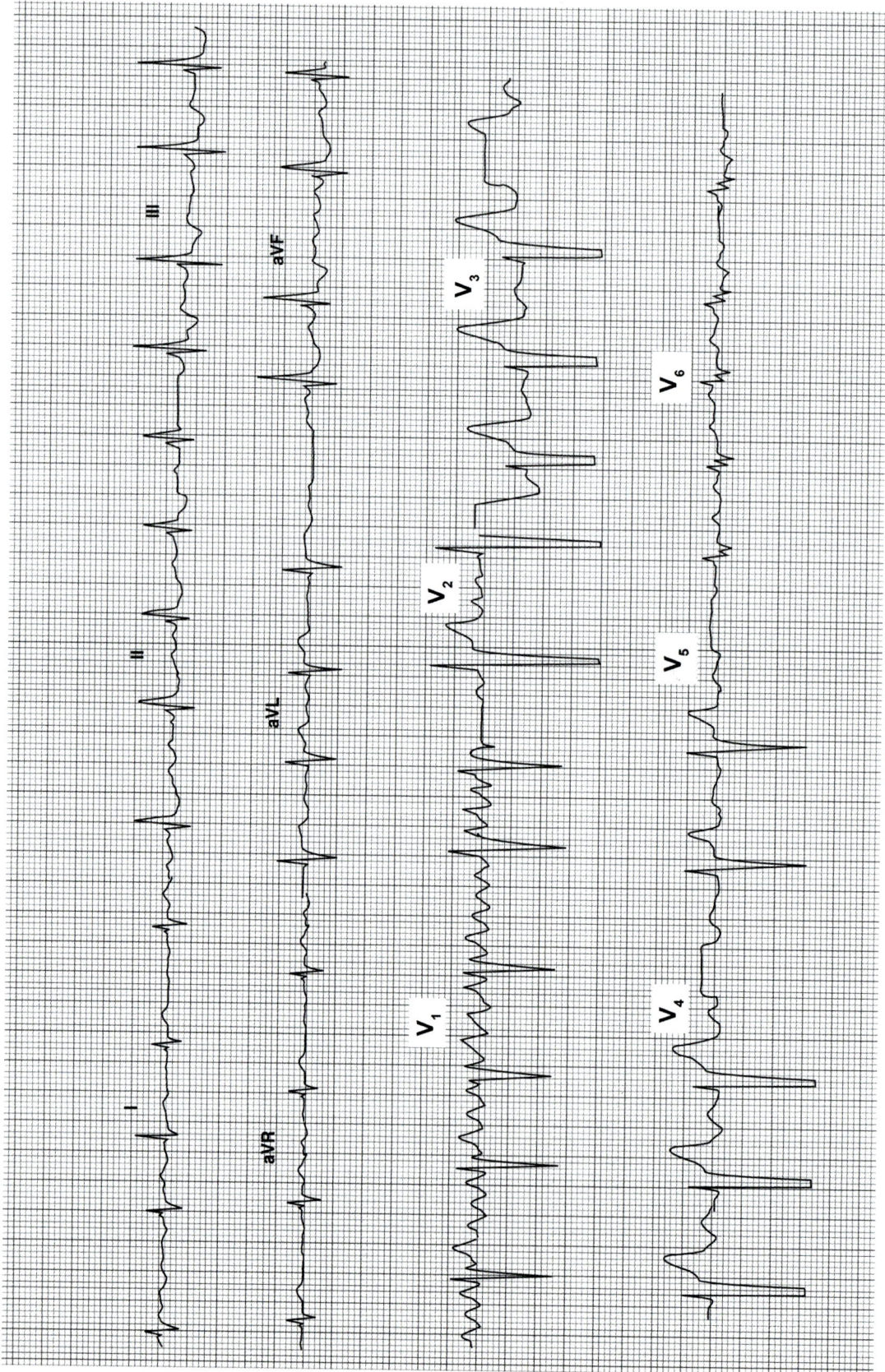

ECG NO. 93

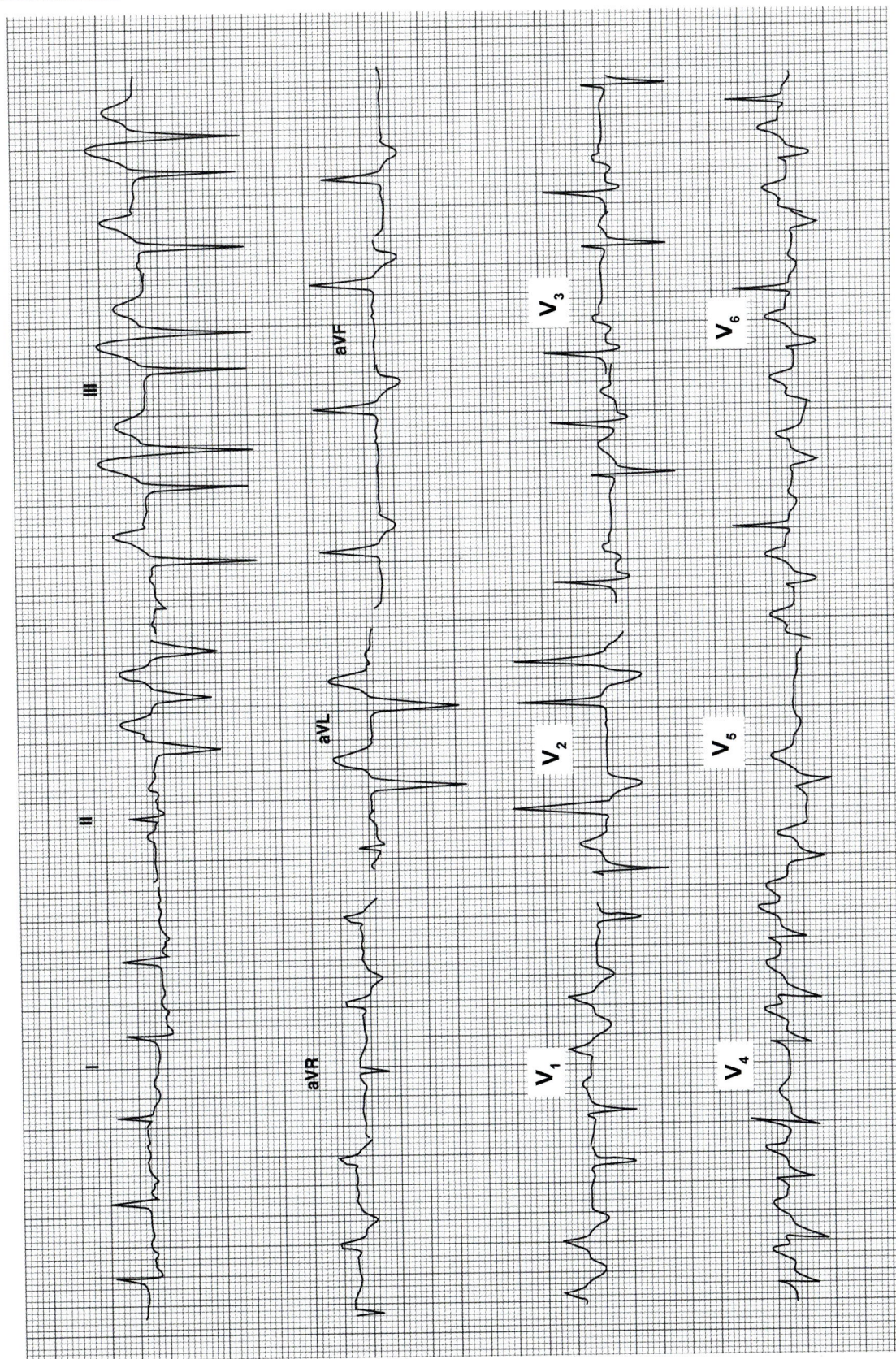

ECG NO. 94

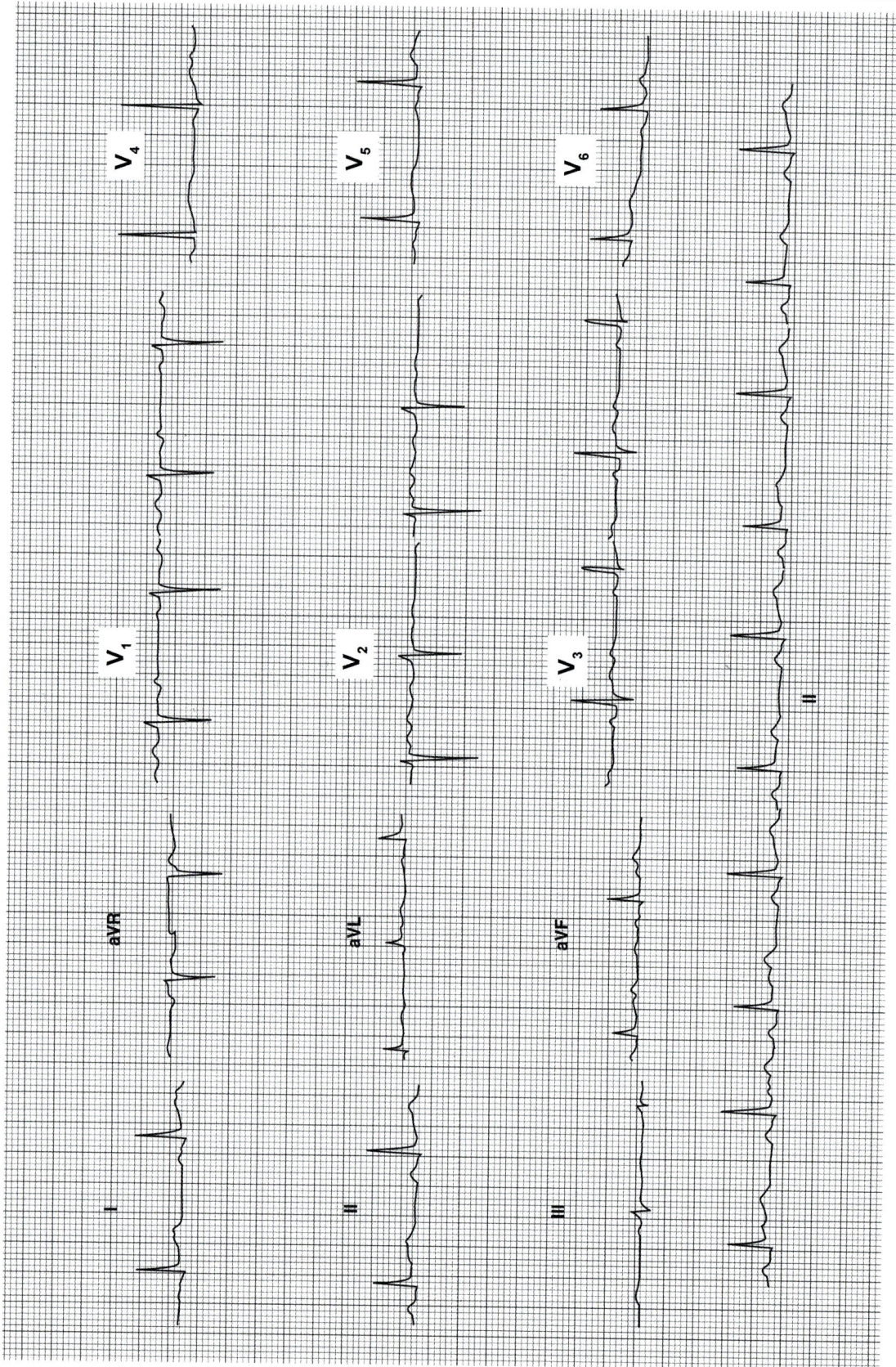

ECG NO. 95

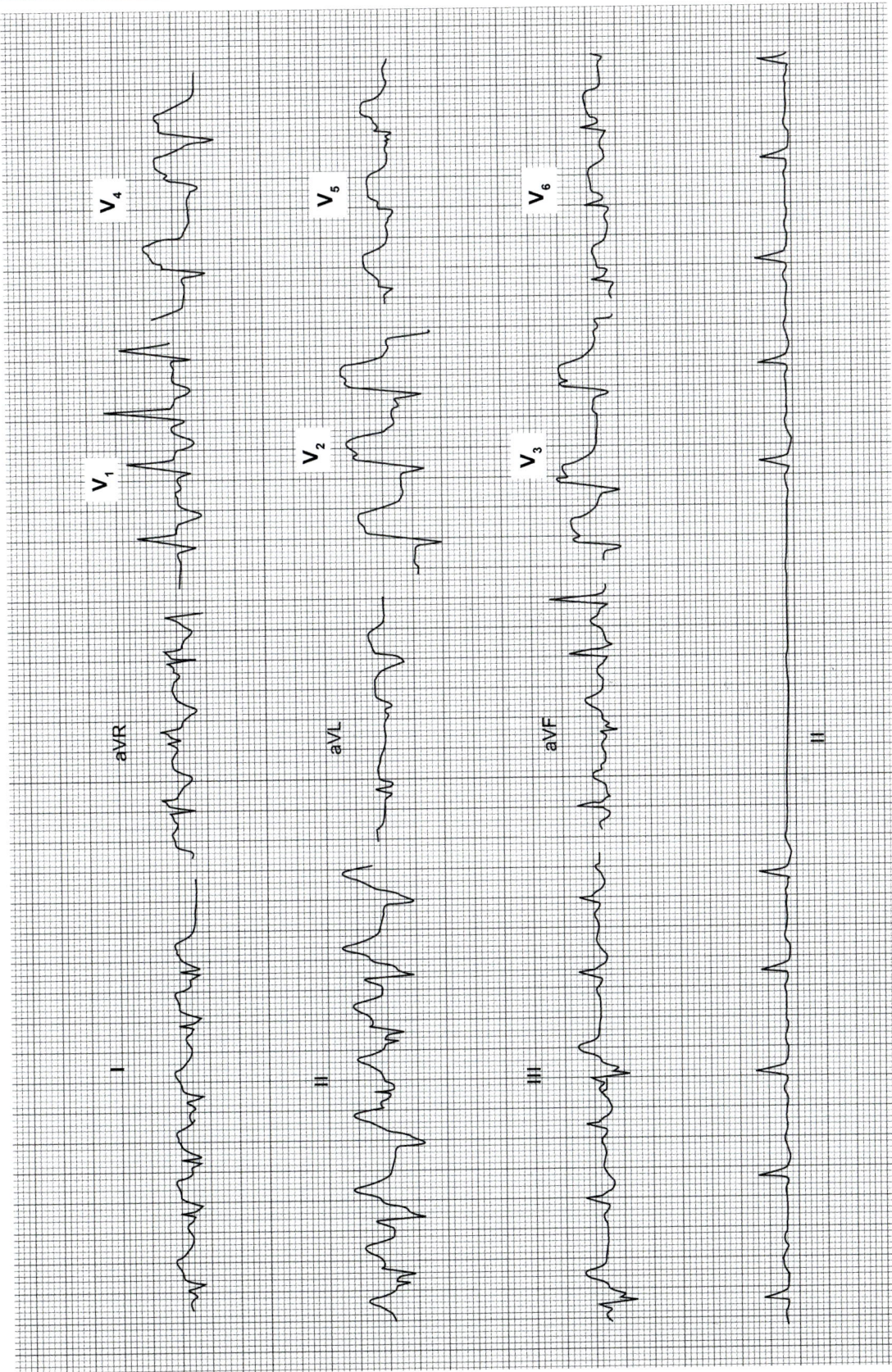

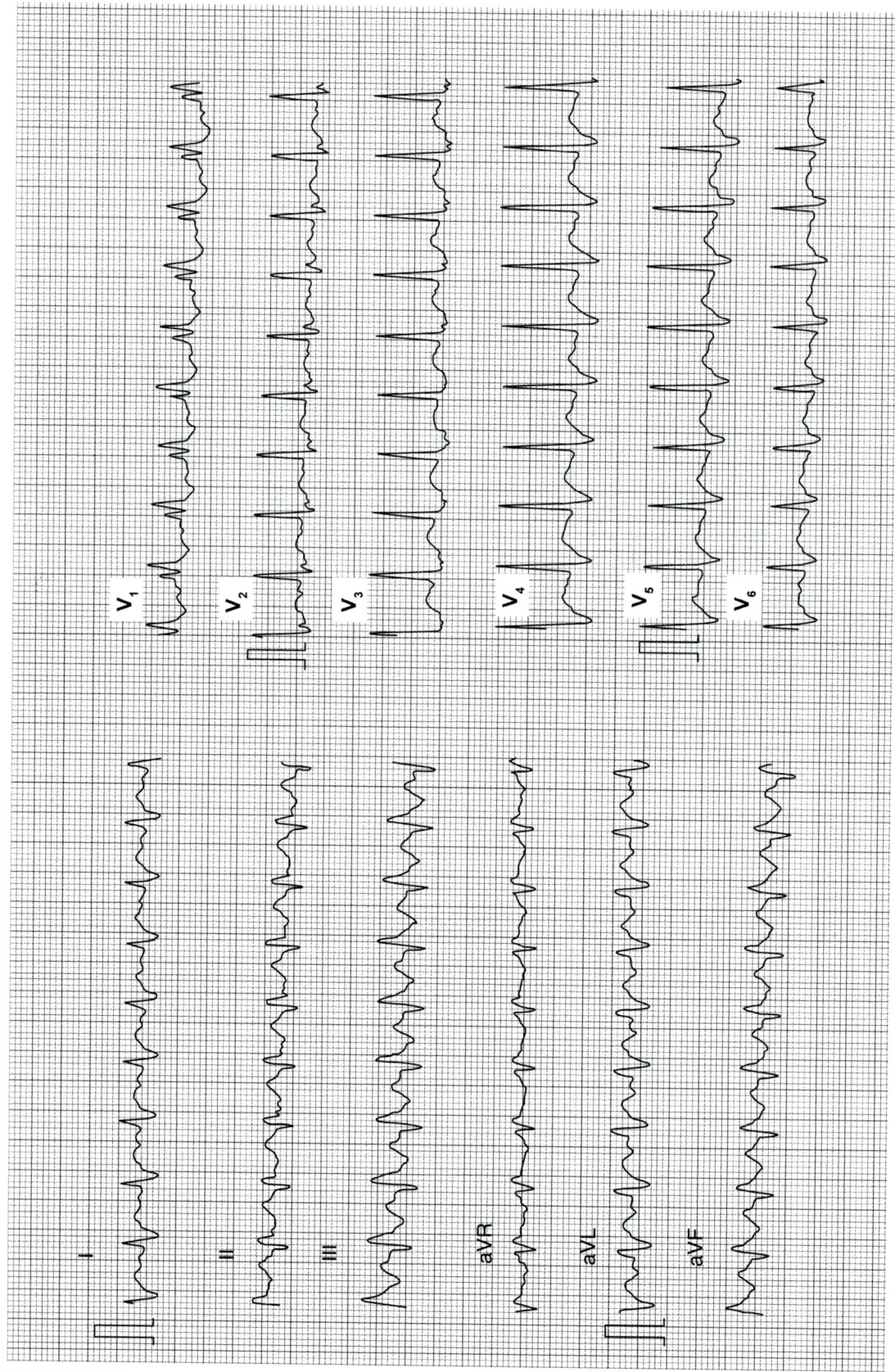

ECG NO. 97

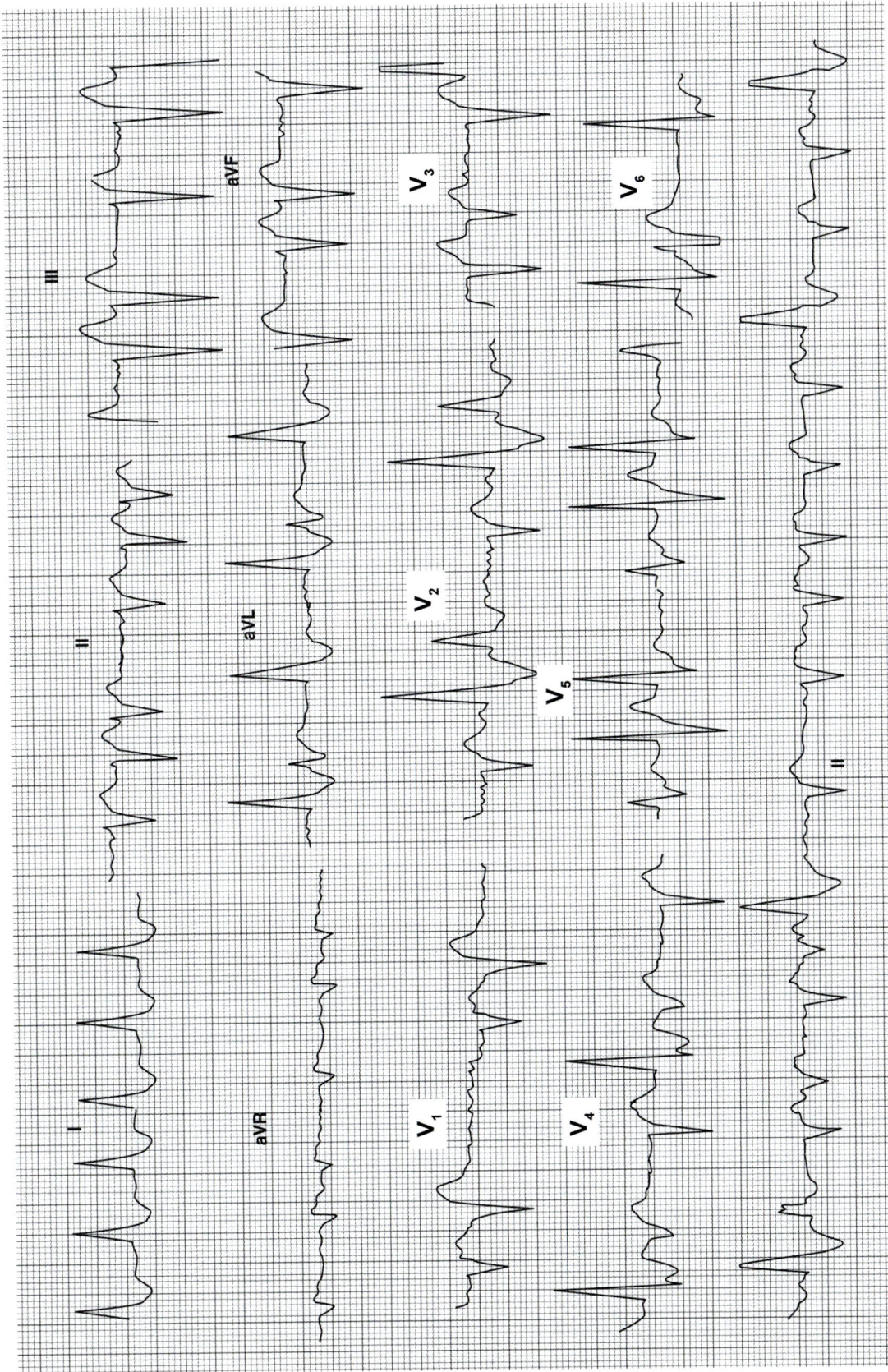

I   II   III   aVR   aVL   aVF   V₁   V₂   V₃   V₄   V₅   V₆   II

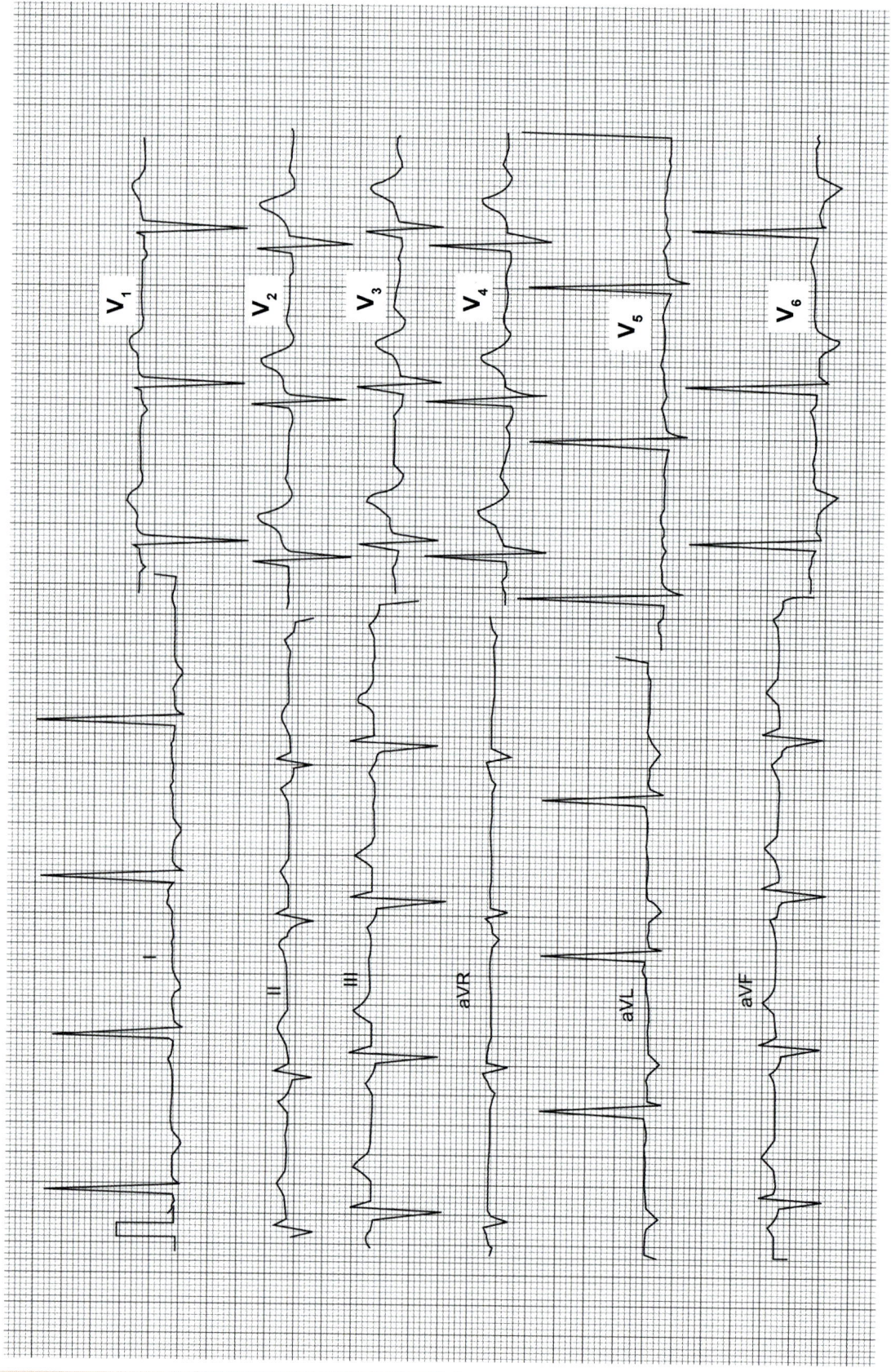

ECG NO. 98

ECG NO. 99

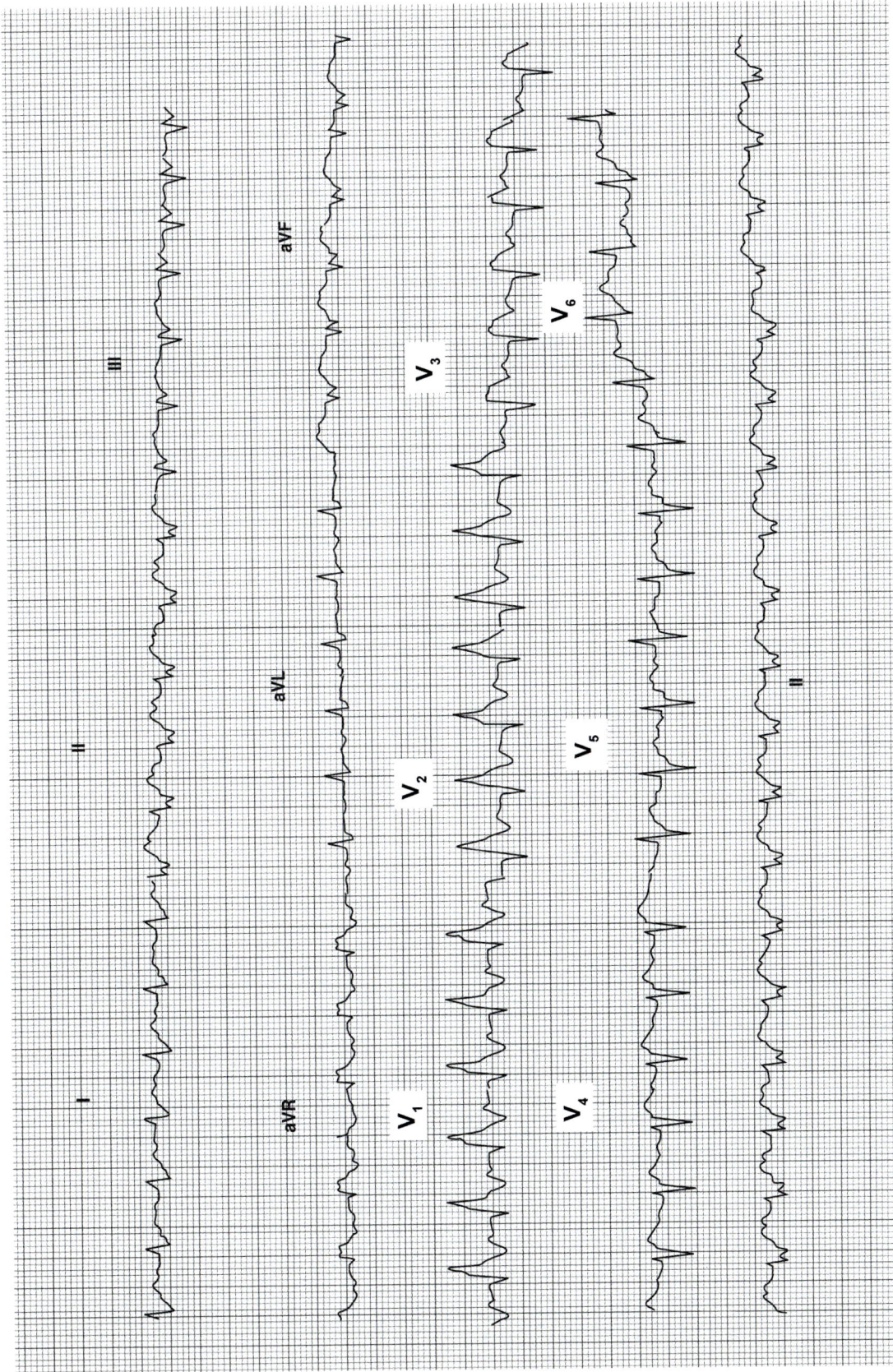

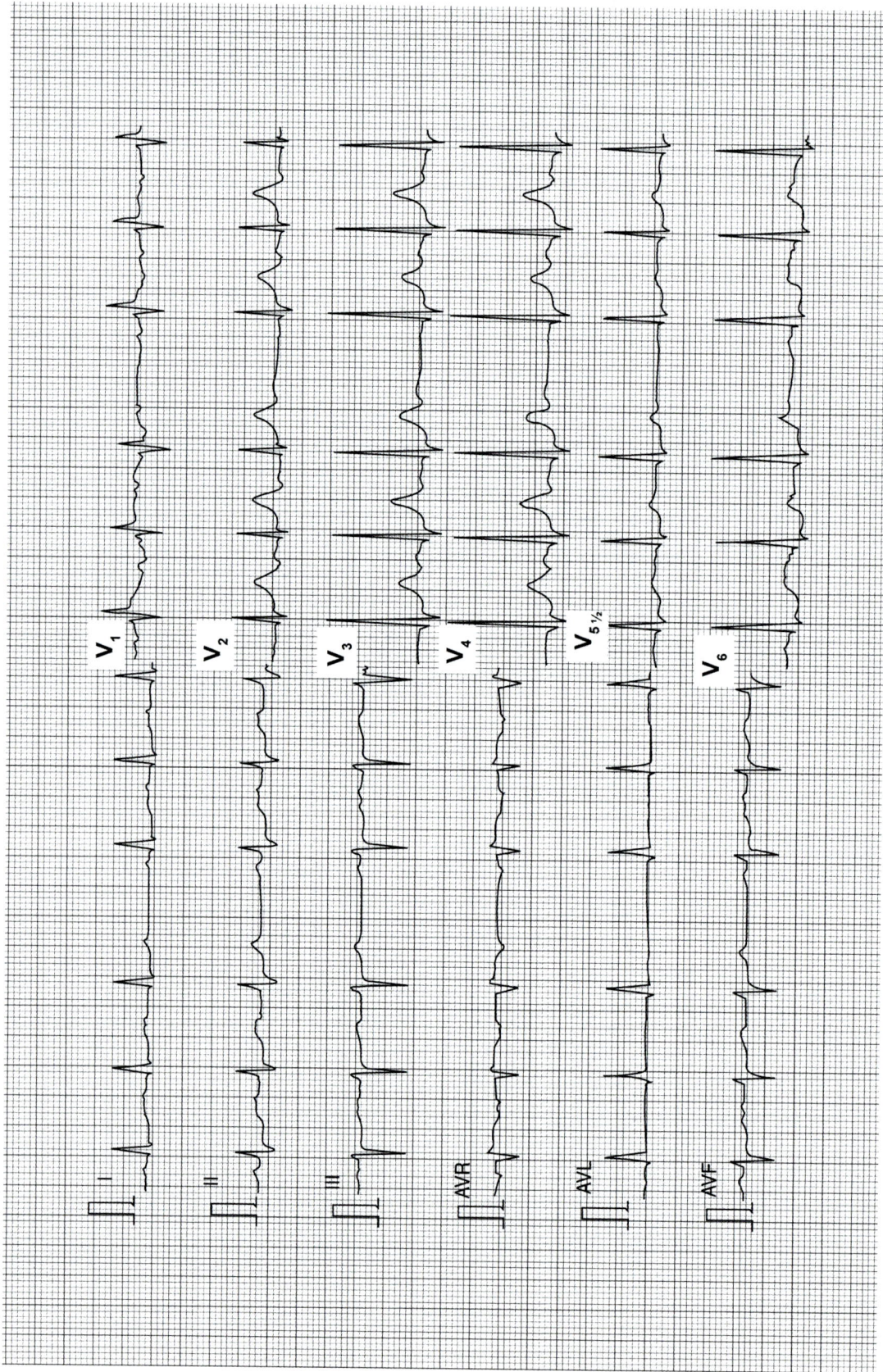

ECG NO. 101

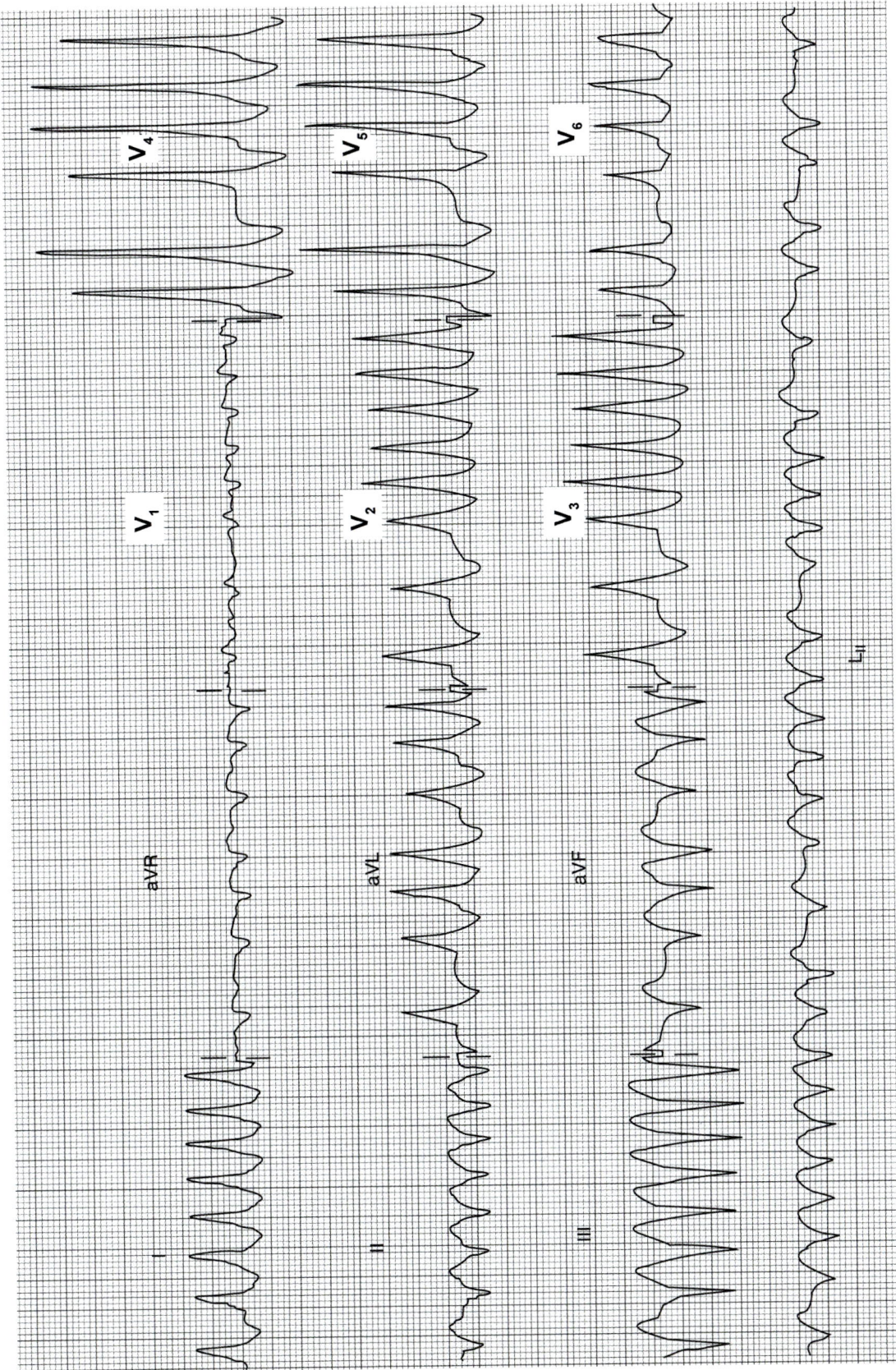

ECG NO. 102

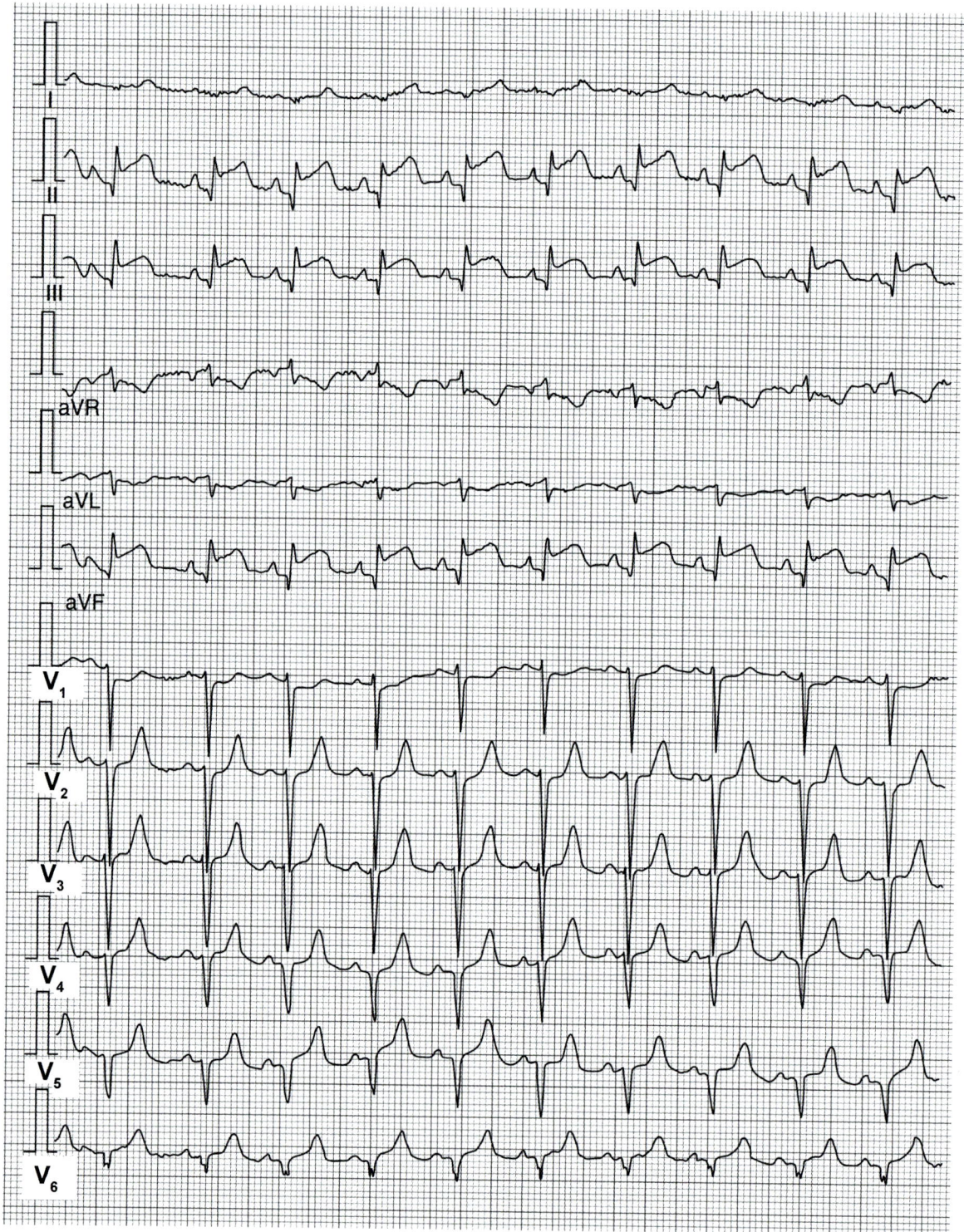

ECG NO. 103

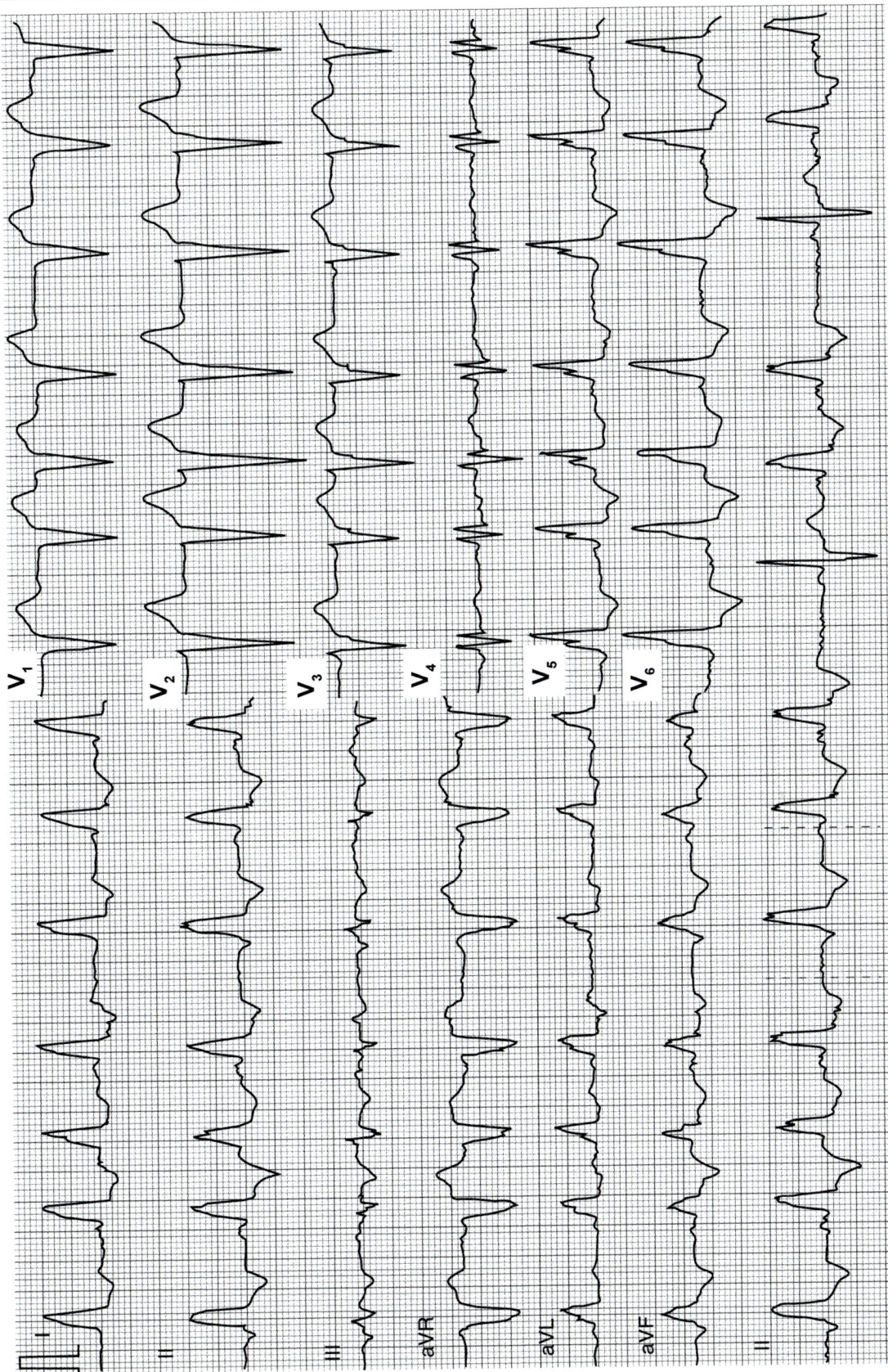

I

II

III

aVR

aVL

aVF

II

V₁

V₂

V₃

V₄

V₅

V₆

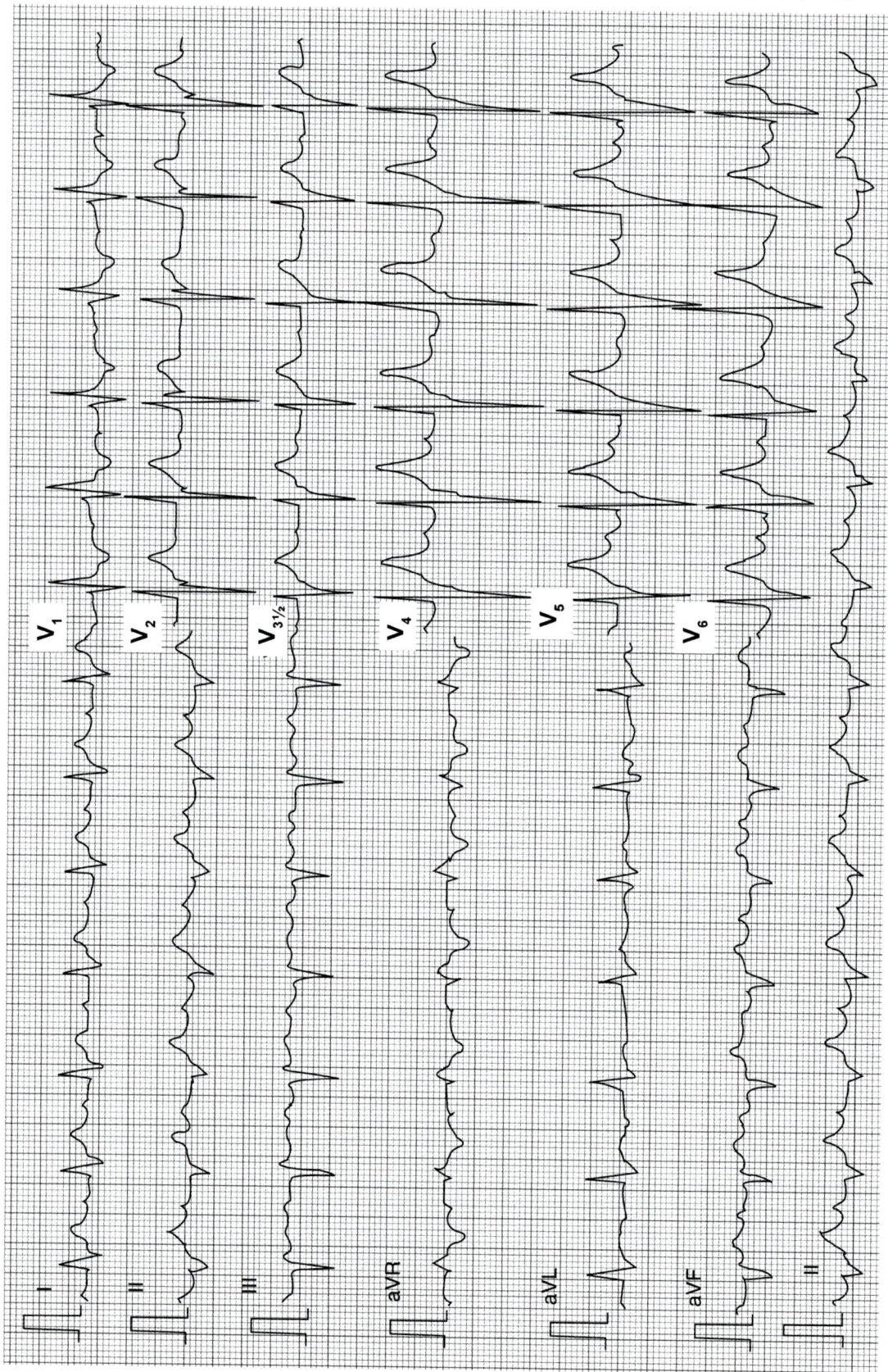

ECG NO. 104

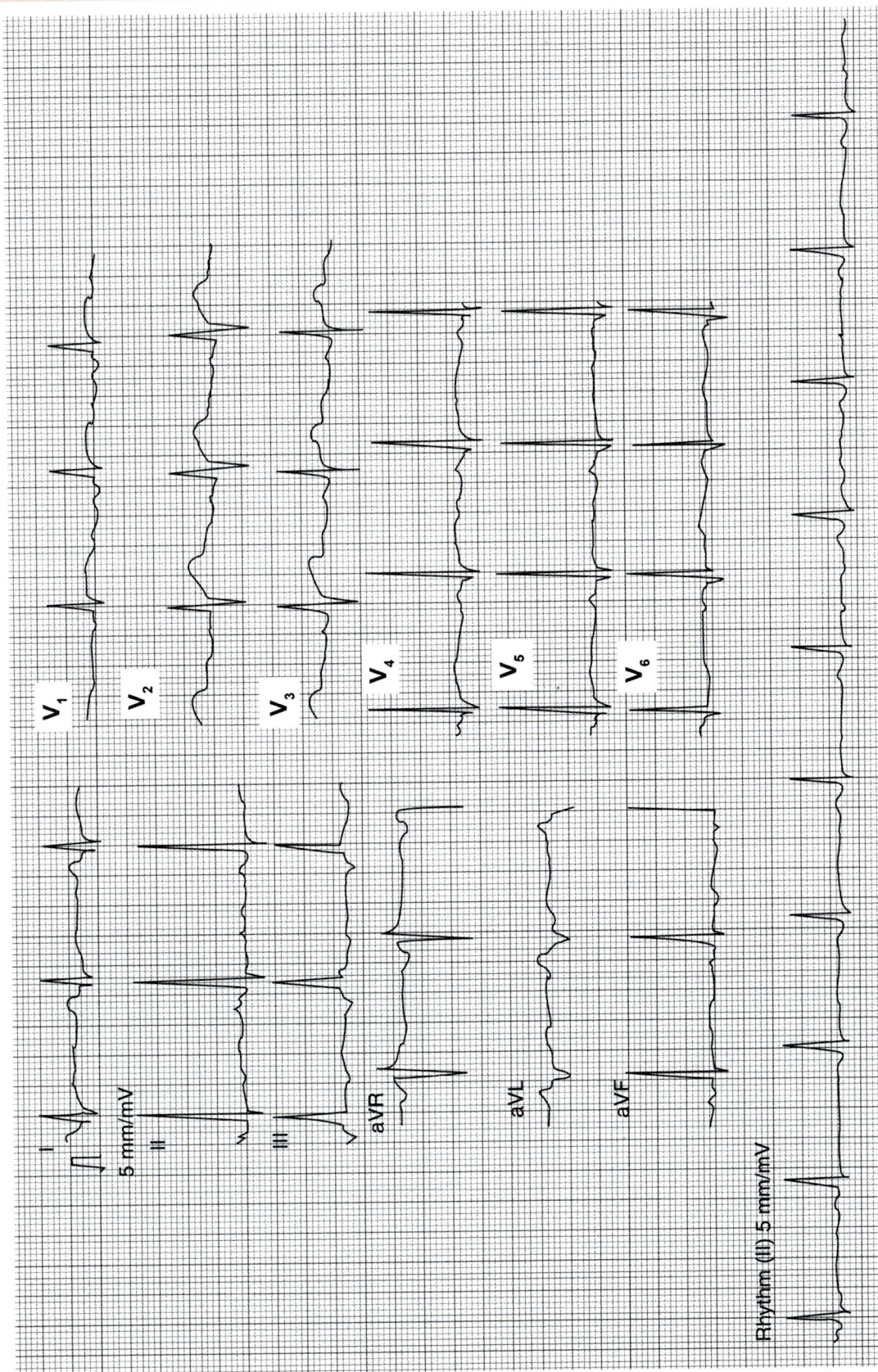

ECG NO. 105

I

5-mm/mV

II

III

aVR

aVL

aVF

V₁

V₂

V₃

V₄

V₅

V₆

Rhythm (II) 5 mm/mV

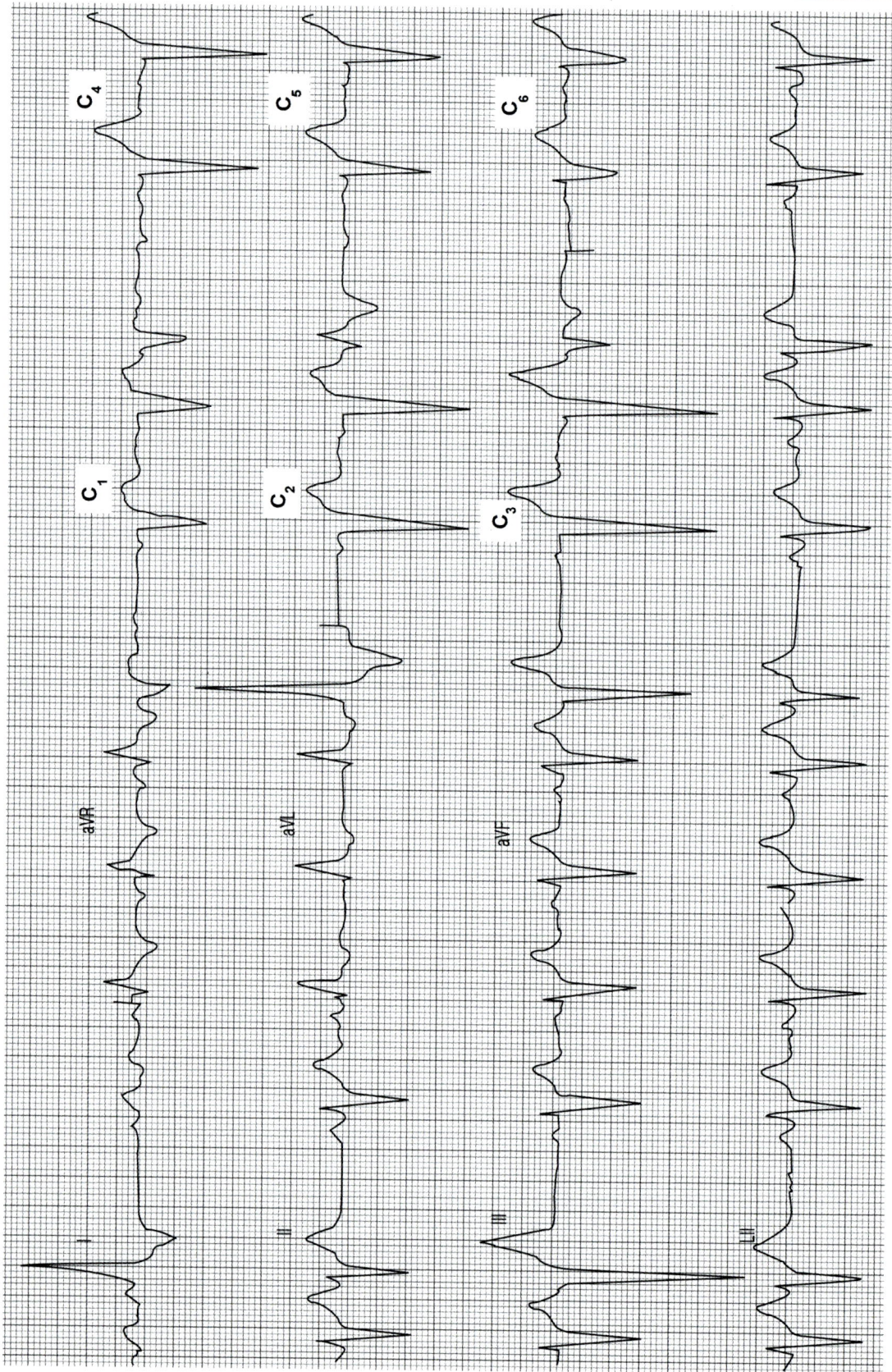

ECG NO. 107

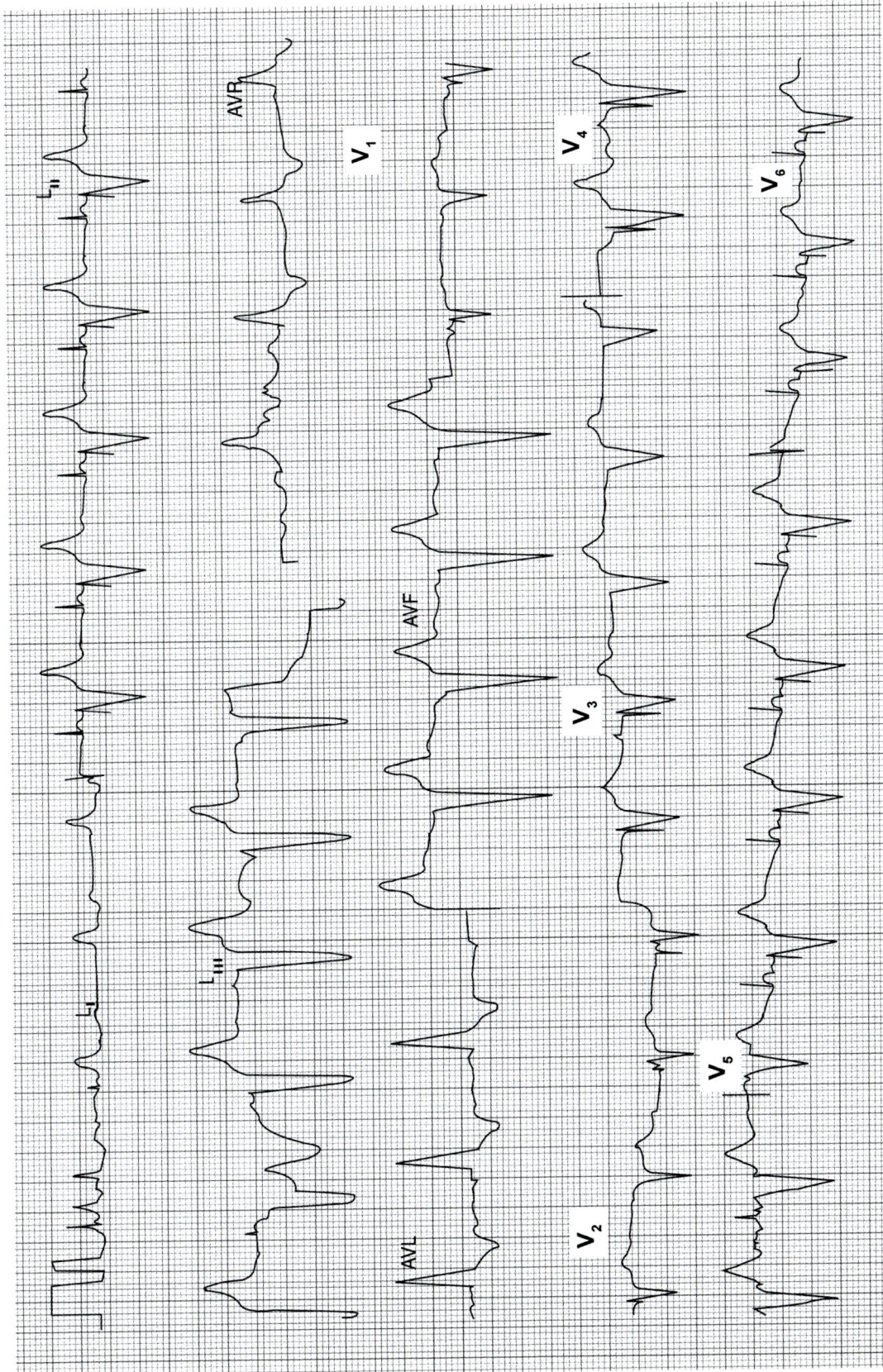

ECG NO. 108

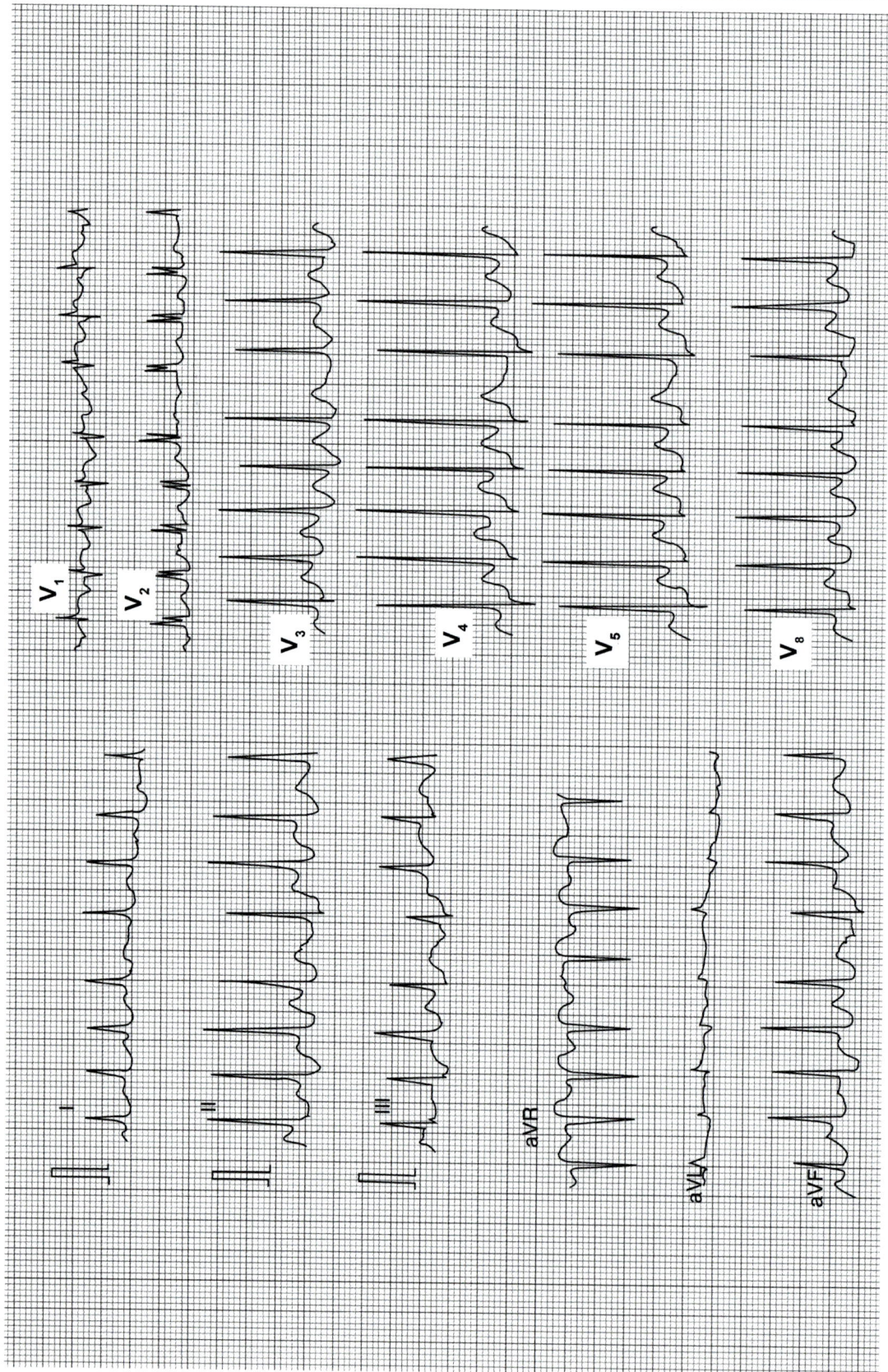

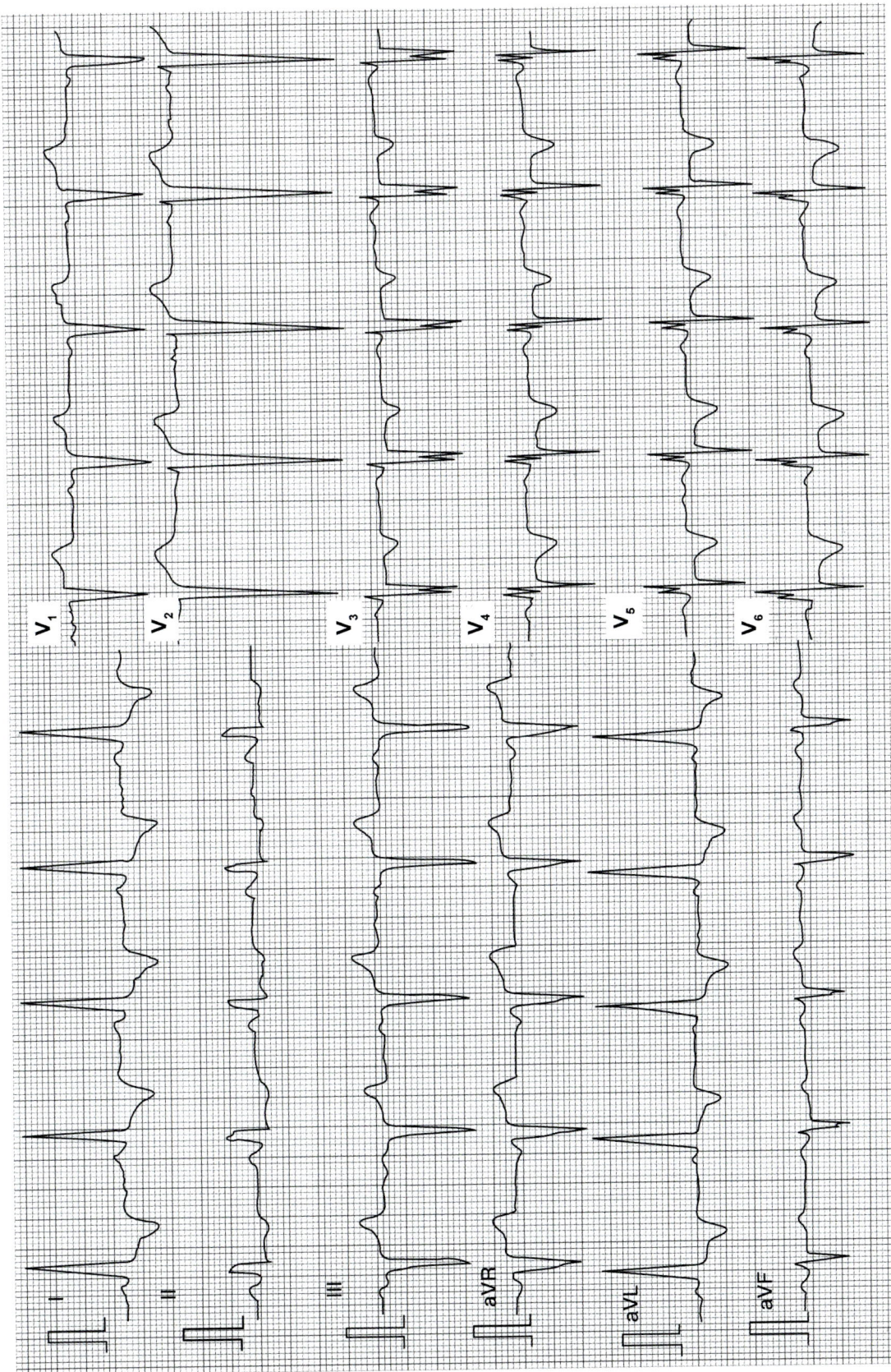

ECG NO. 109

V₁

V₂

V₃

V₄

V₅

V₆

I

II

III

aVR

aVL

aVF

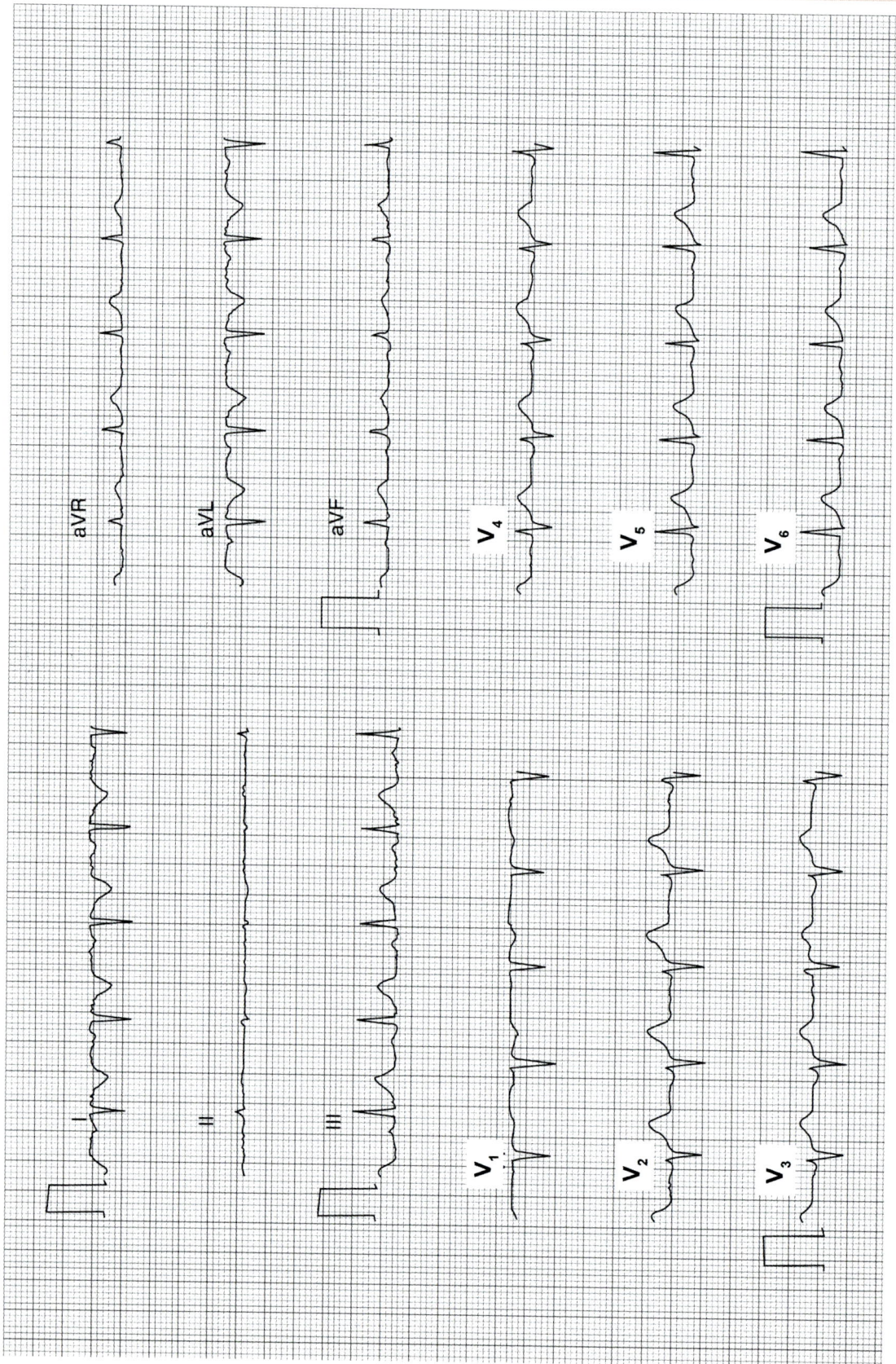

ECG NO. 110

aVR

aVL

aVF

V4

V5

V6

I

II

III

V1

V2

V3

ECG NO. 111

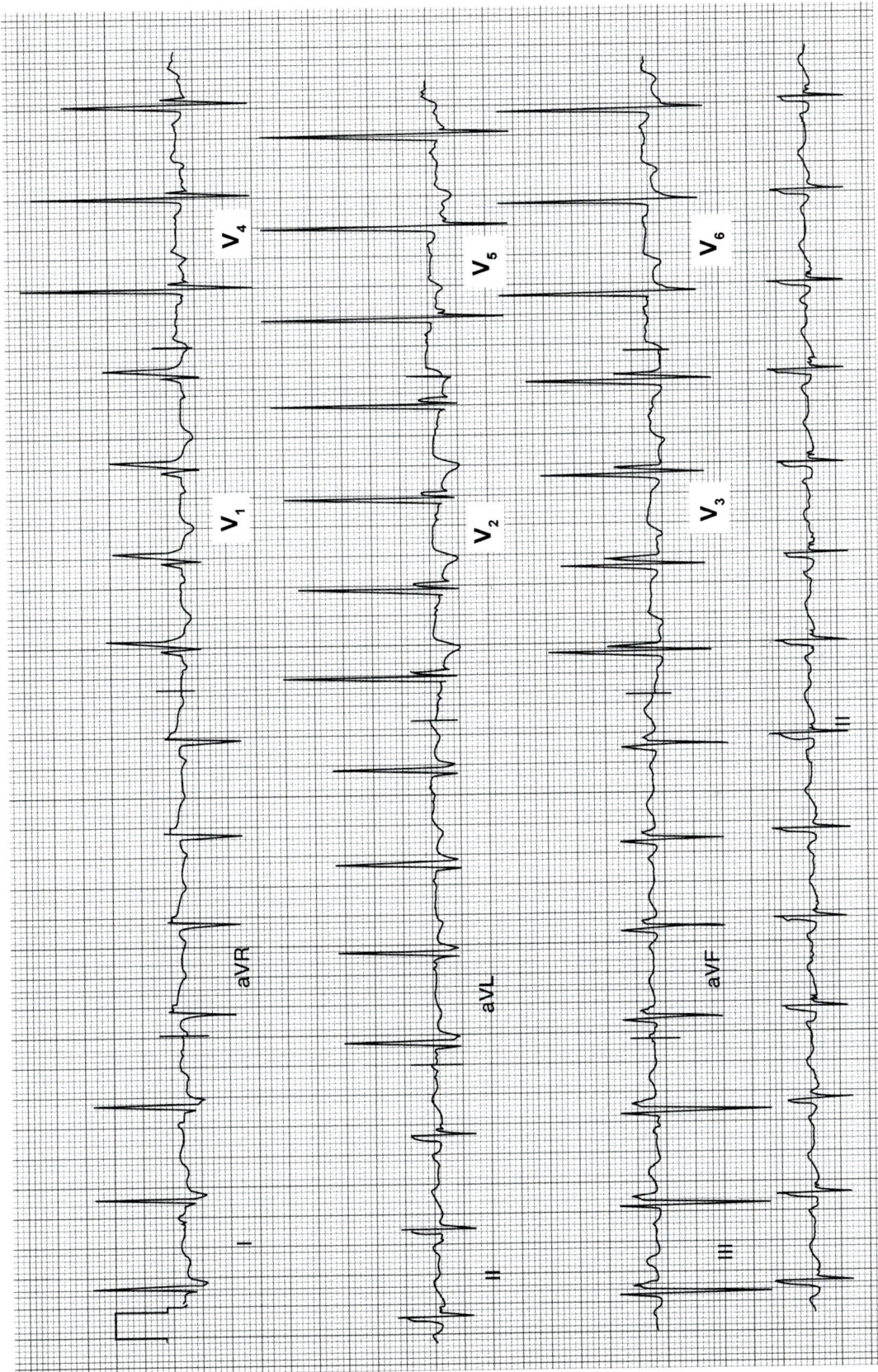

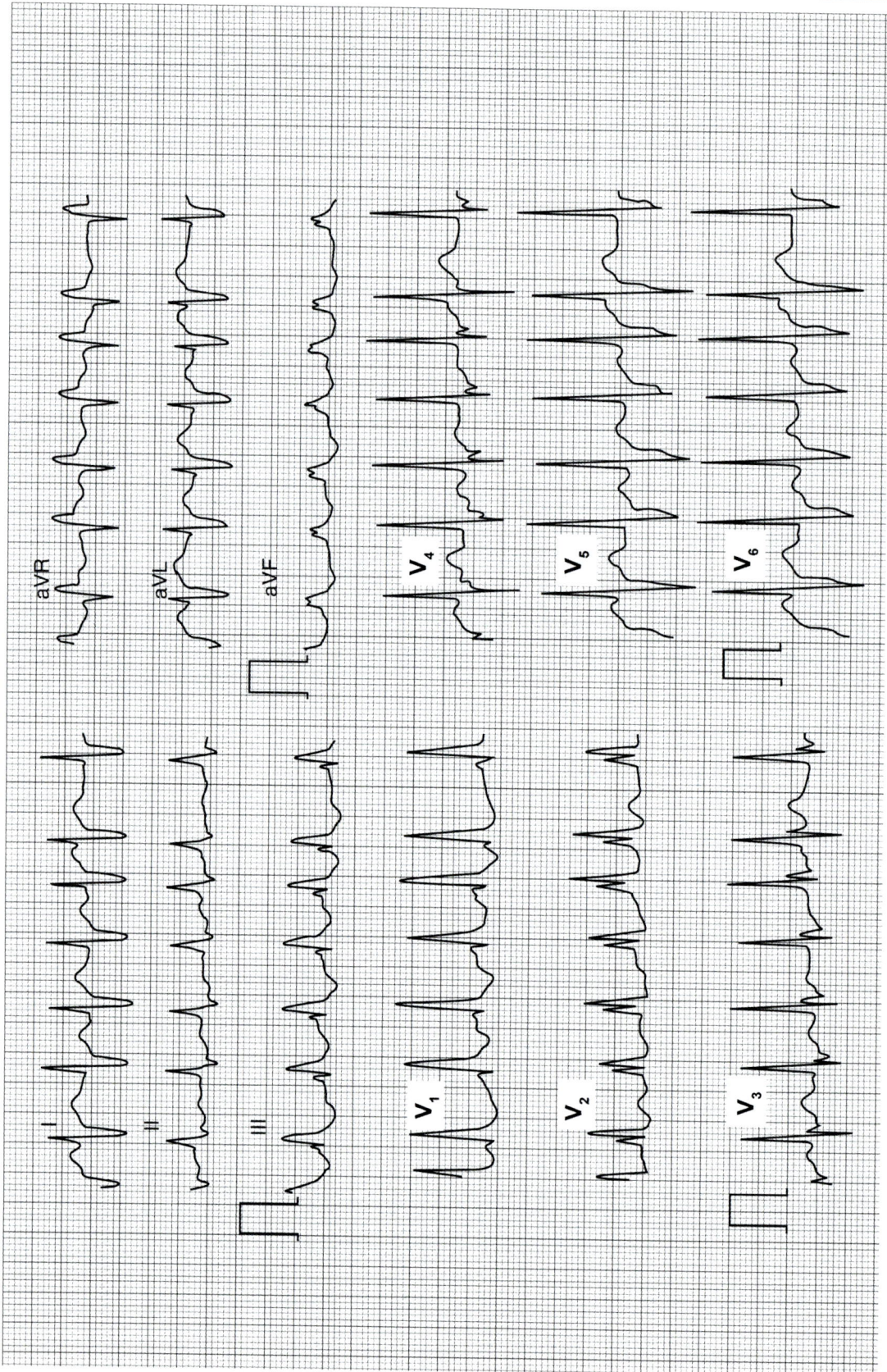

ECG NO. 112

I

II

III

aVR

aVL

aVF

V_1

V_2

V_3

V_4

V_5

V_6

ECG NO. 113

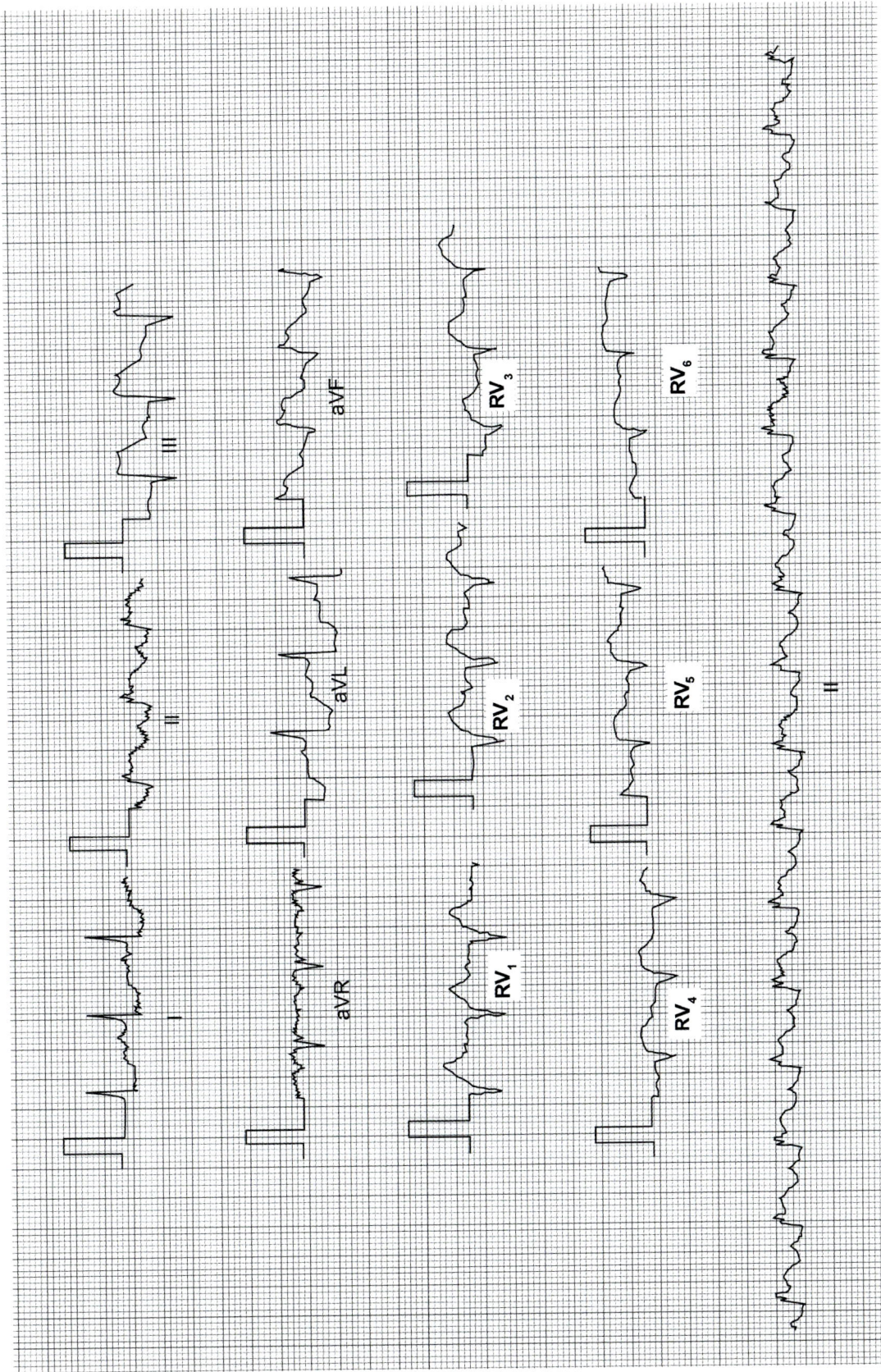

ECG NO. 114

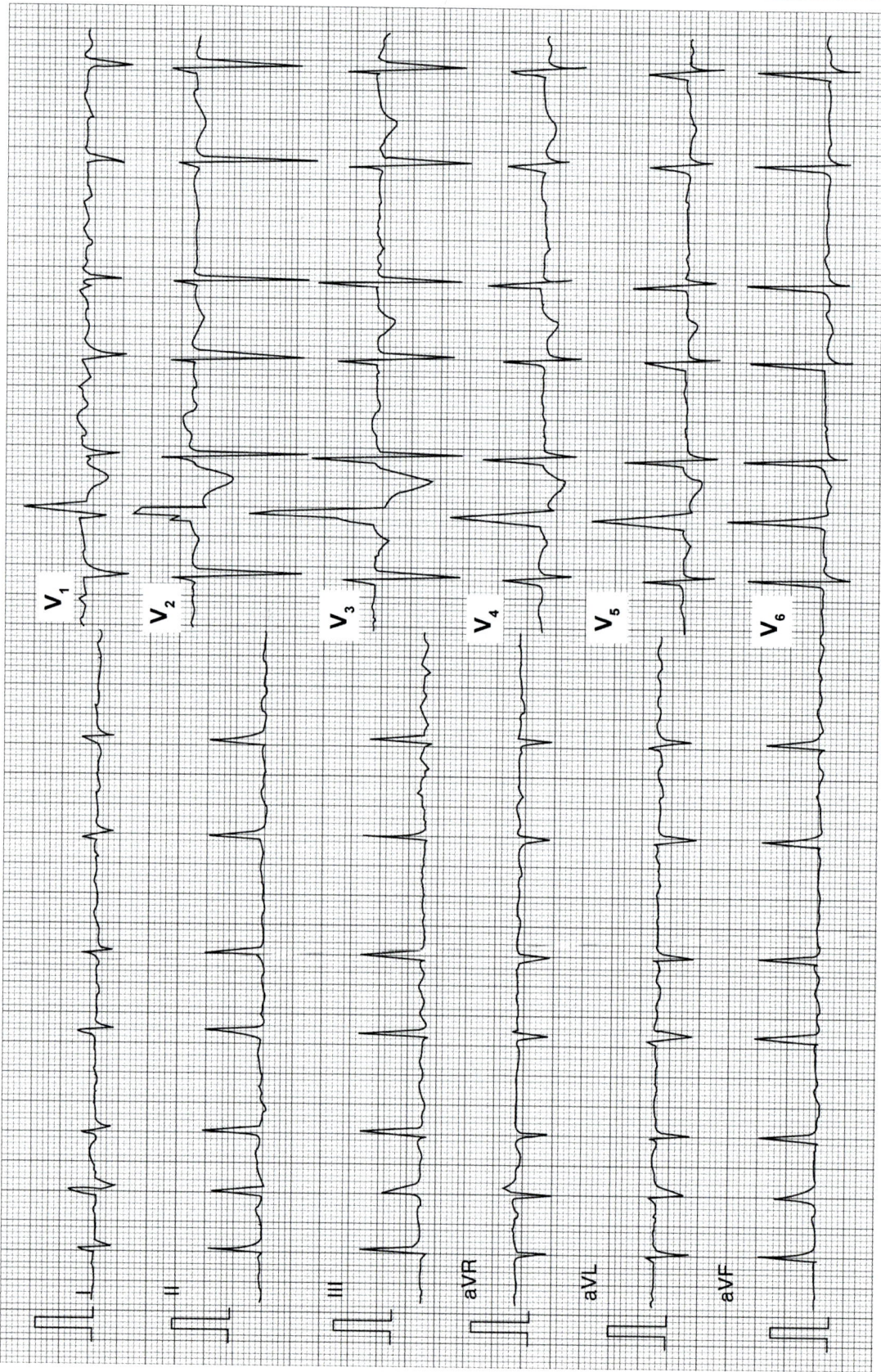

V₁
V₂
V₃
V₄
V₅
V₆

I
II
III
aVR
aVL
aVF

ECG NO. 115

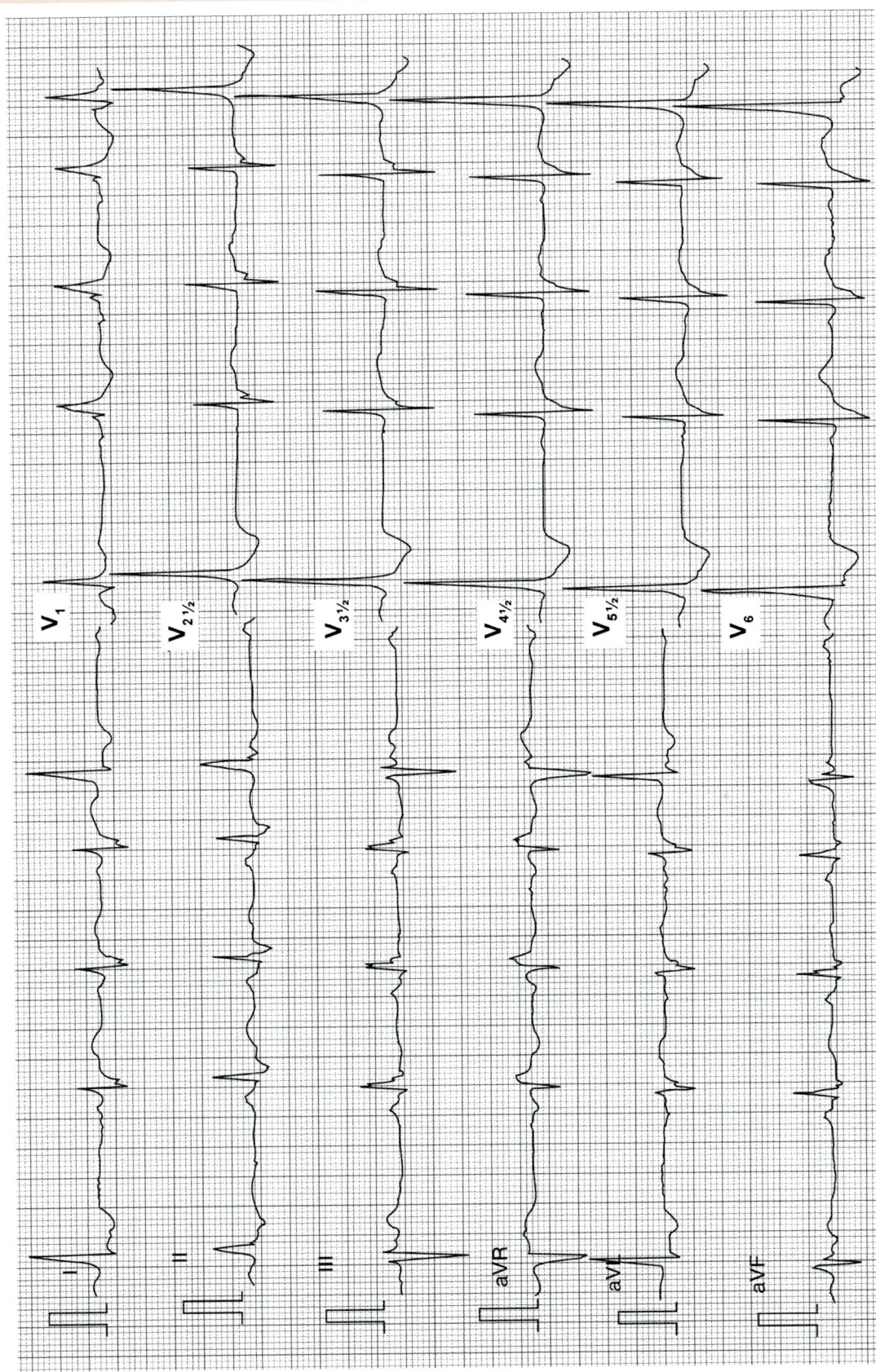

V₁

V₂½

V₃½

V₄½

V₅½

V₆

I

II

III

aVR

aVL

aVF

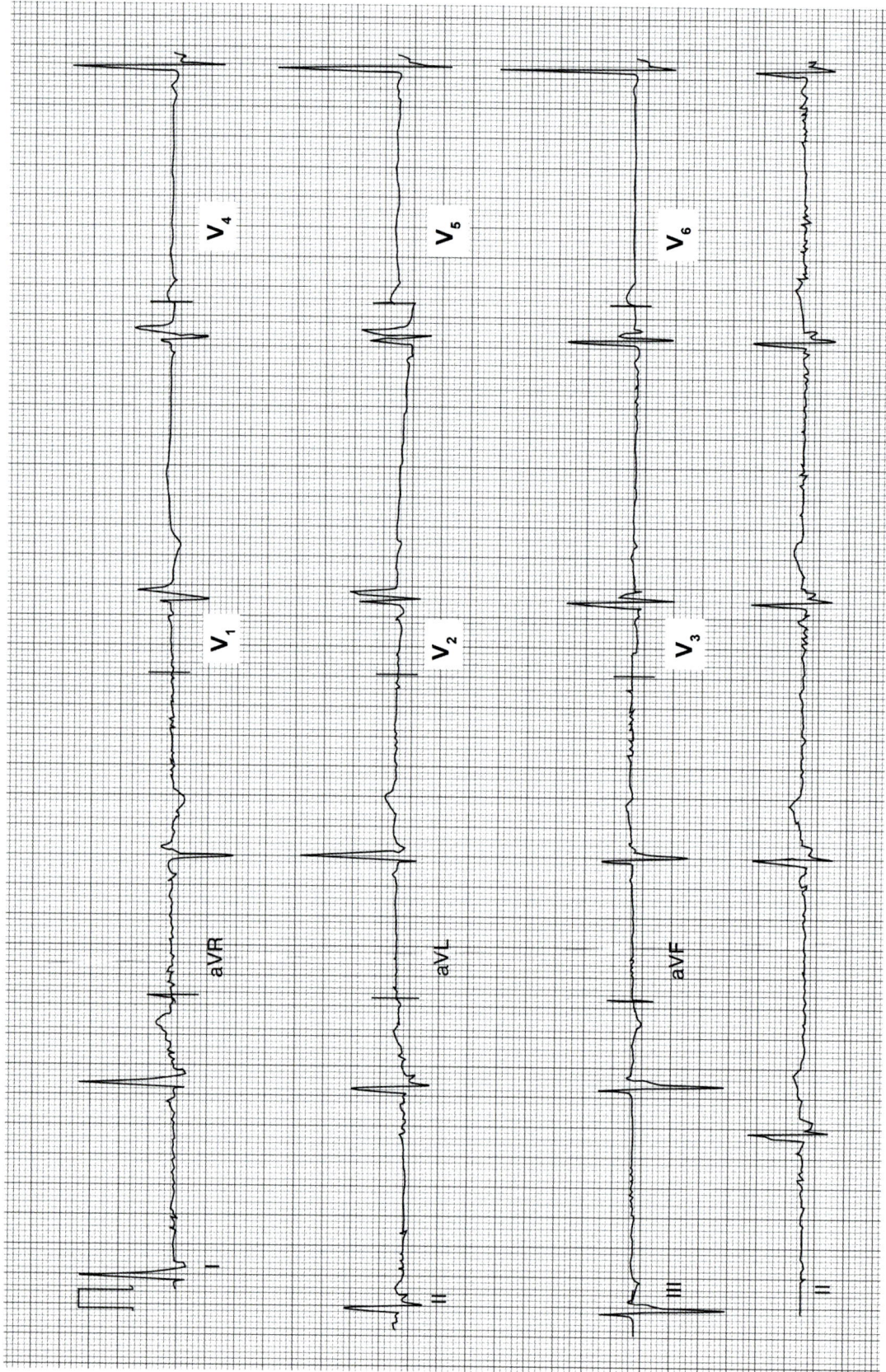

ECG NO. 117

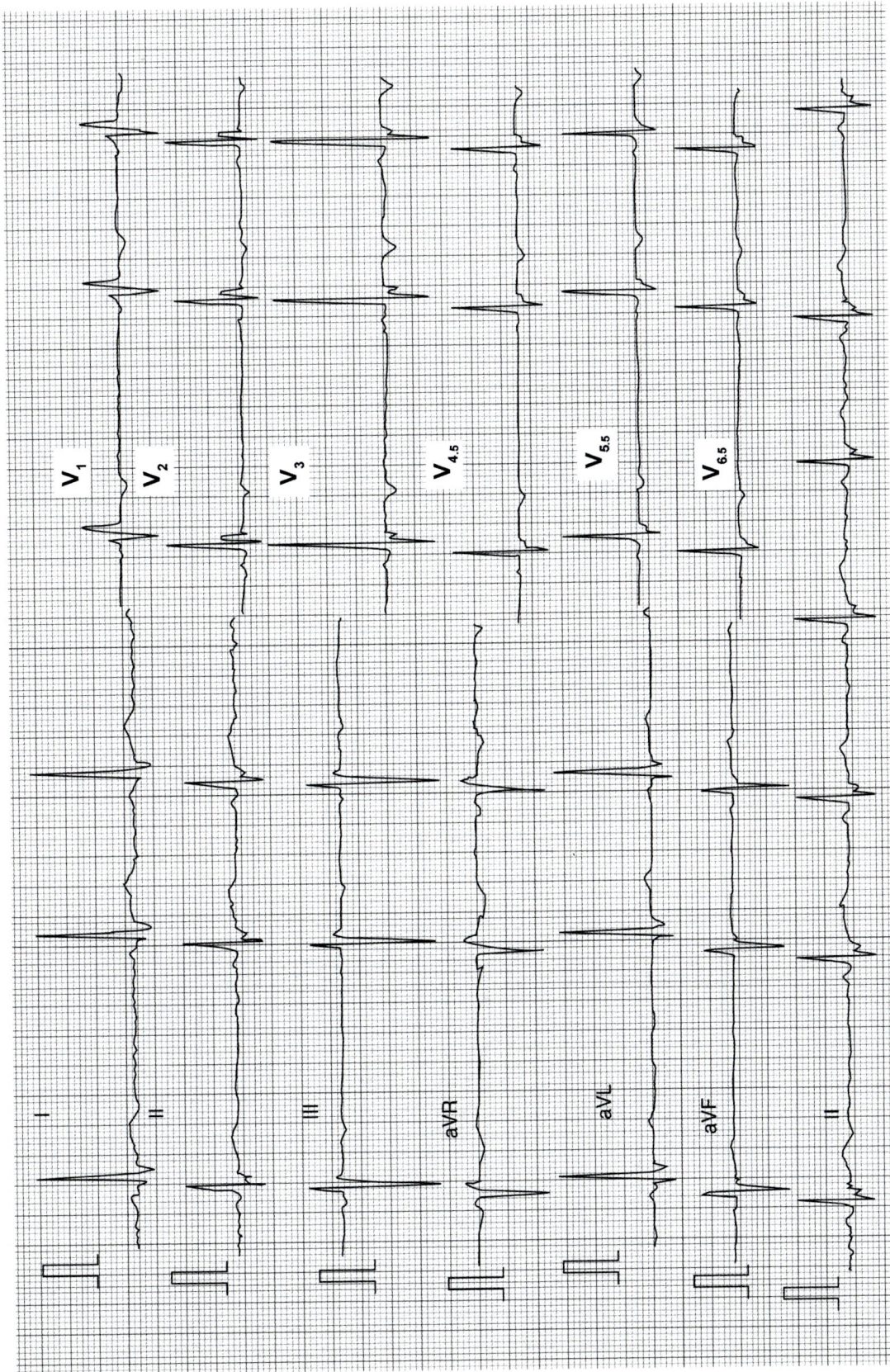

ECG NO. 118

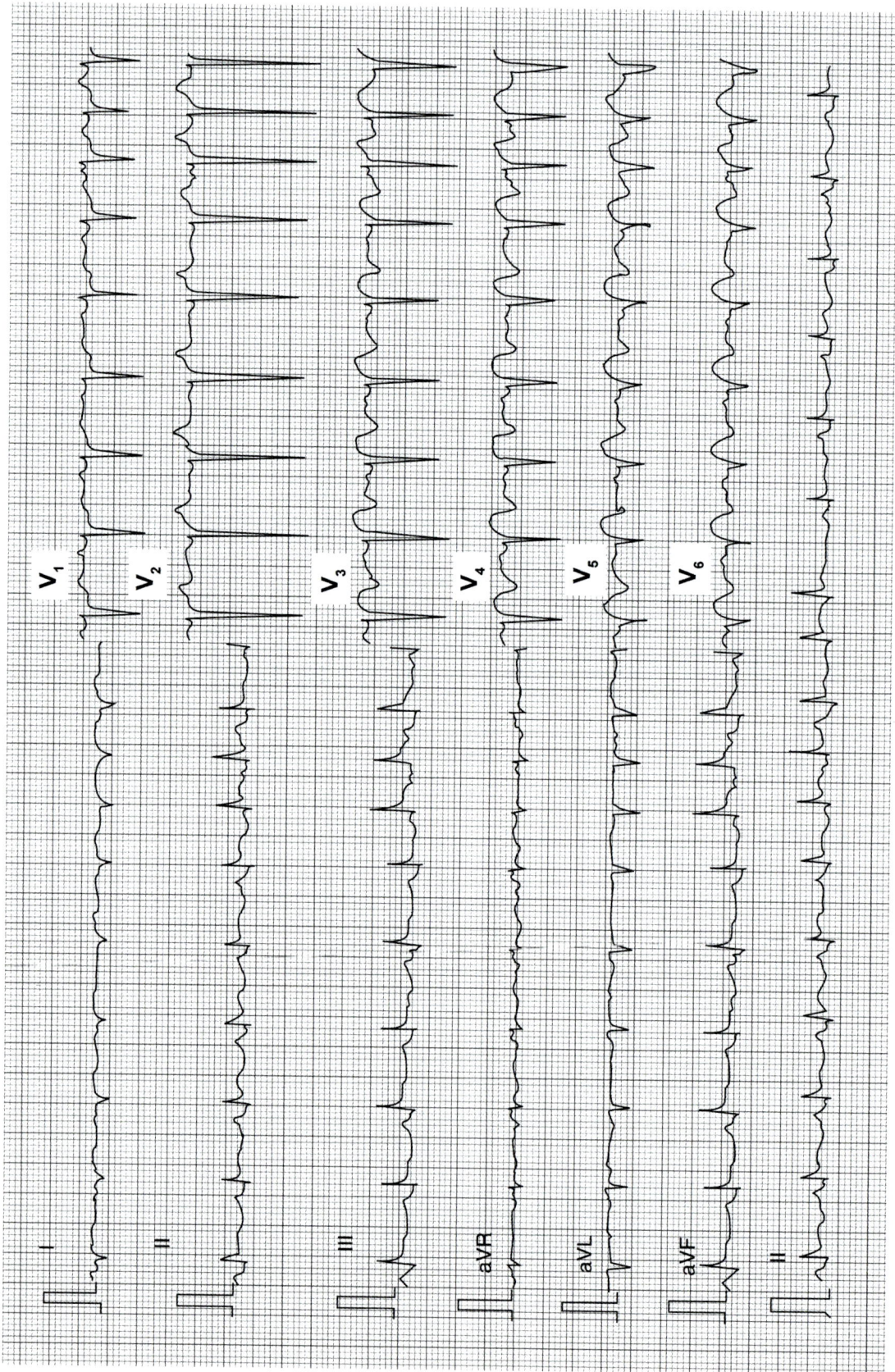

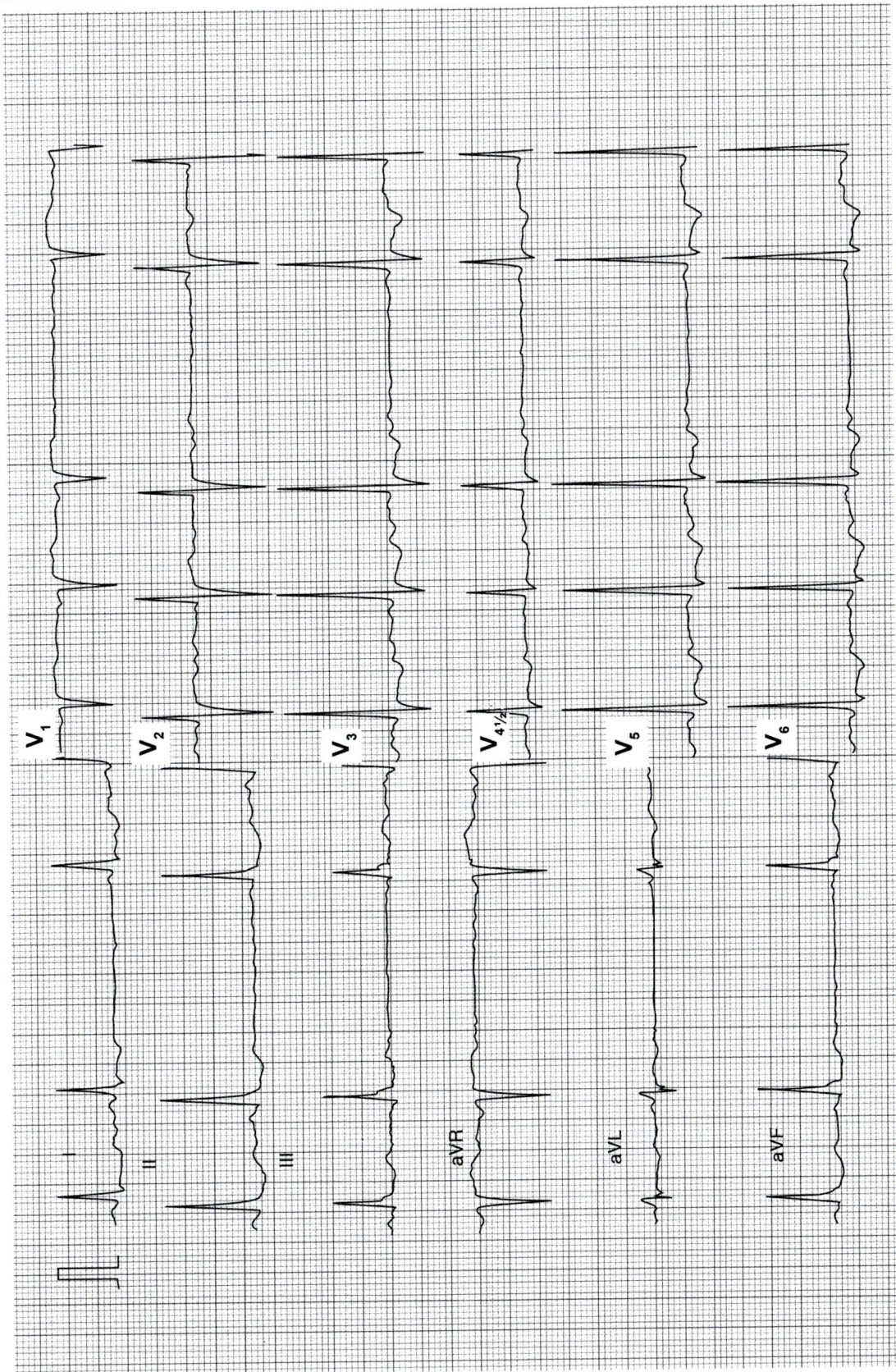

ECG NO. 119

V₁

V₂

V₃

V₄½

V₅

V₆

I

II

III

aVR

aVL

aVF

ECG NO. 120

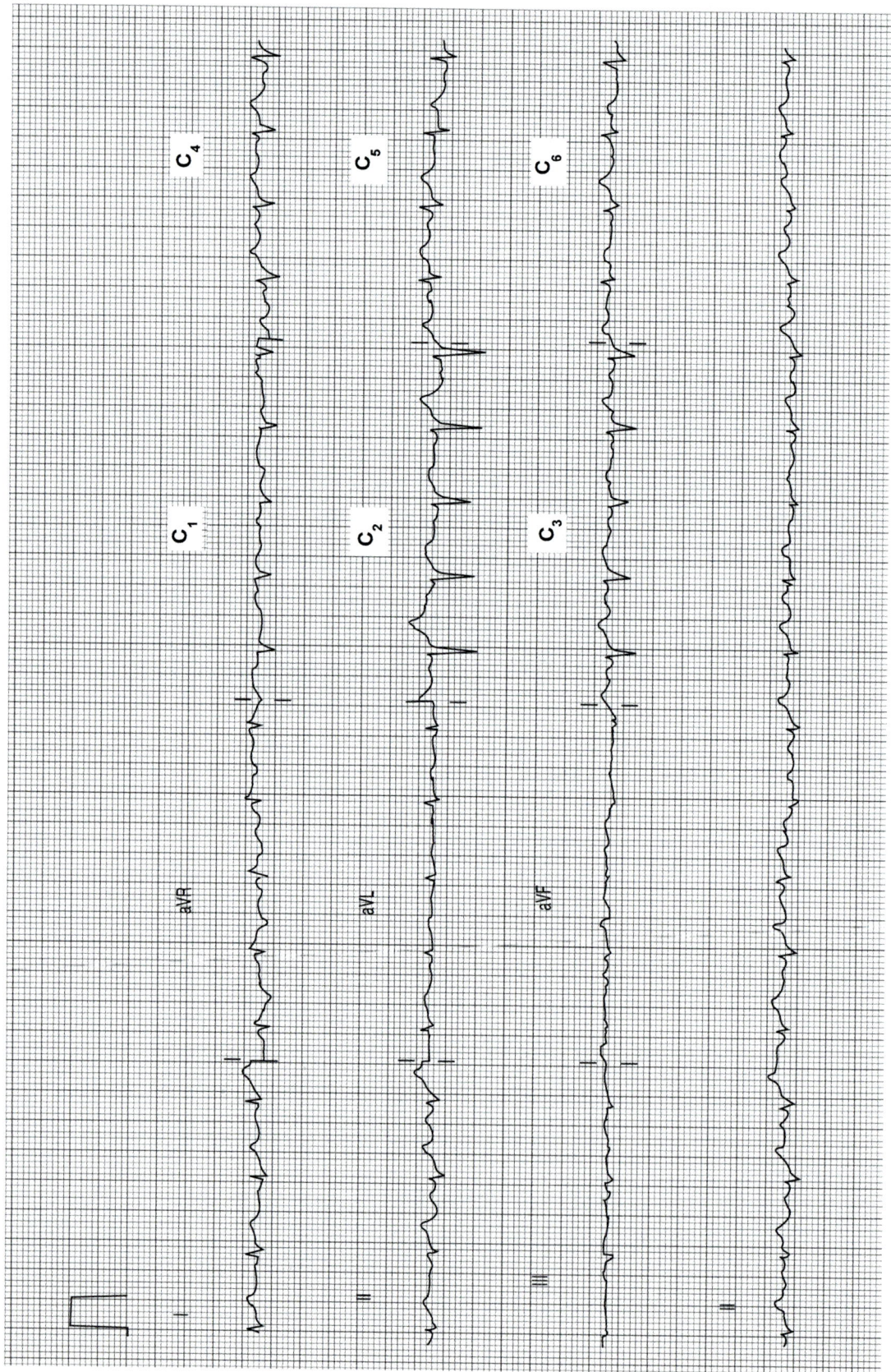

ECG NO. 121

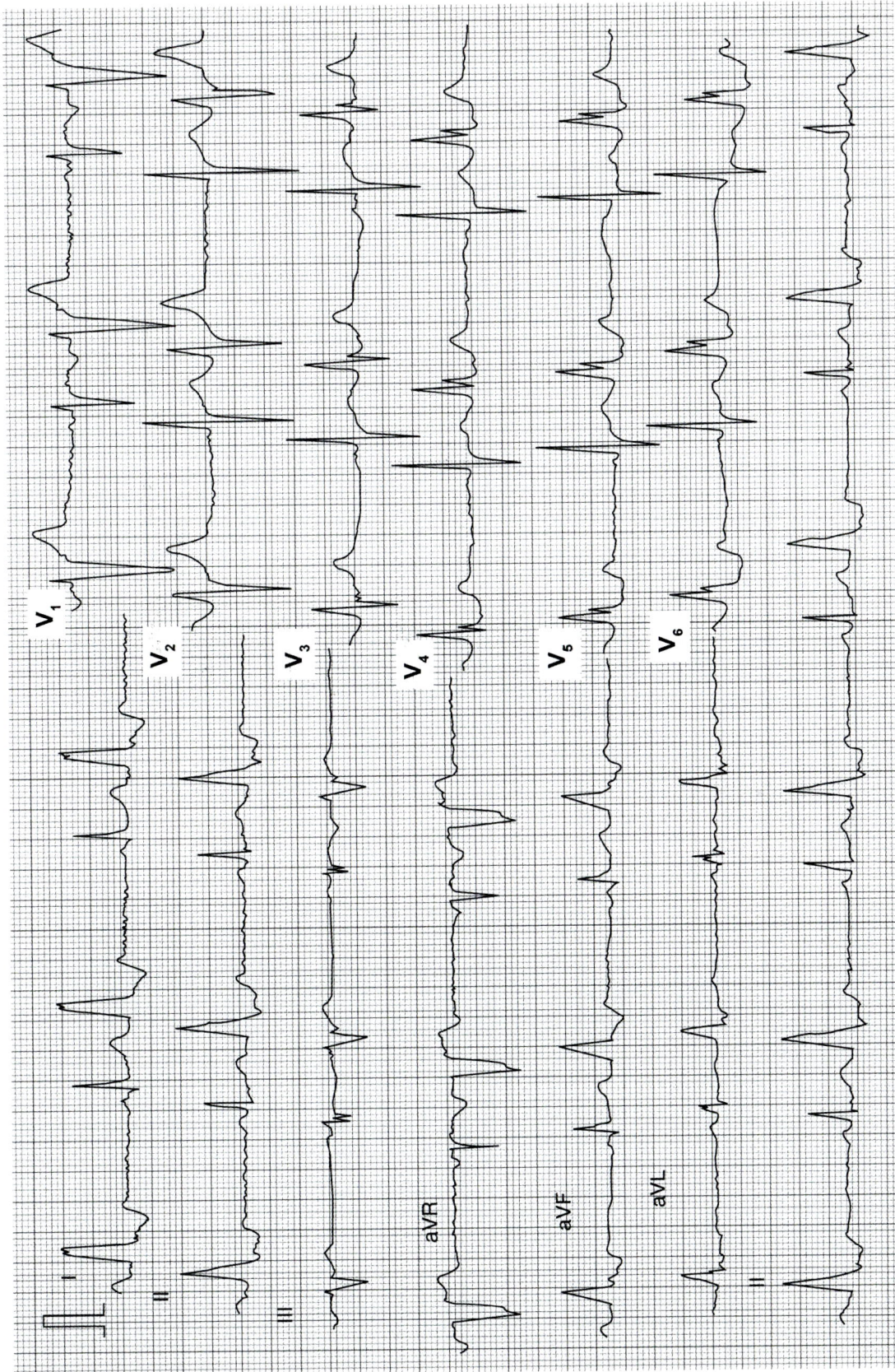

I

II

III

aVR

aVF

aVL

V₁

V₂

V₃

V₄

V₅

V₆

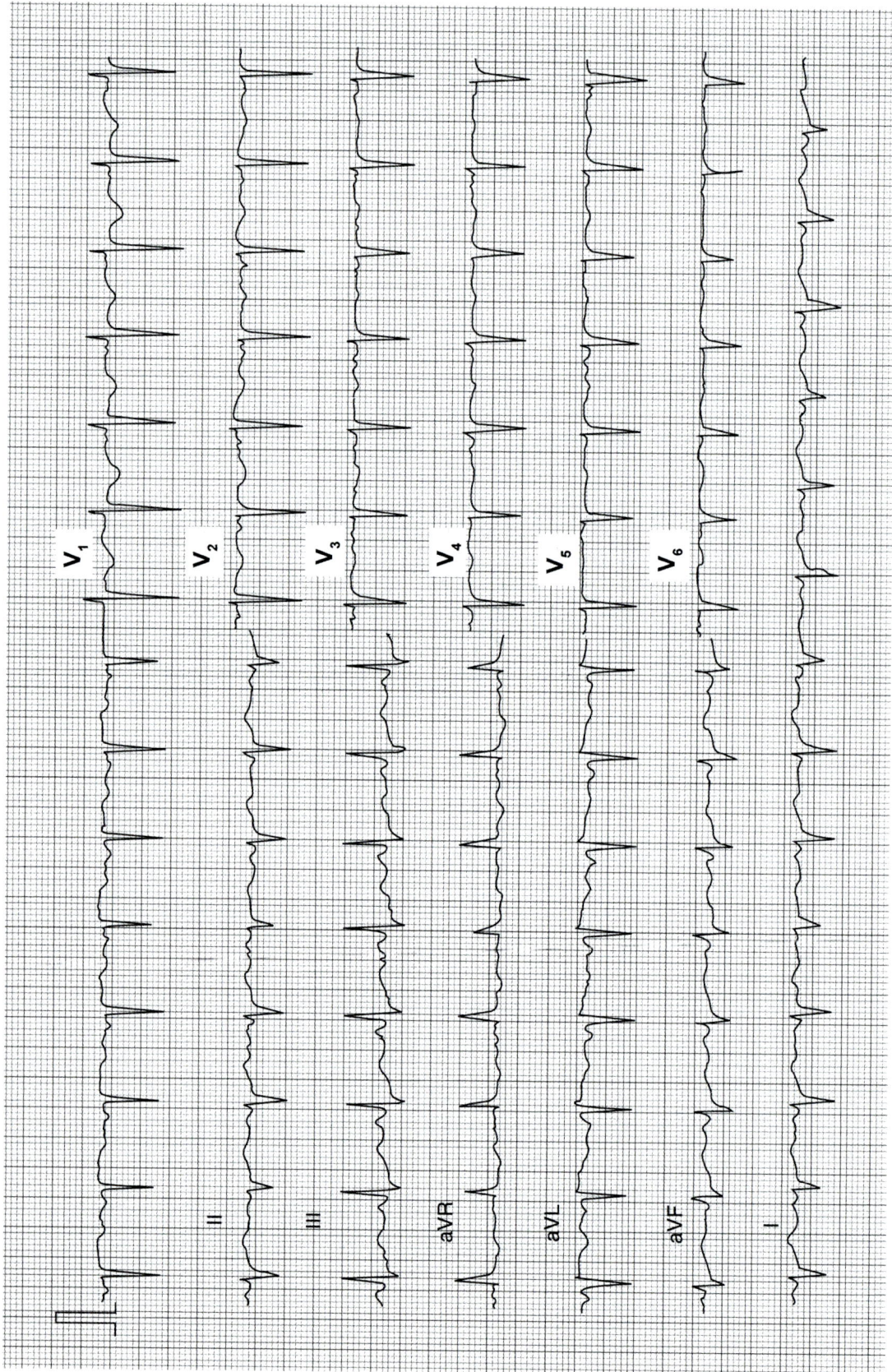

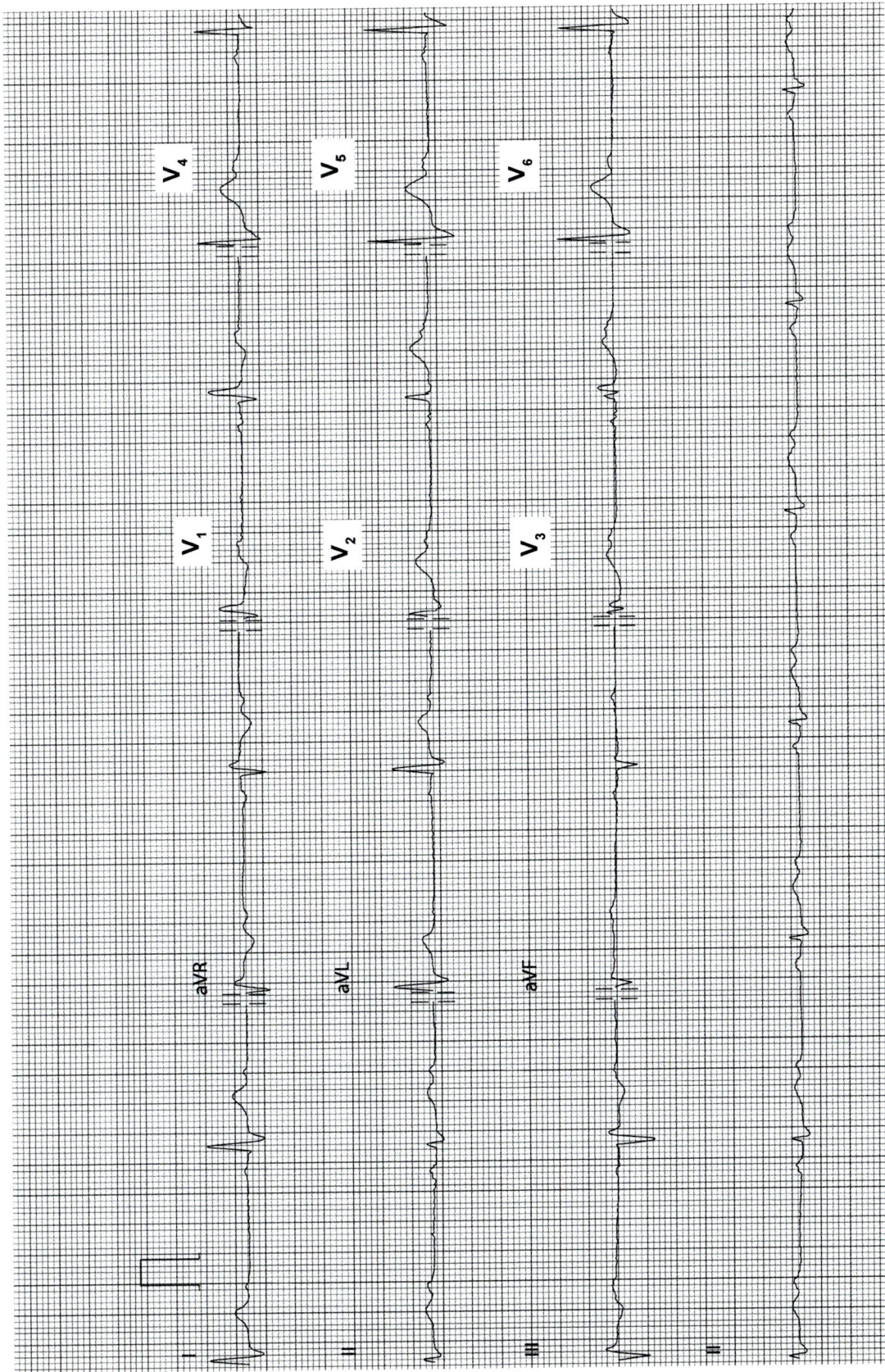

ECG NO. 123

ECG NO. 124

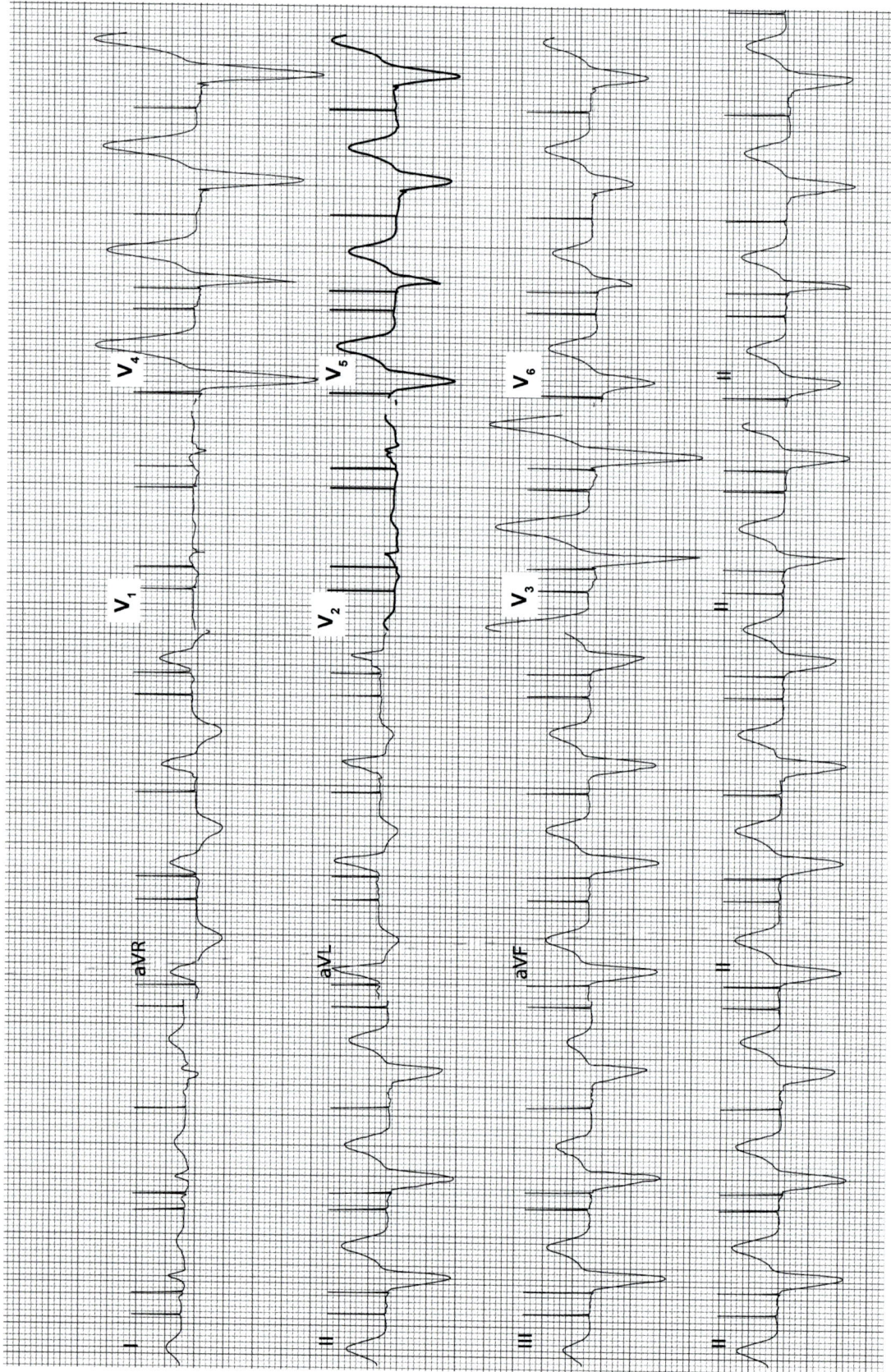

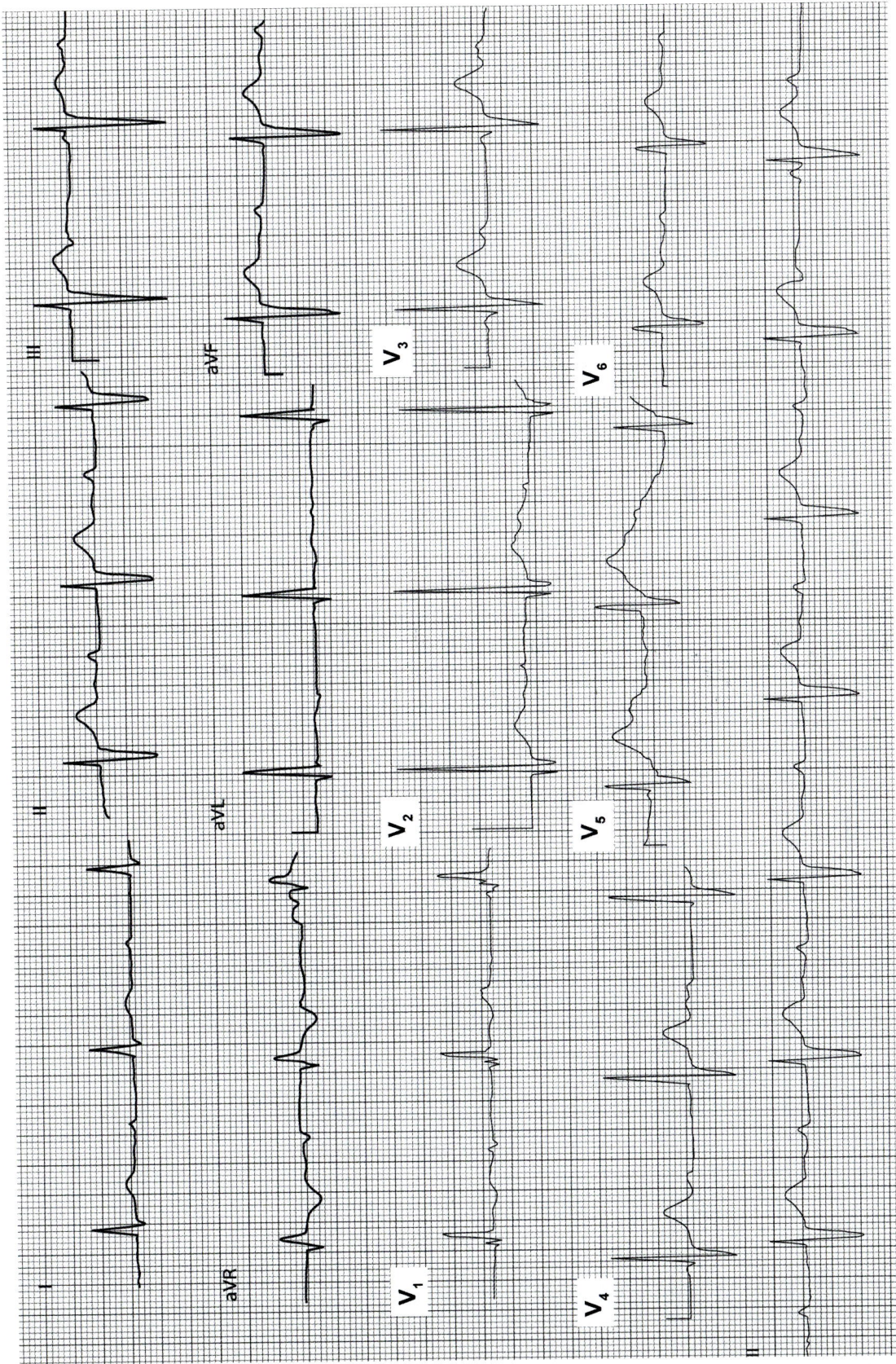

ECG NO. 125

ECG NO. 126

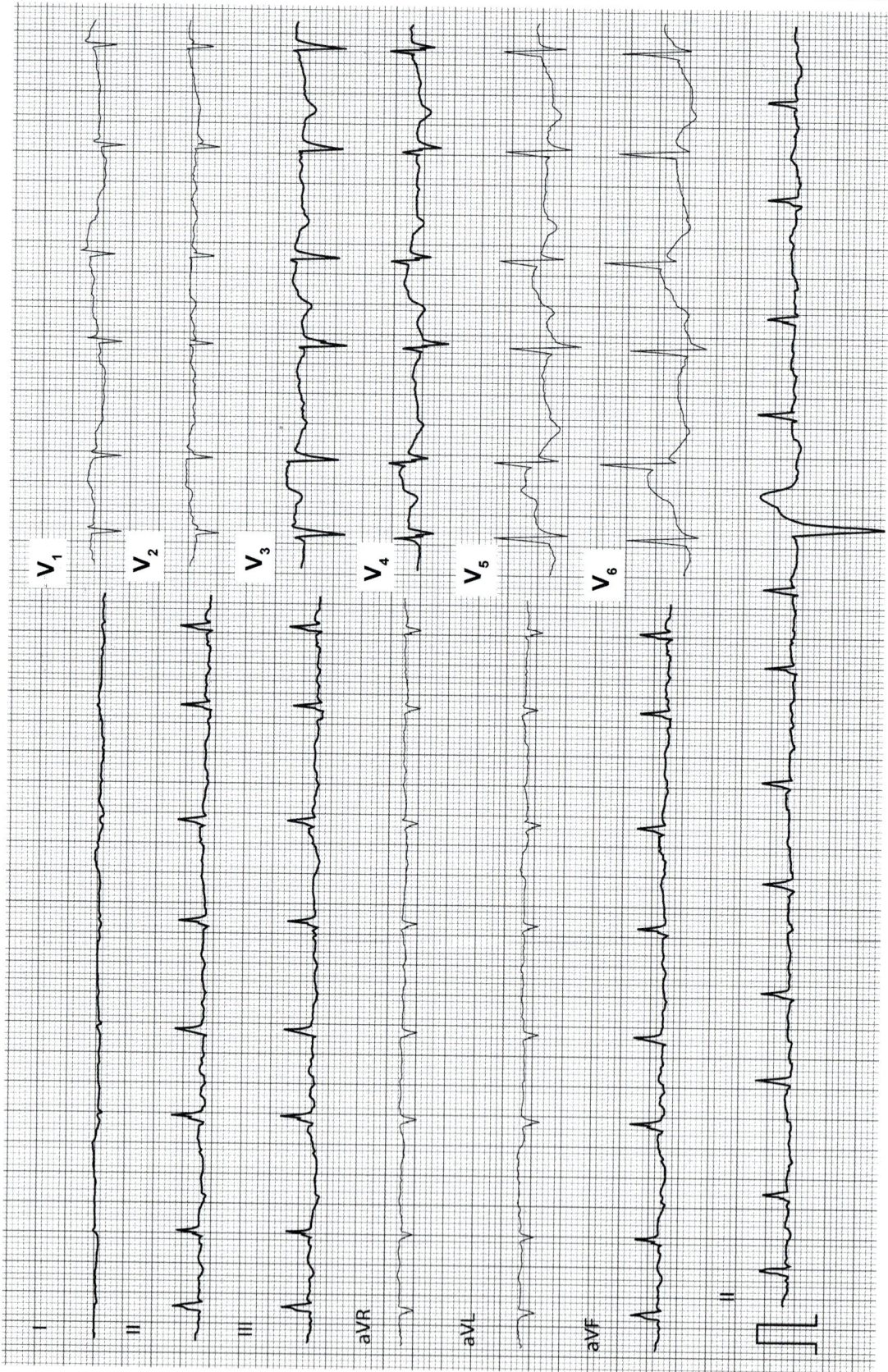

I

II

III

aVR

aVL

aVF

V₁

V₂

V₃

V₄

V₅

V₆

ECG NO. 127

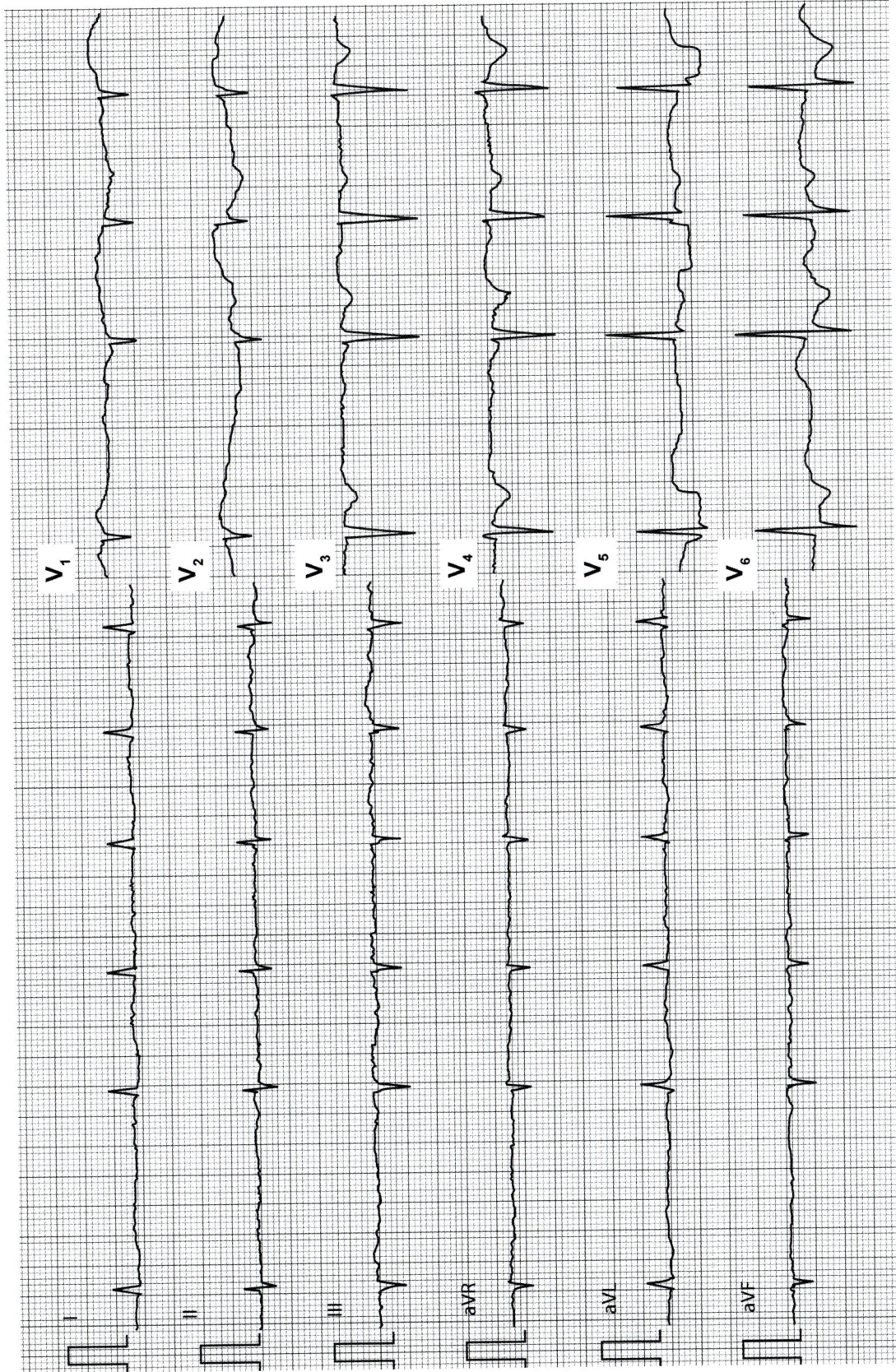

I

II

III

aVR

aVL

aVF

V₁

V₂

V₃

V₄

V₅

V₆

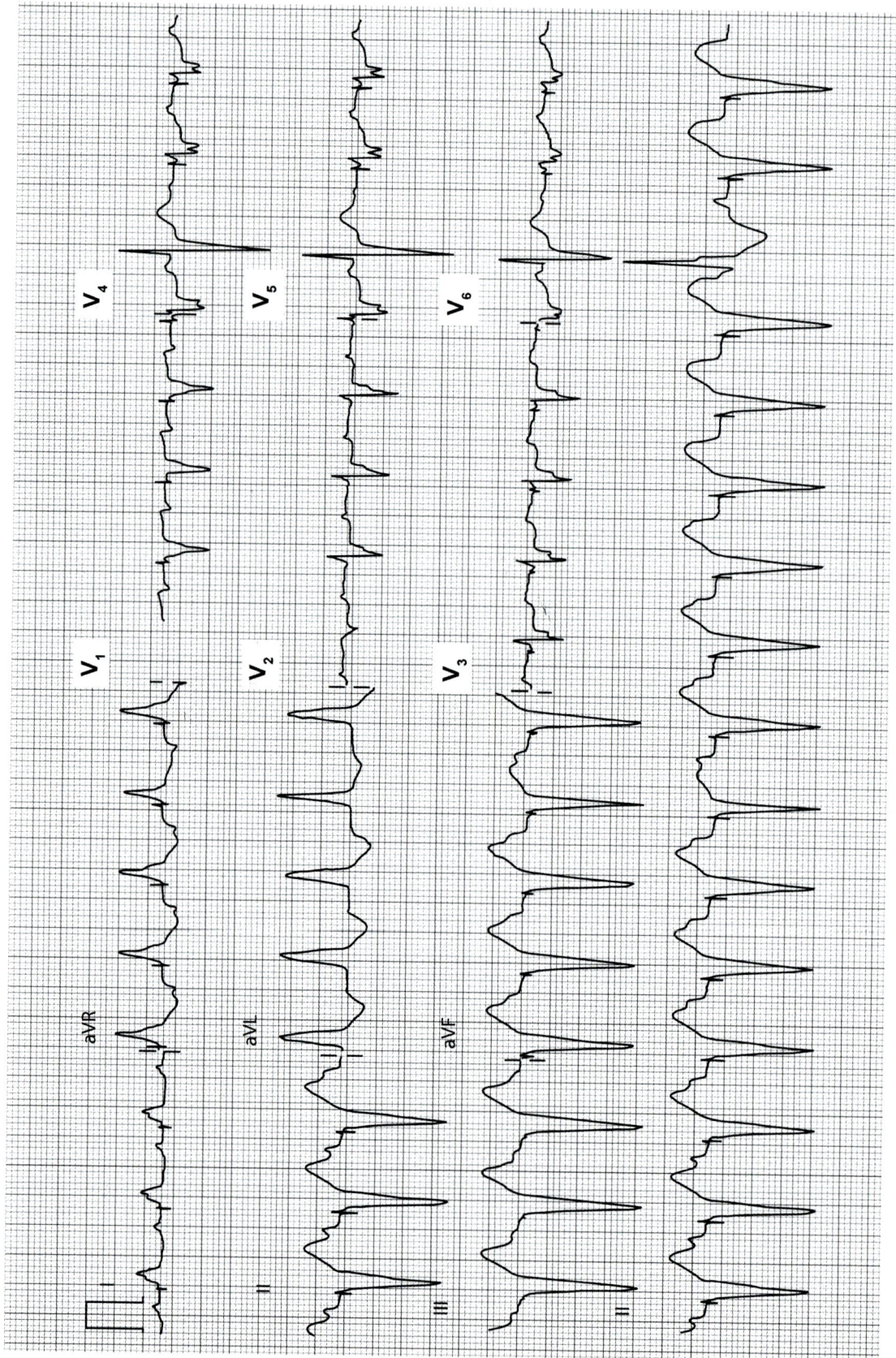

ECG NO. 129

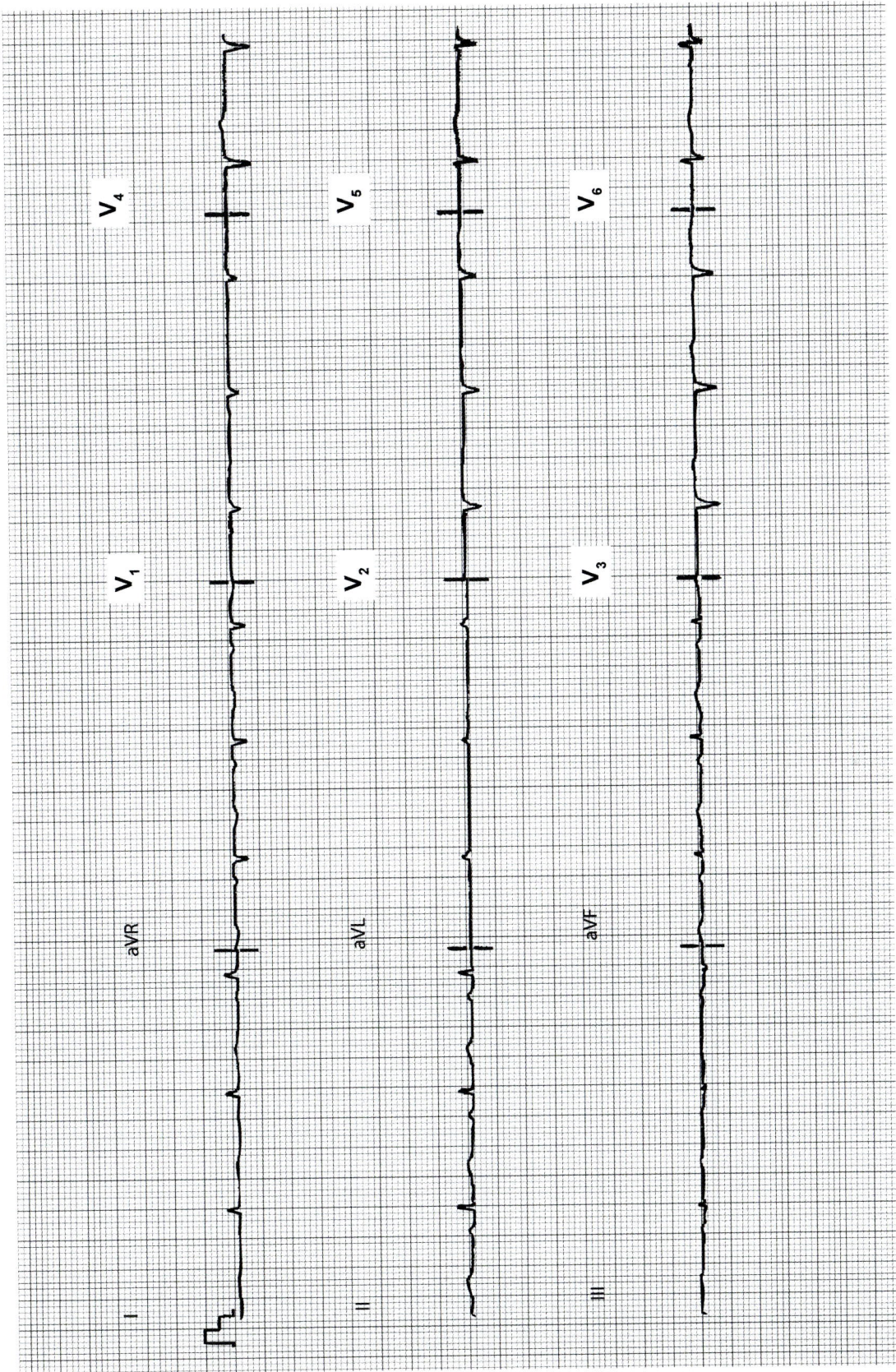

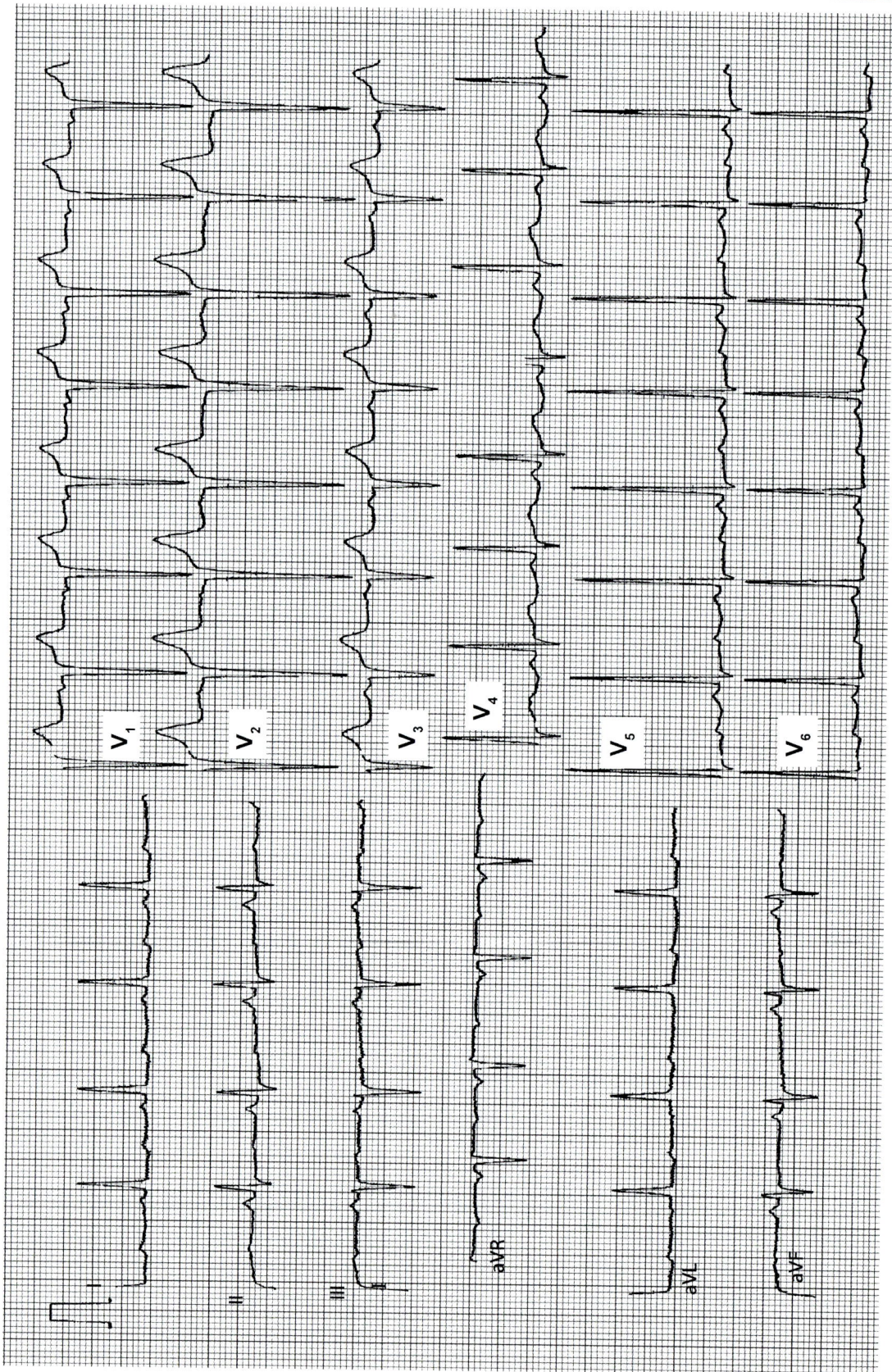

V₁

V₂

V₃

V₄

V₅

V₆

I

II

III

aVR

aVL

aVF

ECG NO. 131

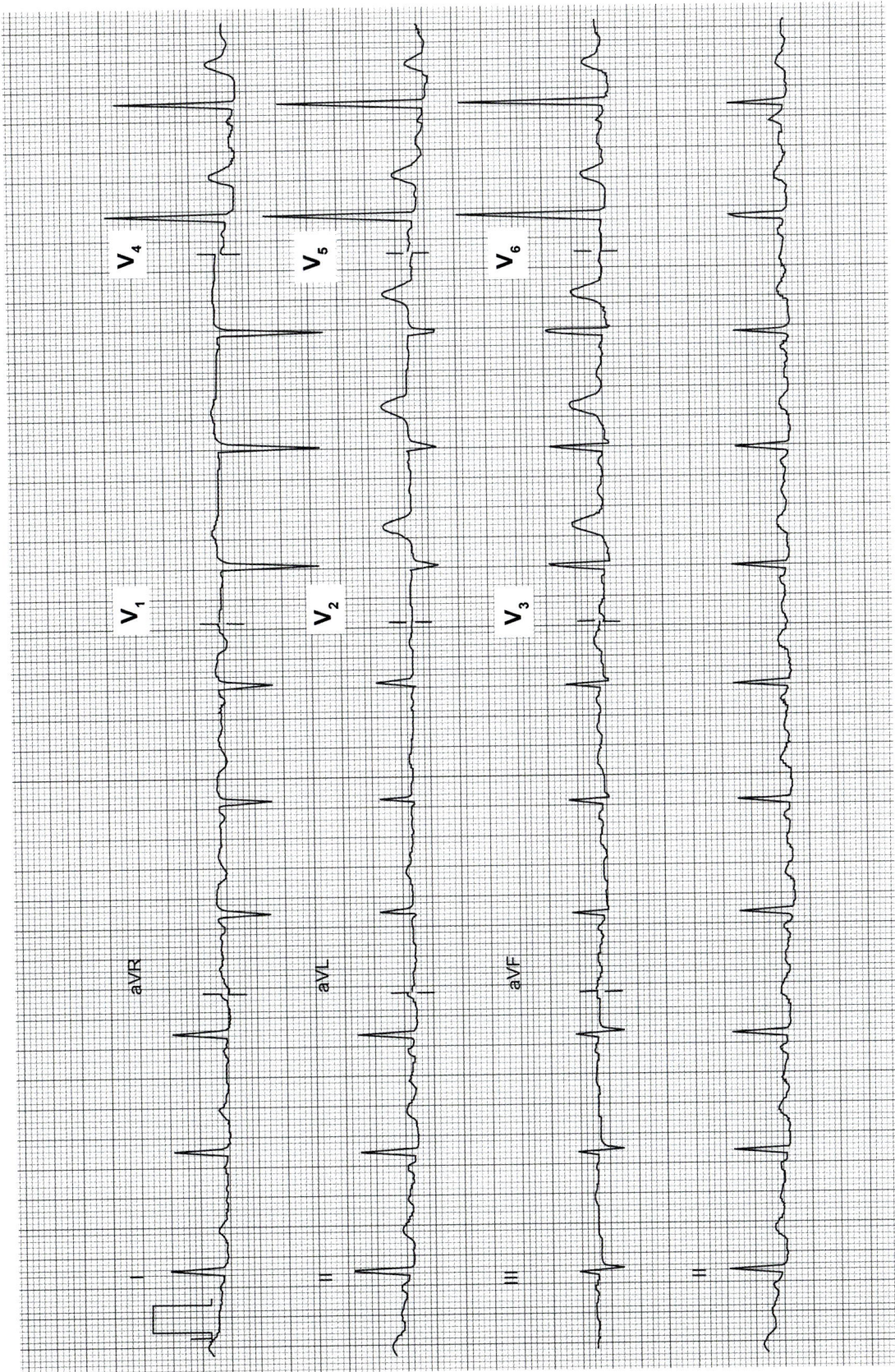

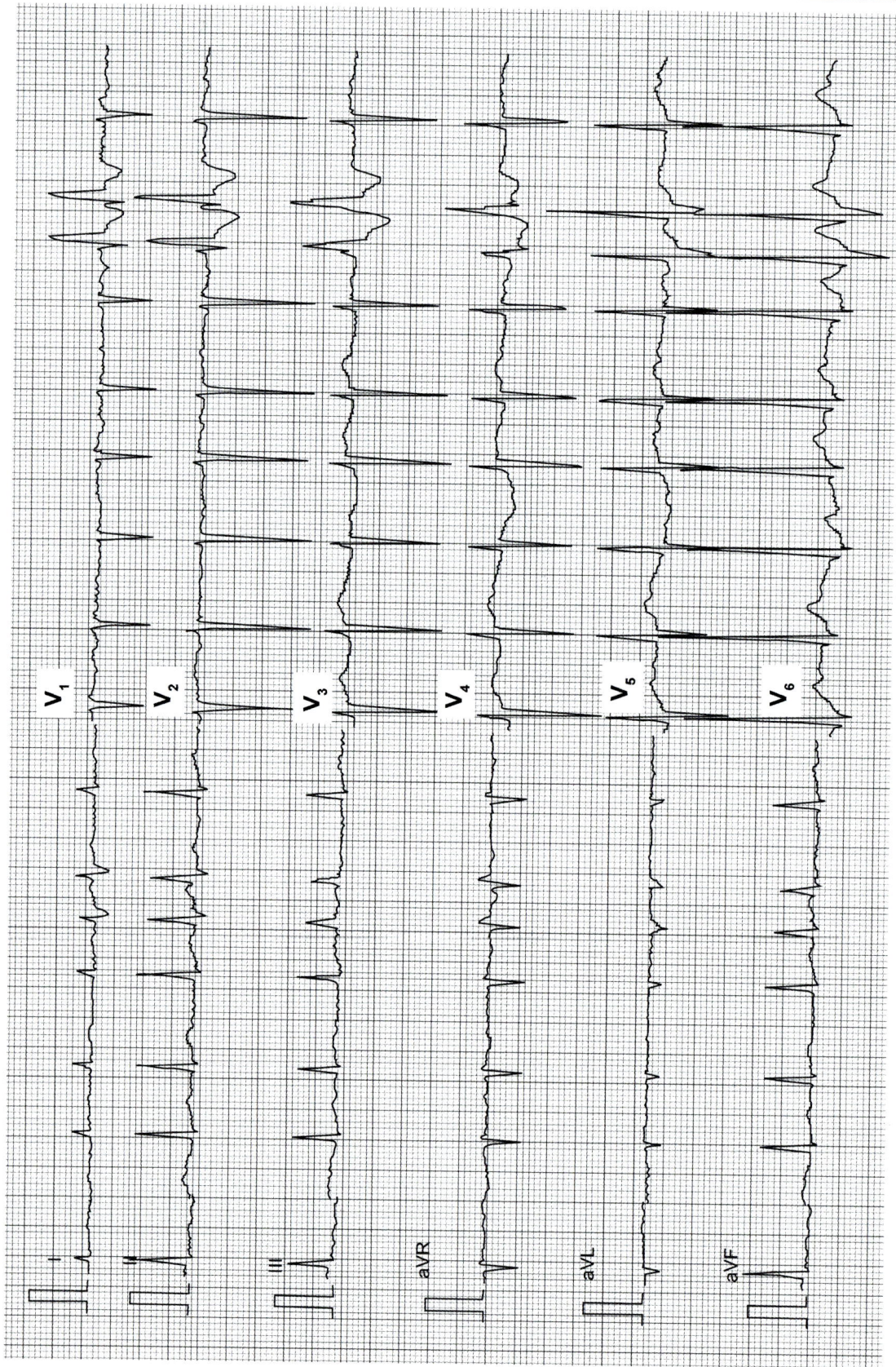

ECG NO. 133

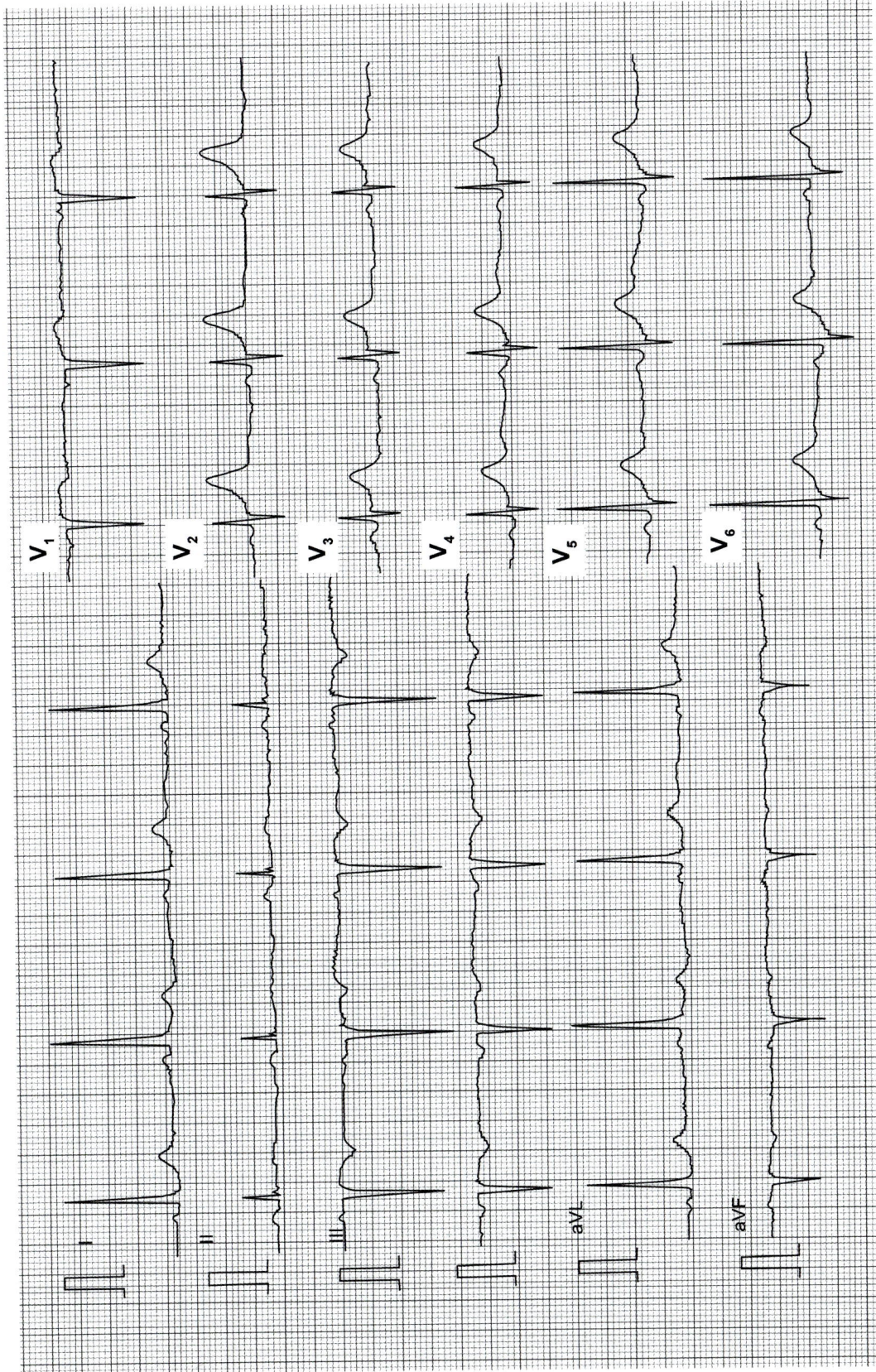

ECG NO. 134

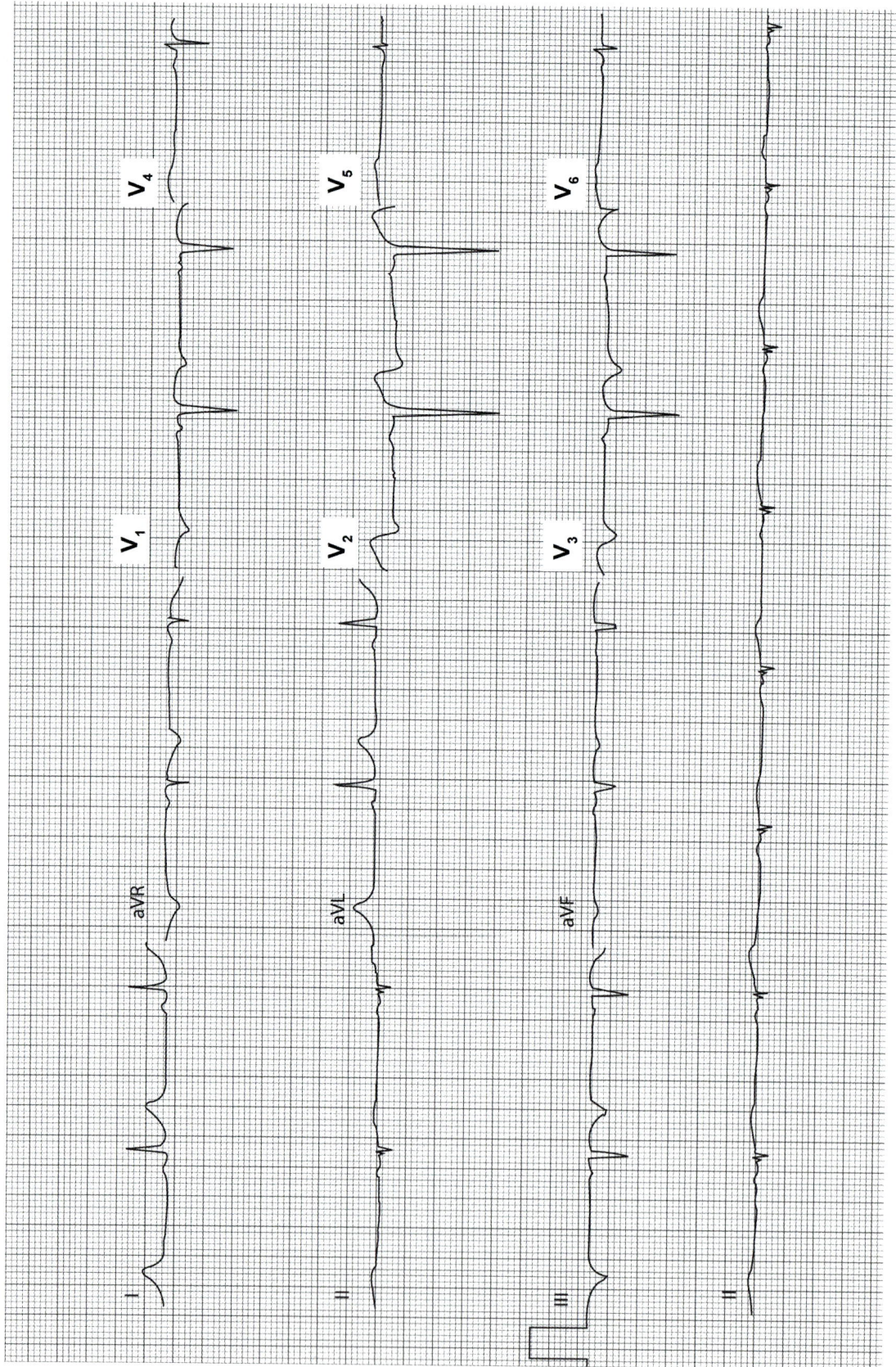

ECG NO. 135

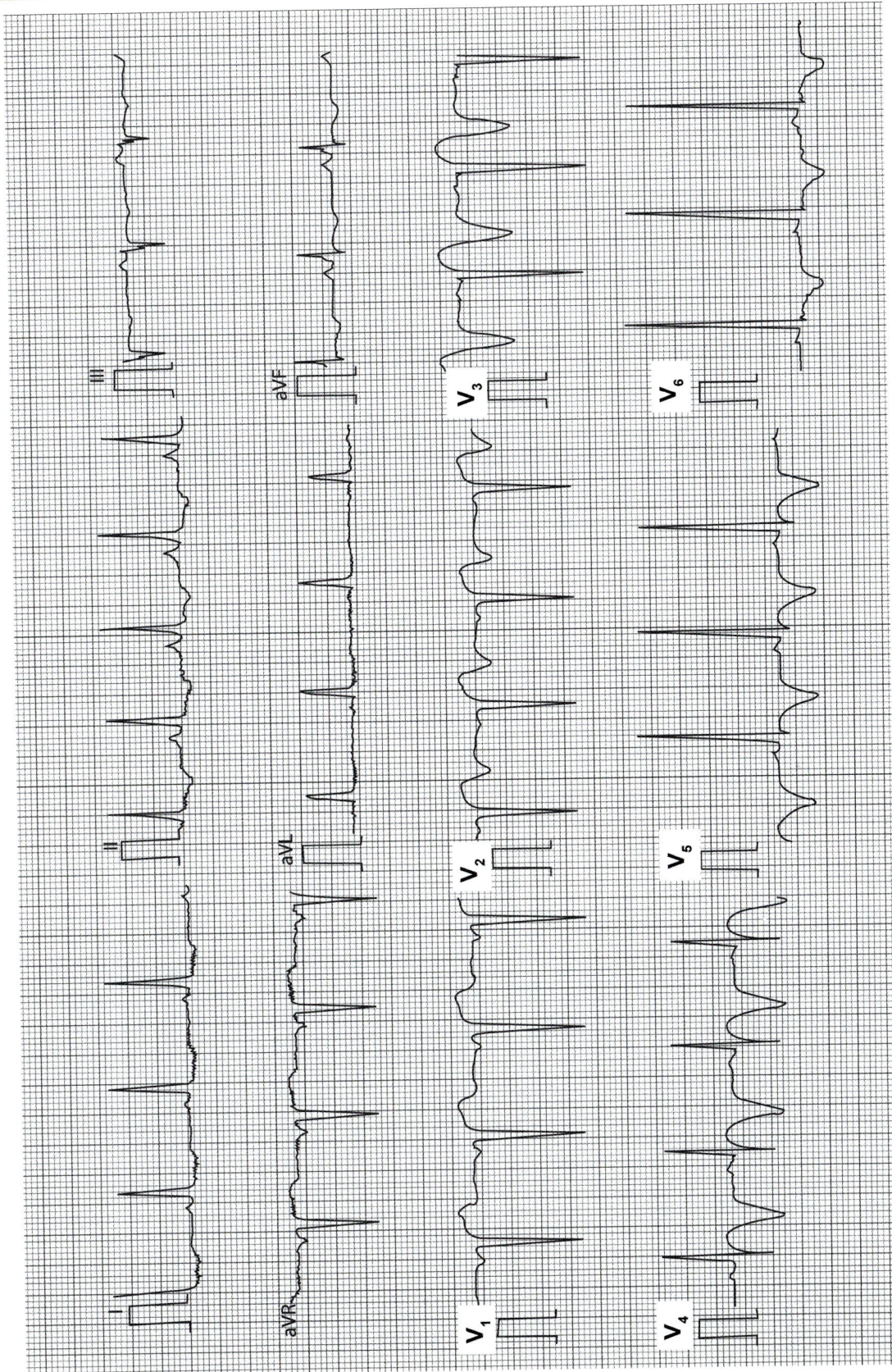

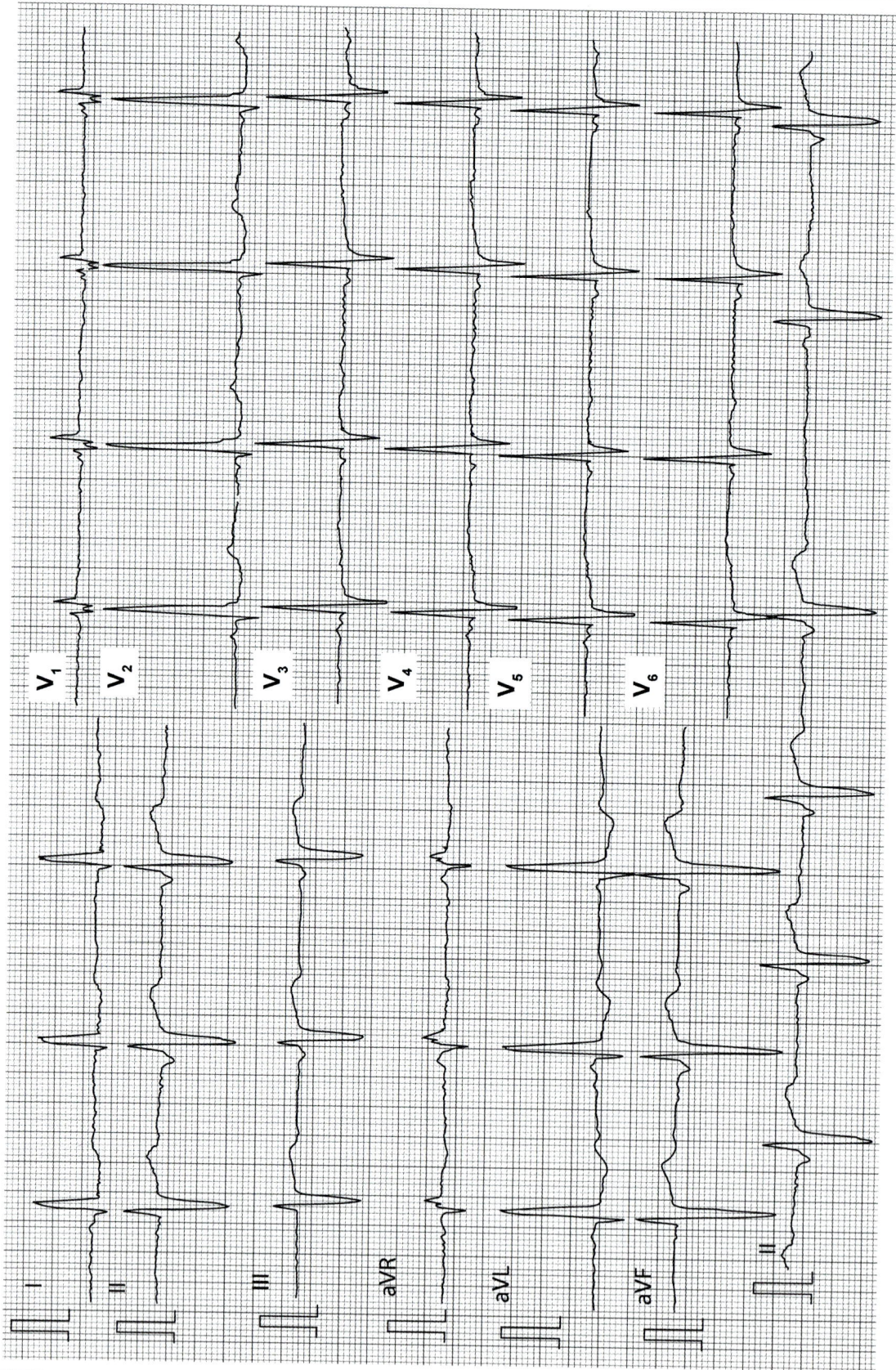

ECG NO. 136

ECG NO. 137

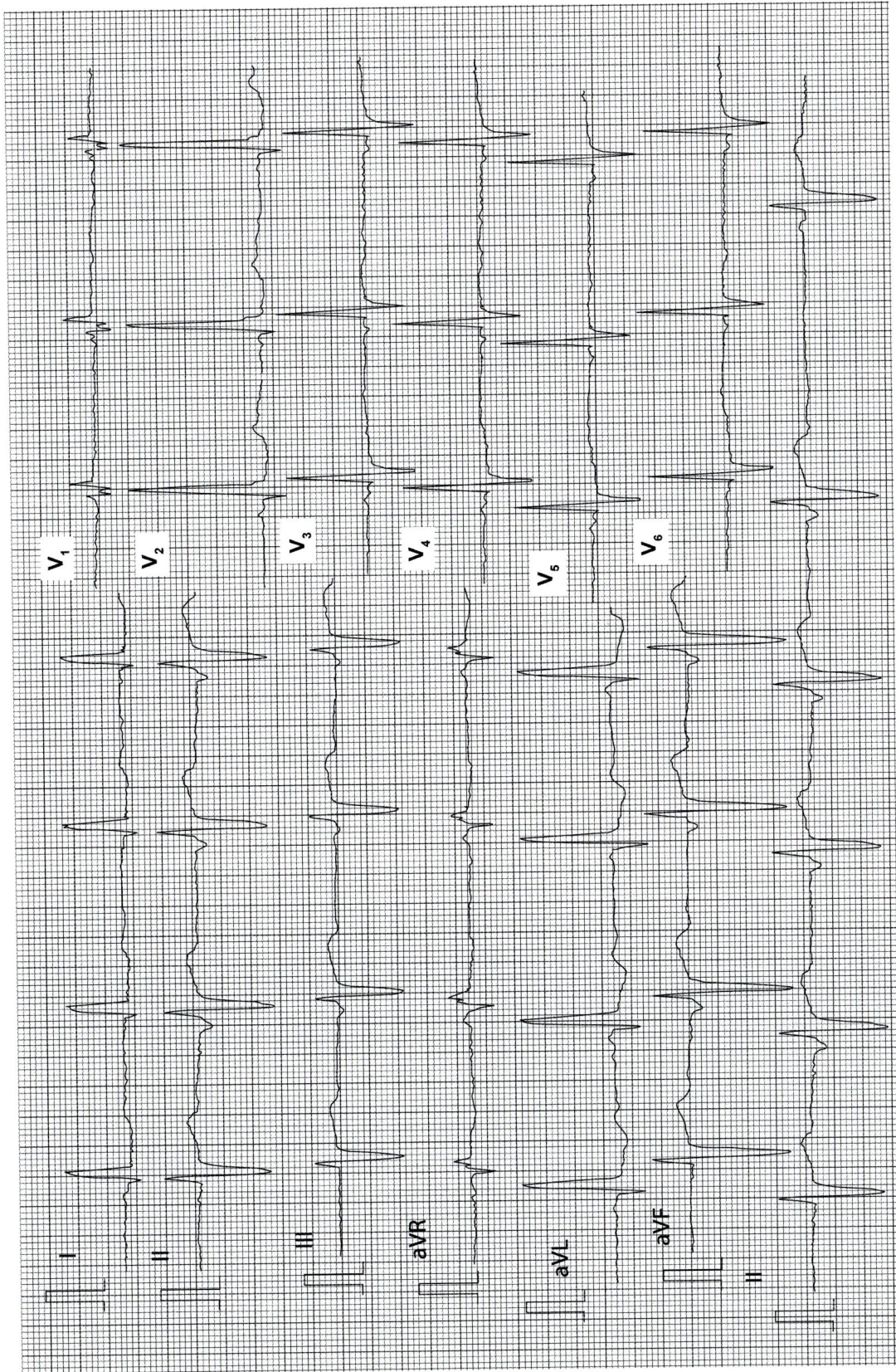

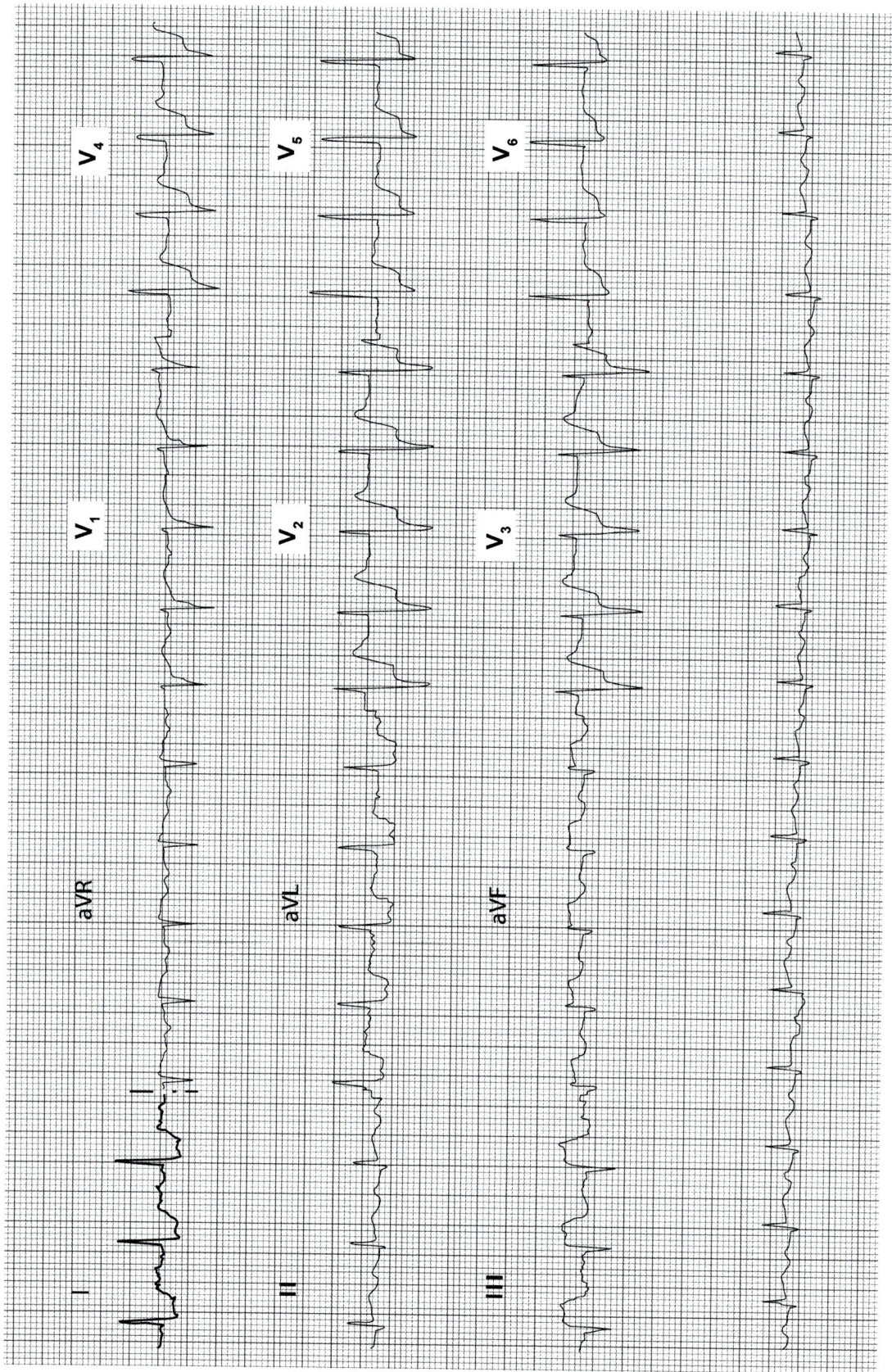

ECG NO. 138

ECG NO. 139

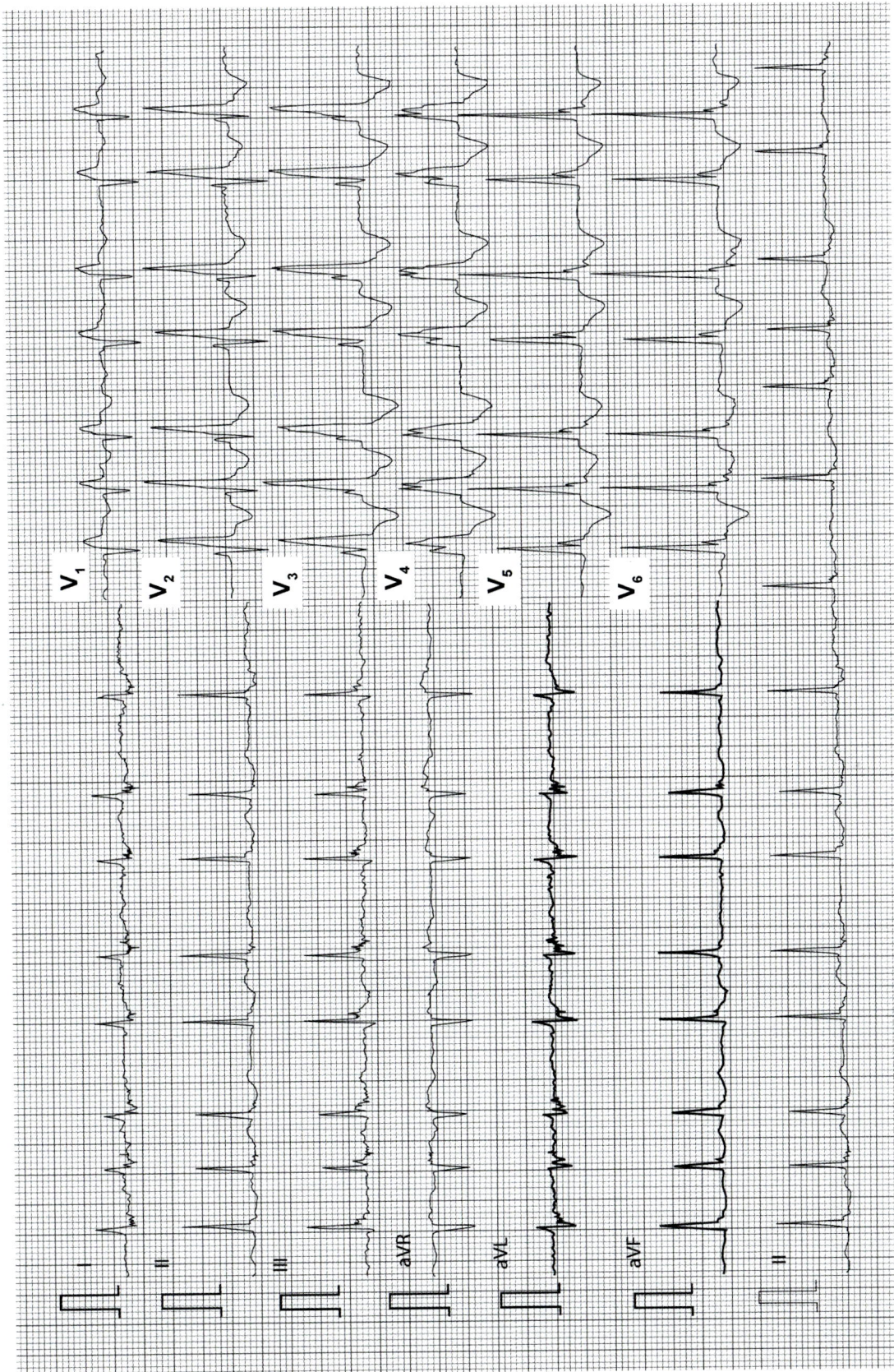

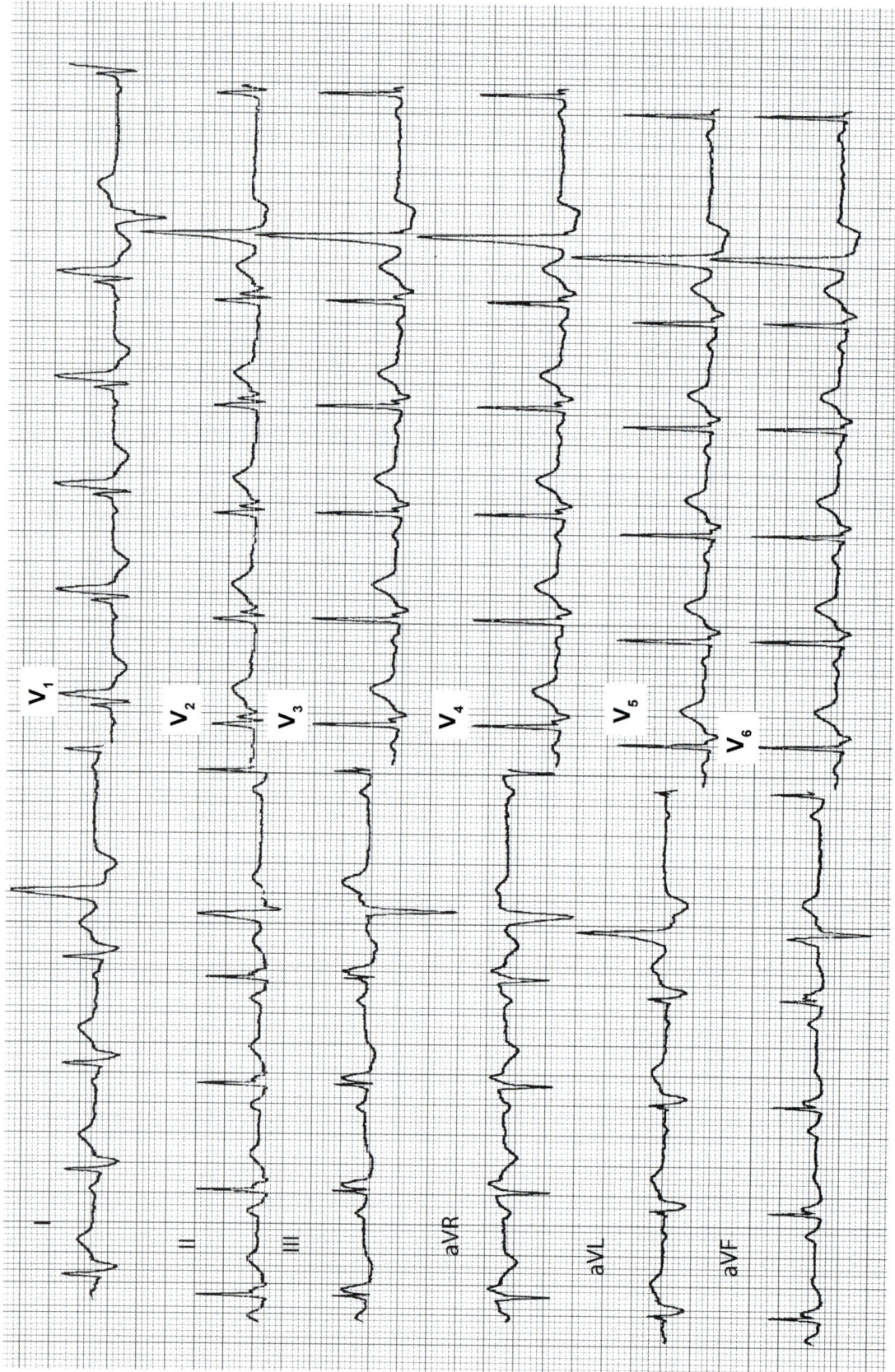

ECG NO. 140

ECG NO. 141

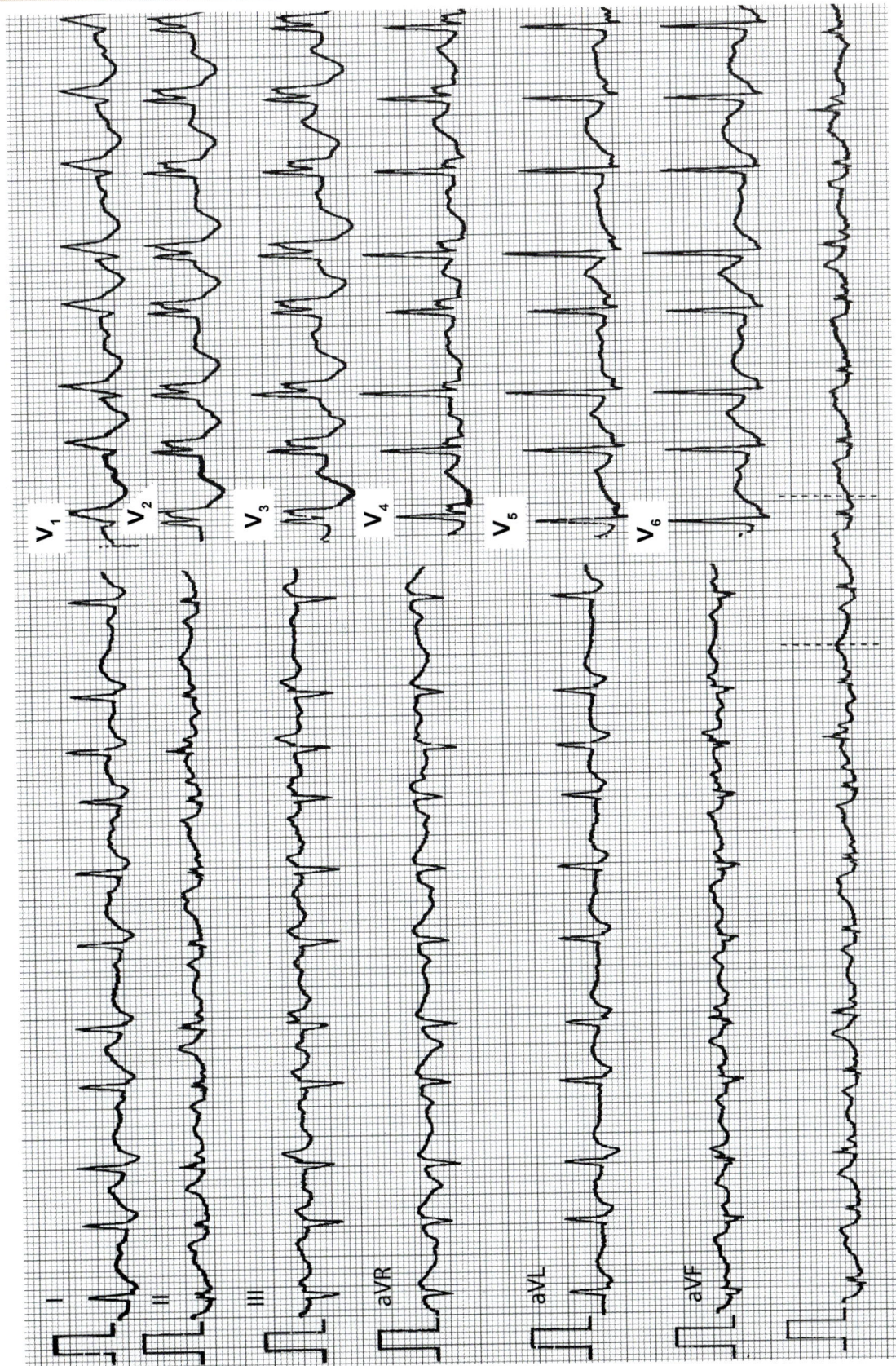

V₁ V₂ V₃ V₄ V₅ V₆

I II III aVR aVL aVF

ECG NO. 142

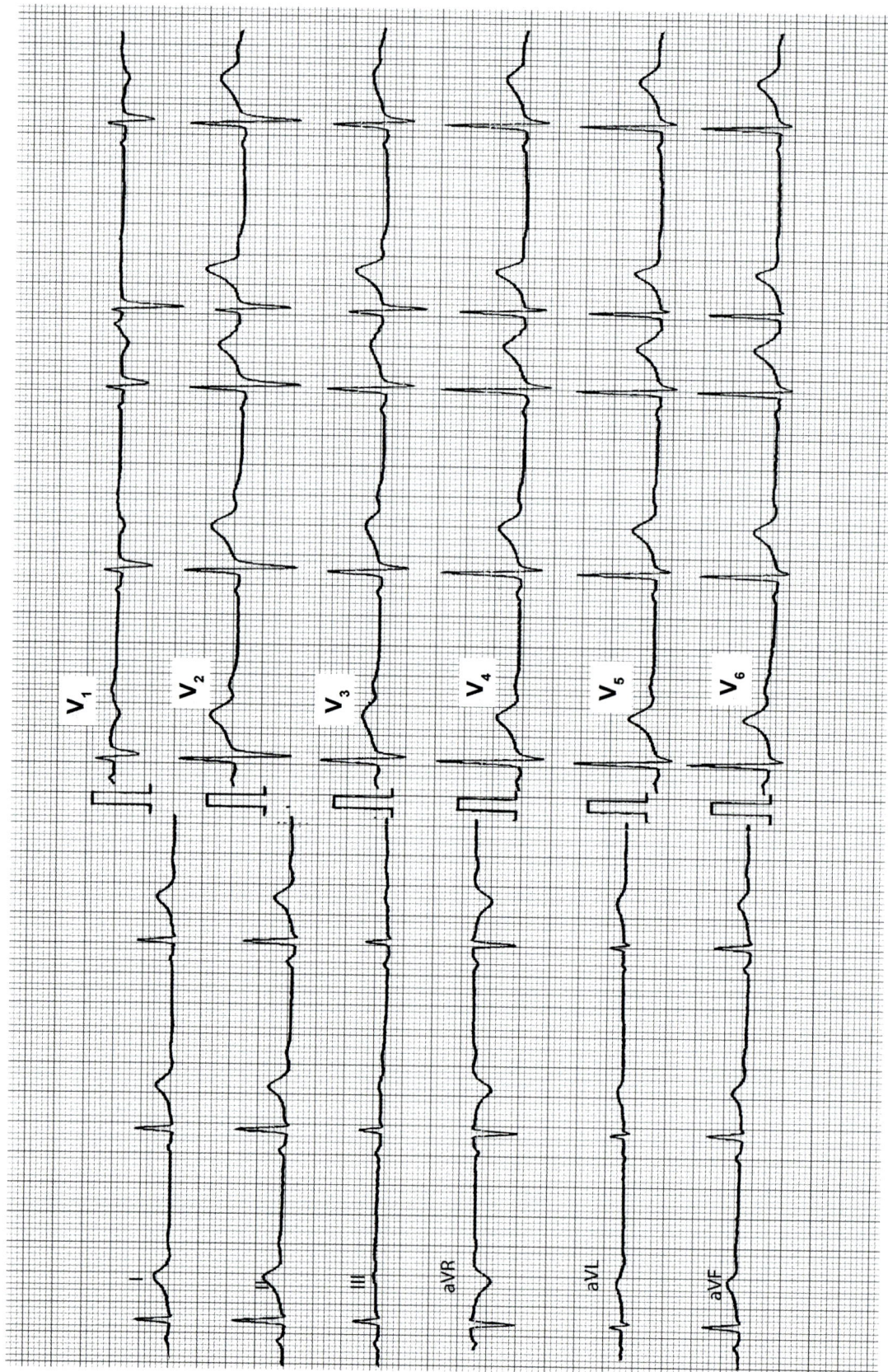

V$_1$

V$_2$

V$_3$

V$_4$

V$_5$

V$_6$

I

III

aVR

aVL

aVF

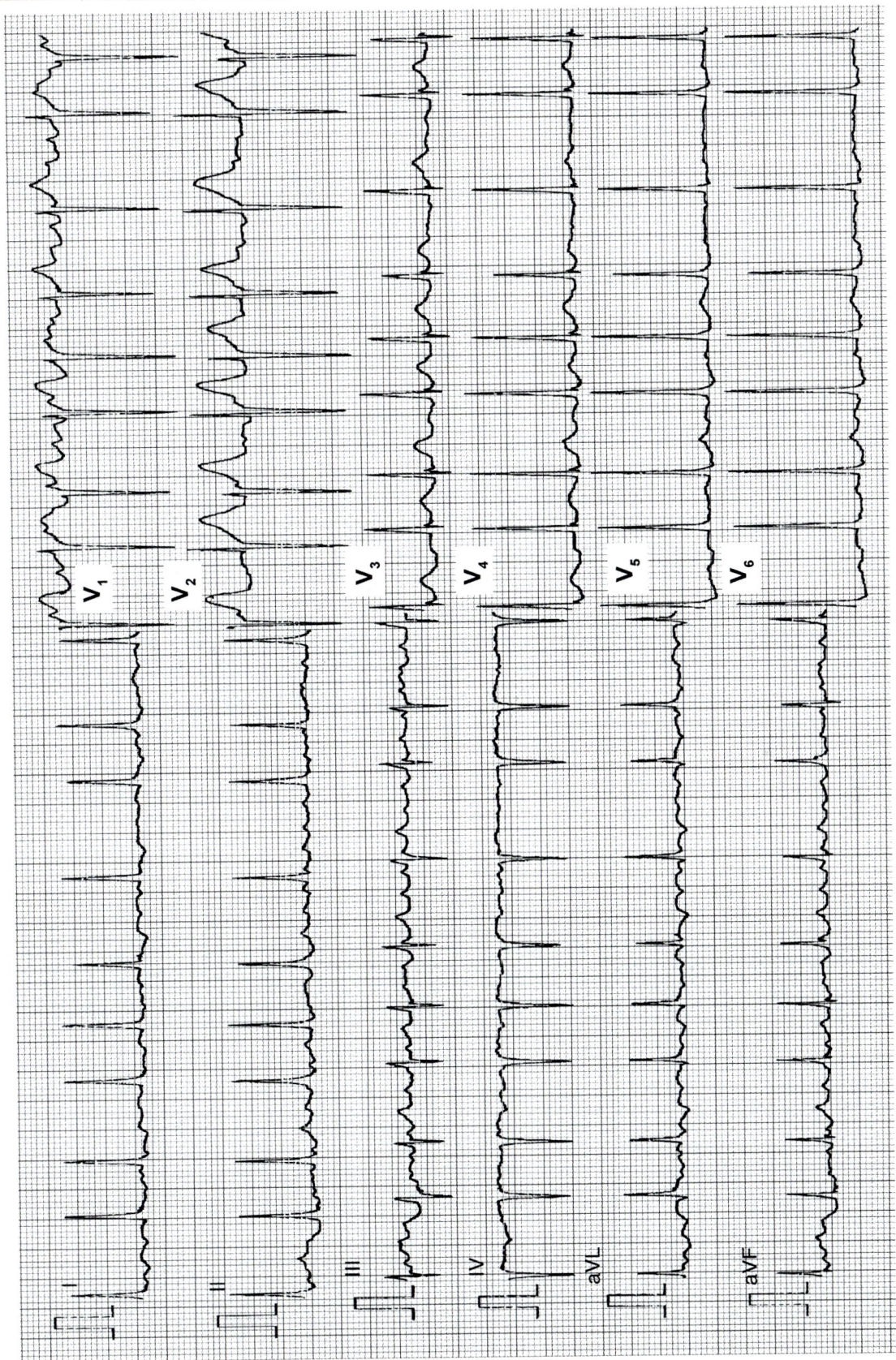

ECG NO. 143

V₁
V₂
V₃
V₄
V₅
V₆

I
II
III
IV
aVL
aVF

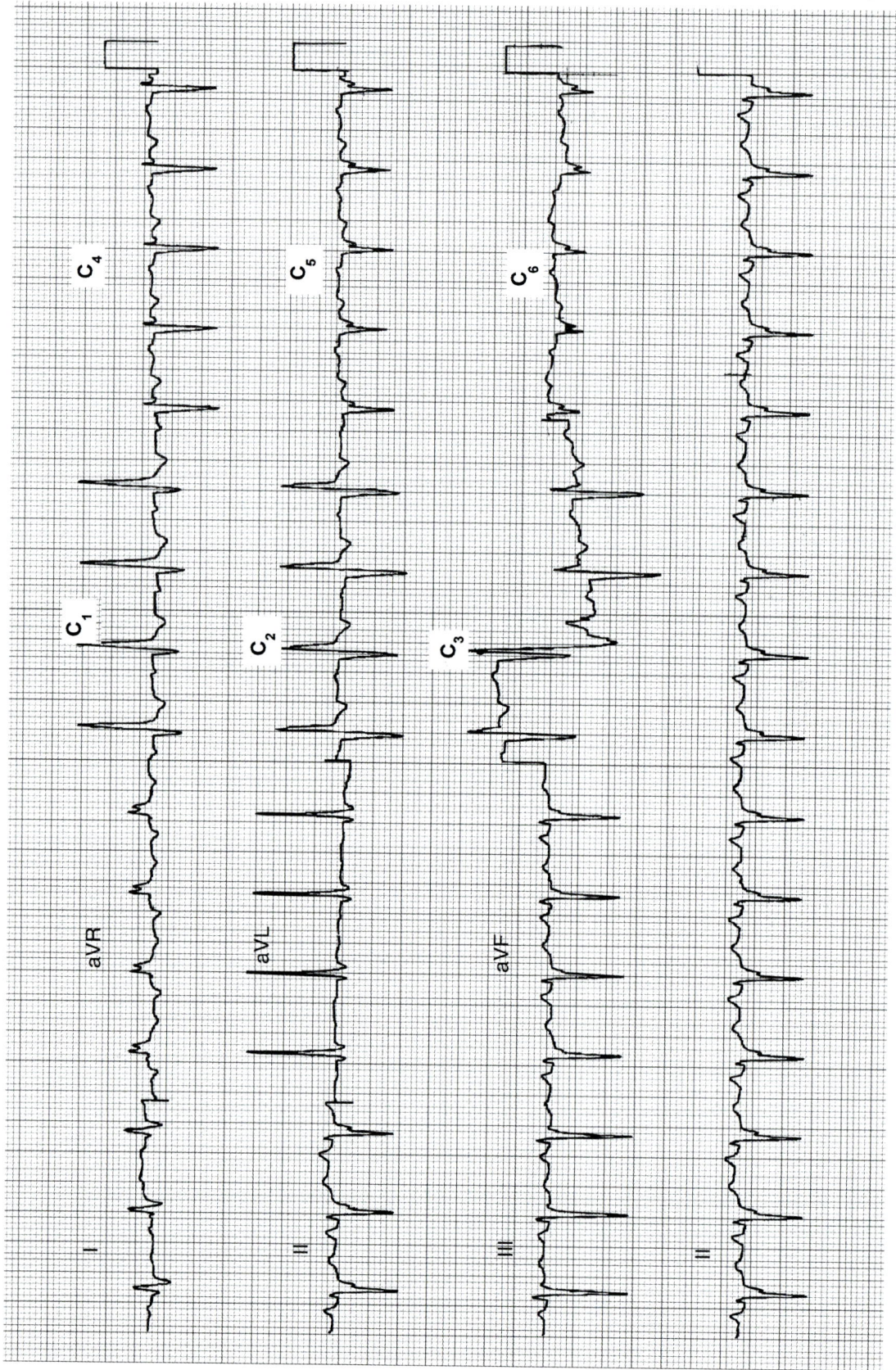

ECG NO. 145

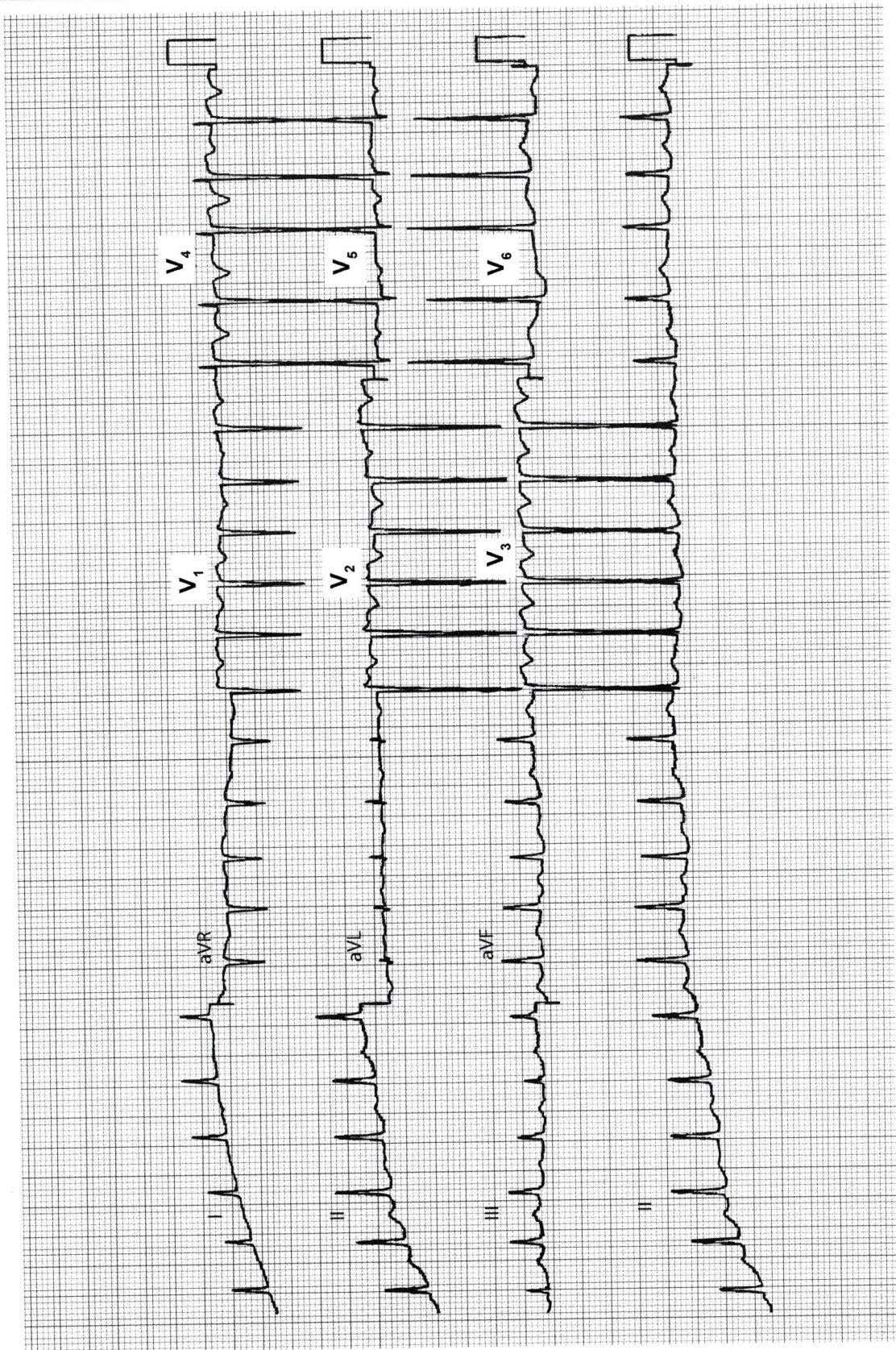

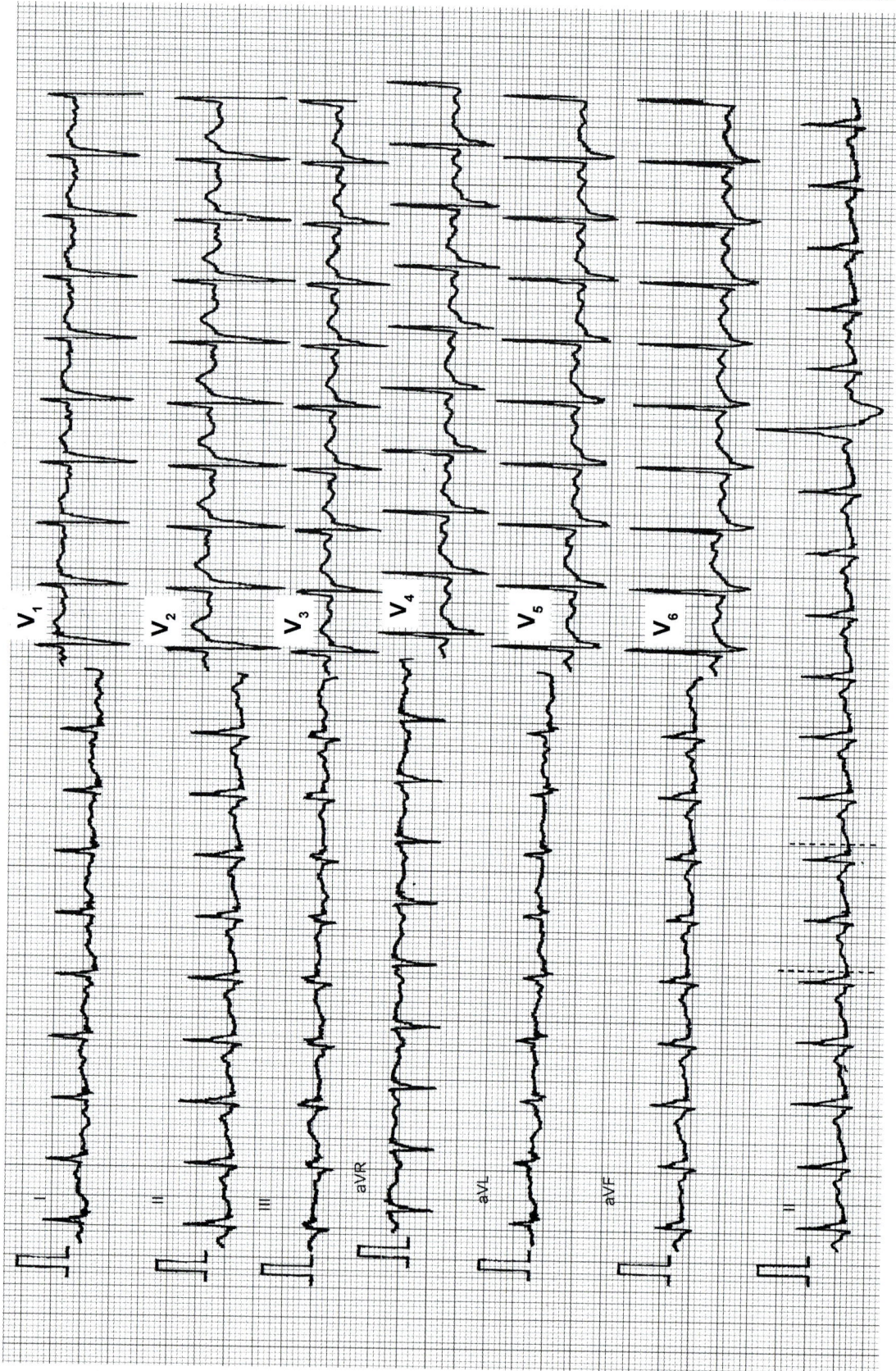

ECG NO. 146

ECG NO. 147

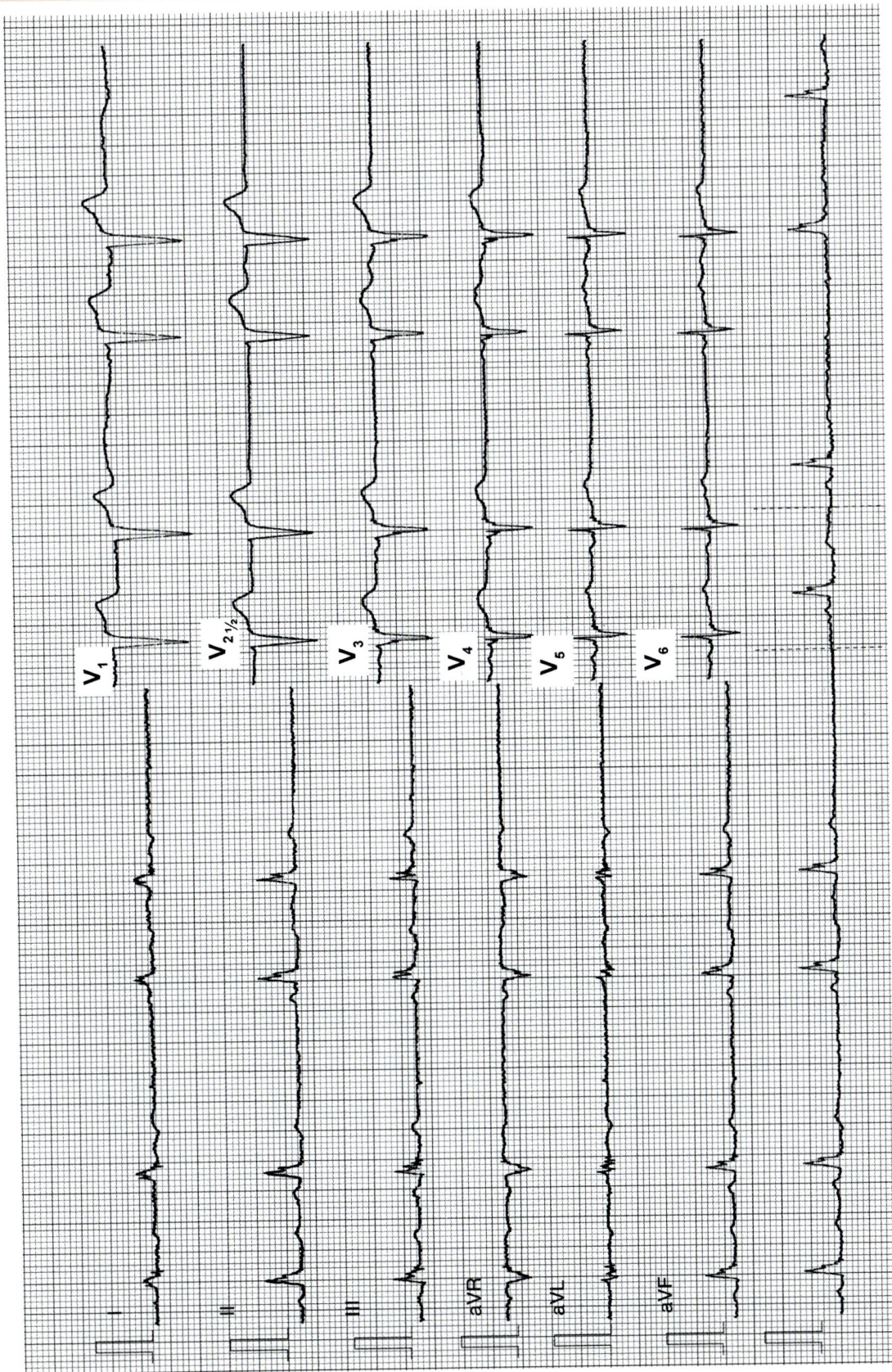

V₁
V₂½
V₃
V₄
V₅
V₆

I
II
III
aVR
aVL
aVF

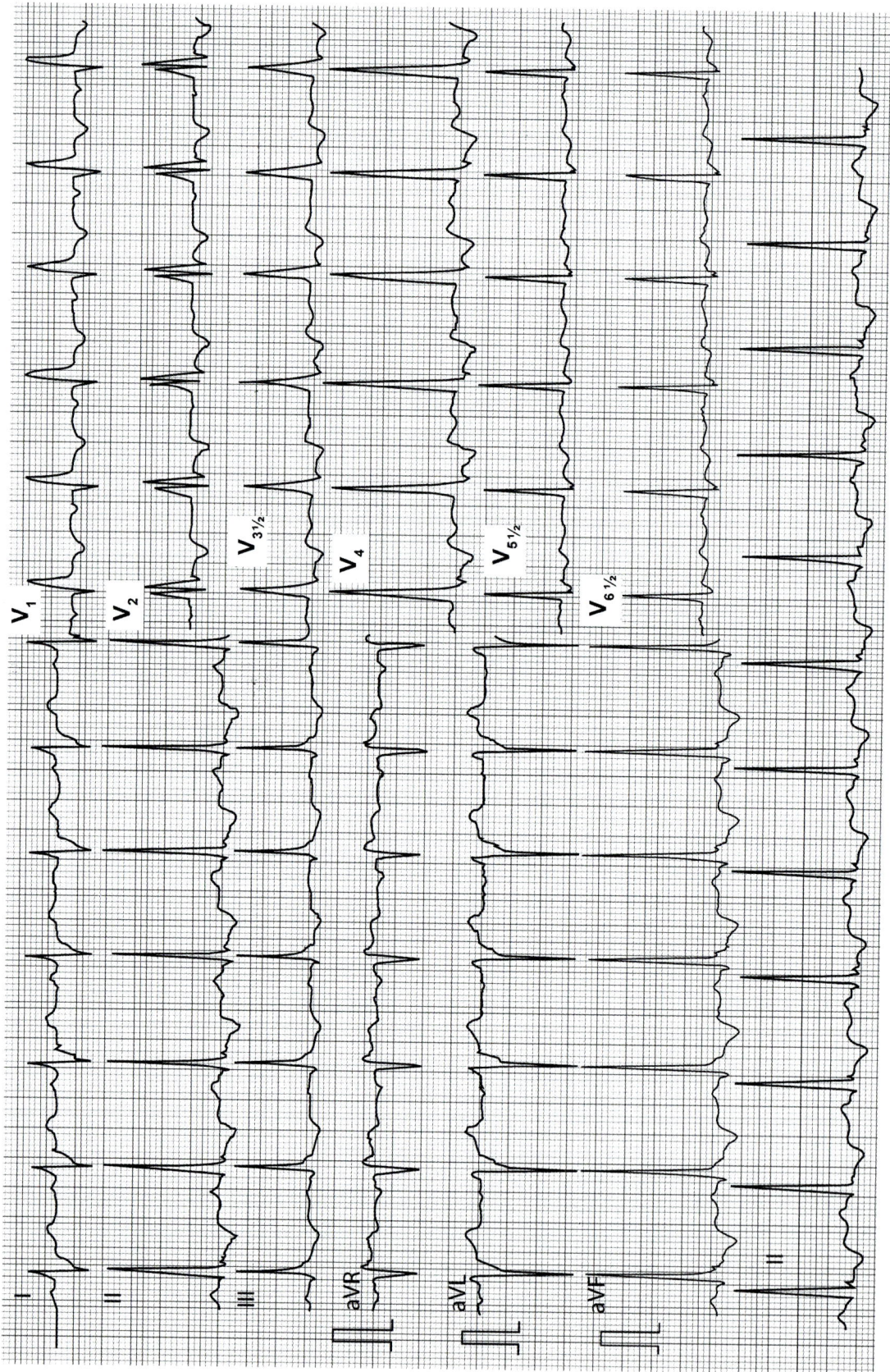

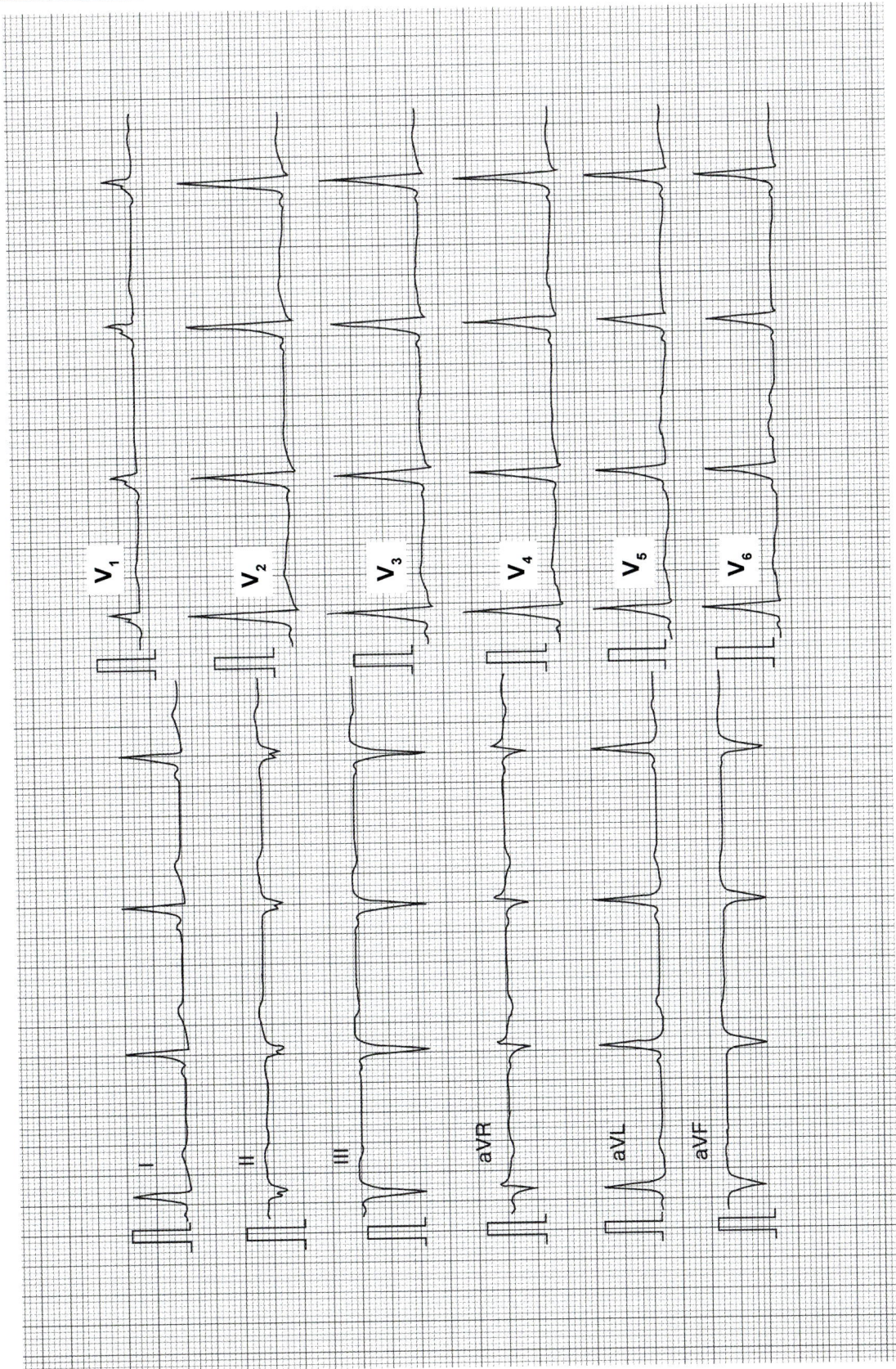

ECG NO. 149

V₁ V₂ V₃ V₄ V₅ V₆

I II III aVR aVL aVF

ECG NO. 150

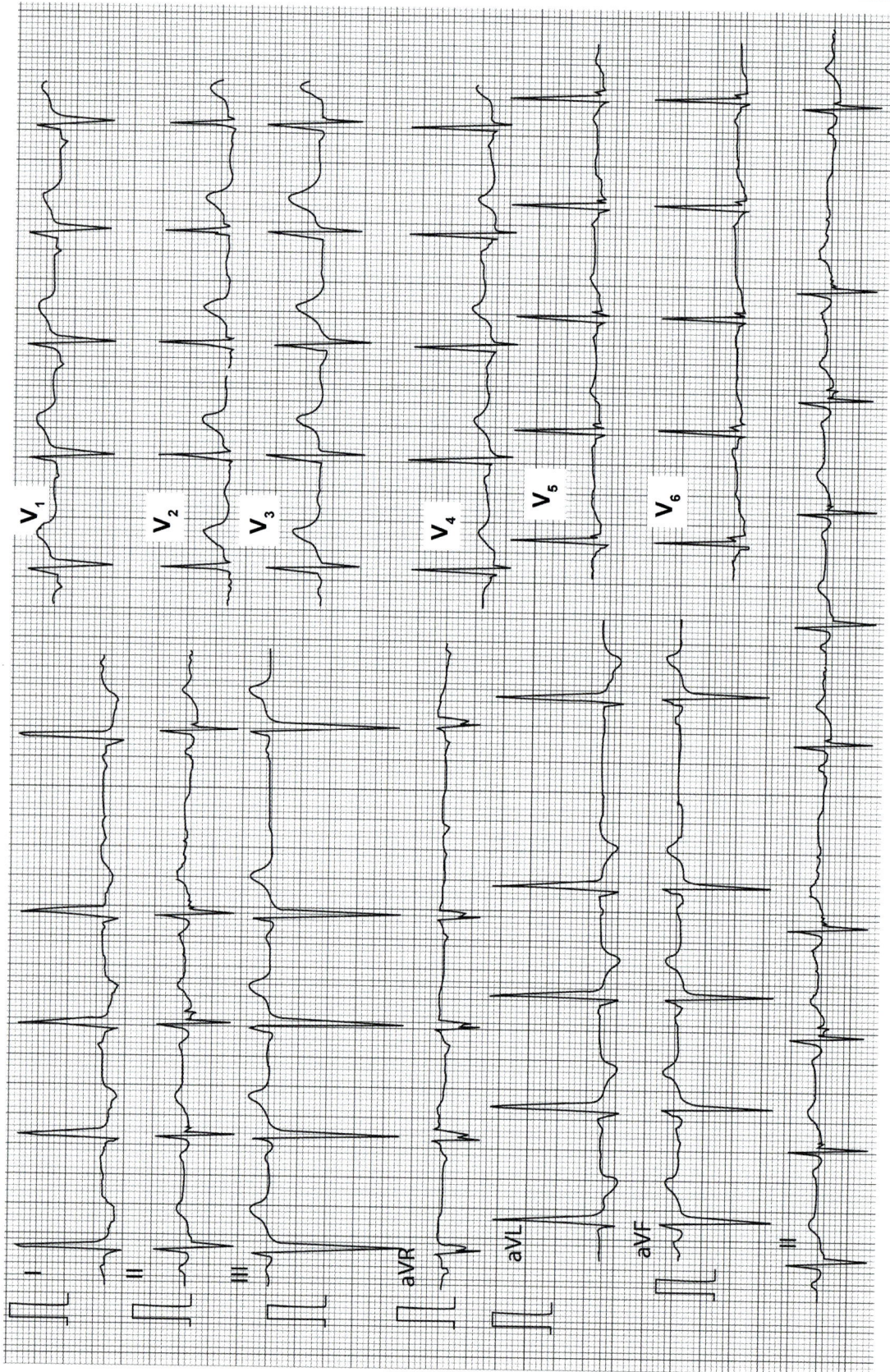

FINDINGS OF ECG TRACINGS

1. This ECG shows:
- Atrial rate—75/min.
- Ventricular rate—50/m.
- There is complete dissociation between P and QRS.

Diagnosis: Complete heart block.

2. This ECG shows:
- P wave—absent.
- RR interval—irregular (rhythm irregular).
- Heart rate >100/minute.

Diagnosis: Fast atrial fibrillation.

3. This ECG shows:
- Pacemaker spike followed by QRS.
- In some leads, there are no spikes which indicates demand pacemaker.

Diagnosis: Demand ventricular pacemaker.

4. This ECG shows:
- Tall R in lead I, deep S/QS in lead III (indicates left axis deviation).
- Pathological Q in lead III and aVF.
- Tall R (19 mm) in aVL (left ventricular hypertrophy).
- U wave in V_4 and V_5.

Diagnosis: Old inferior myocardial infarction, left ventricular hypertrophy with hypokalemia.

5. This ECG shows:
- $SV_1 + RV_6 > 35$ (here 48).
- T inversion in V_2 to V_6.

Diagnosis: Left ventricular hypertrophy with strain.

Q. Is there any other criteria of LVH in this ECG?
Ans. Yes. There is tall R (33 mm) in V_5 (R>25 in V_5 indicates LVH).

Q. What is the differential diagnosis in this type of ECG?
Ans. Hypertrophic cardiomyopathy (echocardiogram should be done to confirm the diagnosis).

6. This ECG shows:
- Heart rate—150/min.
- P, QRS and T—normal.
- Rhythm—regular

Diagnosis: Sinus tachycardia.

7. This ECG shows:
- Heart rate—107/min.
- ST elevation in V_2 to V_5 and pathological Q in V_1 to V_5.
- Pathological Q in lead II, III and aVF.

Diagnosis: Acute anterior and old inferior myocardial infarction with sinus tachycardia.

8. This ECG shows:
- Tall P in lead II and III (P pulmonale).
- Old Q in lead II, III and aVF.
- Tall R in V_1.
- Poor R wave progression in V_5 and V_6.

Diagnosis: Right atrial hypertrophy (P pulmonale) with right ventricular hypertrophy with old inferior myocardial infarction.

9. This ECG shows:
- Short P-R interval (0.08).
- Delta wave in V_2 to V_6.
- Deep S in V_1.
- (Q in lead III and aVF—confuses with old inferior myocardial infarction).

Diagnosis: WPW syndrome type B.

10. This ECG shows:
- P wave—absent.
- Rhythm is irregular (R-R interval is irregular).
- ST depression in lead I, II, V_4 to V_6 (thumb impression or reversed tick appearance).

Diagnosis: Atrial fibrillation with digoxin effect.

11. This ECG shows:
- ST elevation in V_2 to V_4.
- Pathological Q in V_1 to V_4.
- T inversion in lead I, aVL, V_2 to V_6.

Diagnosis: Acute anteroseptal myocardial infarction.

12. This ECG shows:
- ST elevation in V_2 to V_6.
- Pathological Q in V_1 to V_6.

Diagnosis: Acute extensive anterior myocardial infarction.

13. This ECG shows:
- Tall R in lead I and deep S in lead III (indicates left axis deviation).
- Deep T inversion in V_2 to V_6.

- Also T inversion in lead I, II and aVL.

Diagnosis: Subendocardial myocardial infarction (also left axis deviation and lateral ischemia).

14. This ECG shows:
- Pacemaker spike in V_4 to V_6.
- No spike in other leads.

Diagnosis: Demand ventricular pacemaker.

15. This ECG shows:
- Pacemaker spike in almost all the leads.

Diagnosis: Ventricular pacemaker.

16. This ECG shows:
- P wave—absent.
- Flutter wave in V_1 to V_3.
- Rhythm—irregular
- Ventricular ectopic (in some leads).

Diagnosis: Atrial flutter fibrillation with multiple ventricular ectopics.

17. This ECG shows:
- P wave—absent.
- QRS normal and narrow.
- Rhythm—irregular (RR irregular).
- Rate—high >100/minute

Diagnosis: Fast atrial fibrillation.

Differential Diagnosis: SVT with variable block.

18. This ECG shows:
- M pattern (RSR' pattern) in V_5 to V_6.
- QRS—wide (0.16 second).
- Pathological Q in V_1 to V_3 (may be old antero-septal myocardial infarction).

Diagnosis: Left bundle branch block.

19. This ECG shows:
- M pattern (RSR' pattern) in V_5 to V_6.
- QRS—wide (0.16 second).
- Pathological Q in V_1 to V_2 (may be old myocardial infarction).

Diagnosis: Left bundle branch block.

20. This ECG shows:
- Multiple ventricular ectopics.
- Ventricular bigeminy pattern (every normal beat followed by an ectopic).
- Pathological Q in lead II, III, aVF and in V_1 to V_3.

Diagnosis: Old inferior and anteroseptal myocardial infarction with multiple ventricular ectopics (bigeminy pattern).

21. This ECG shows:
- PP interval–120/min, regular.
- RR interval—58/min, regular.
- There is dissociation between P and QRS.

Diagnosis: Complete heart block.

22. This ECG shows:
- ST elevation in V_1 to V_5 with upward convexity.
- P-absent and rhythm is irregular in II, III, aVL and aVF.

Diagnosis: Acute anterior myocardial infarction with paroxysmal atrial fibrillation.

23. This ECG shows:
- Tall R in lead III and deep S in lead I (indicates left axis deviation).
- Tall P in lead II (indicates right atrial hypertrophy)
- Tall R in V_1 and V_2.
- Multiple ventricular ectopics.

Diagnosis: Right ventricular hypertrophy with right atrial hypertrophy with multiple ventricular ectopics.

24. This ECG shows:
- Pathological Q in lead II, III and aVF.
- Tall R in V_1.
- Wide QRS (0.16 sec) and M pattern in V_2.
- Ventricular ectopics.
- Poor R wave progression in V_5 and V_6.

Diagnosis: Old inferior myocardial infarction with right bundle branch block with ventricular ectopics.

25. This ECG shows:
- Pathological Q in lead II, III and aVF with ST elevation in lead III and aVF.
- Atrial rate (PP interval)—100/min.
- Ventricular rate (RR interval)—50/min.
- Complete dissociation between P and QRS.

Diagnosis: Acute inferior myocardial infarction with complete heart block.

26. This ECG shows:
- Wide P (P mitrale) in lead II.
- P wave is absent in some leads.
- Rhythm is irregular.
- Multiple ventricular ectopics.

Diagnosis: Left atrial hypertrophy (mitral stenosis) with atrial fibrillation with multiple ventricular ectopics.

27. This ECG shows:
    - Low voltage tracing.
    - P wave is absent.
    - There are some fibrillary f waves in lead I and II.
    - Rhythm—irregular.
    - Pathological Q in V_1 to V_4.

Diagnosis: Old anteroseptal myocardial infarction with atrial fibrillation with low voltage tracing.

28. This ECG shows:
    - Multiple ventricular ectopics.
    - Tall R in lead I, deep S in lead III (indicates left axis deviation).
    - RSR′ / M pattern in V_1 to V_3.

Diagnosis: Right bundle branch block with left anterior hemiblock (bifascicular block) with multiple ventricular ectopics.

29. This ECG shows:
    - P wave is absent, some fibrillary f waves in lead III.
    - Rhythm is irregular.
    - Few flutter waves in V_1.
    - Left ventricular hypertrophy (voltage is half in V_2 to V_6).

Diagnosis: Atrial flutter fibrillation with left ventricular hypertrophy.

30. This ECG shows:
    - Pathological Q and ST elevation in V_1 to V_3.

Diagnosis: Acute anteroseptal myocardial infarction.

31. This ECG shows:
    - ST elevation in lead III and aVF.
    - RSR′/ M pattern in V_1 and V_2 with wide QRS (0.16 second).
    - P is absent.
    - Rhythm is irregular.
    - Tall R in lead III, deep S in lead I.

Diagnosis: Acute inferior myocardial infarction with atrial fibrillation with right bundle branch block with left posterior hemiblock.

32. This ECG shows:
    - Multiple atrial ectopics with bigeminy pattern in lead II.

- RSR′ in V_1 and V_2 with QRS—0.12 second.
- T inverted in V_2 to V_6.

Diagnosis: Atrial ectopics with bigeminy with partial right bundle branch block with anterior ischemia.

33. This ECG shows:
    - P wave is absent.
    - Rhythm is irregular.
    - Pathological Q in lead II, III, aVF and V_1 to V_4.
    - RSR′/ M pattern in V_5 and V_6.

Diagnosis: Old inferior and anteroseptal myocardial infarction with atrial fibrillation with left bundle branch block.

34. This ECG shows:
    - P wave is absent in V_2 to V_6.
    - Rhythm—irregular in V_2 to V_6.
    - P, QRS, T normal in other leads.

Diagnosis: Paroxysmal atrial fibrillation.

35. This ECG shows:
    - Heart rate—180/min.
    - P wave is absent.
    - QRS is normal and narrow.
    - Rhythm—regular.

Diagnosis: Supraventricular tachycardia.

36. This ECG shows:
    - Tall R in lead I, deep S in lead III (indicates left axis deviation).
    - Tall R in aVL (> 11 mm), tall R in V_5 (> 25 mm).
    - S V_1 + R V_6 > 35 mm (here it is 38 mm).

Diagnosis: Left ventricular hypertrophy.

37. This ECG shows:
    - Multiple ventricular ectopics with bigeminy pattern in rhythm lead (L_{II}).
    - P wave is absent.
    - Rhythm—irregular.

Diagnosis: Multiple ventricular ectopics with bigeminy with atrial fibrillation.

38. This ECG shows:
    - QRS—wide in all leads mainly V_5 and V_6.

Diagnosis: Left bundle branch block.

39. This ECG shows:
    - Pathological Q in lead III and aVF.
    - Tall R in V_1 with wide QRS.
    - Deep S in V_5 and V_6 with poor R wave progression.

Diagnosis: Old inferior myocardial infarction with right bundle branch block.

40. This ECG shows:
- Heart rate is 150/min.
- P—absent.
- QRS—normal.
- Pathological Q in V_2 to V_4 and ST elevation.
- Deep S in V_5 and V_6 with poor R wave progression.
- Rhythm is regular.

Diagnosis: Acute anteroseptal myocardial infarction with supraventricular tachycardia.

41. This ECG shows:
- $S V_1 + R V_6 > 35$ mm (here it is 50).
- Tall peaked T wave in V_4 to V_6.
- There is also tall R in V_5.

Diagnosis: Left ventricular hypertrophy with probable hyperkalemia (tall peak T).

42. This ECG shows:
- ST elevation in lead II, III and aVF and also in V_5 and V_6.

Diagnosis: Acute inferior and lateral myocardial infarction.

43. This ECG shows:
- Heart rate—37/min.
- ST elevation in lead I, II, III and aVF.
- Pathological Q in I, II, III, aVF and V_2 to V_6 with ST elevation.
- P wave is absent.

Diagnosis: Acute inferior and anterior myocardial infarction with complete heart block with atrial fibrillation.

44. This ECG shows:
- Pathological Q in lead III and aVF.
- RSR'/ M pattern in V_1 and V_2.
- QRS wide (0.28 second).

Diagnosis: Old inferior myocardial infarction with right bundle branch block.

45. This ECG shows:
- ST elevation with pathological Q in lead II, III and aVF.
- P—absent.
- Rhythm is irregular.
- Occasional ventricular ectopics.

Diagnosis: Acute inferior myocardial infarction with atrial fibrillation with ventricular ectopics.

46. This ECG shows:
- P—absent.
- Rhythm—irregular.
- Heart rate—110/min.

Diagnosis: Fast atrial fibrillation.

47. This ECG shows:
- P—absent.
- Flutter wave in lead II, III, aVR, aVL and aVF.
- Rhythm—irregular.
- Occasional ventricular ectopics.

Diagnosis: Atrial flutter with fibrillation with ventricular ectopics.

48. This ECG shows:
- Atrial rate (P-P interval)—75/min.
- Ventricular rate (R-R interval)—50/min.
- Complete dissociation between atria and ventricle.

Diagnosis: Complete heart block.

49. This ECG shows:
- Tall R in lead III, deep S in lead I (indicate right axis deviation).
- Wide notched P wave in lead II and aVF (P-mitrale).
- Bifid P in V_1 with deeper downward deflection.
- Tall R in V_1 and V_2.

Diagnosis: Left atrial hypertrophy (mitral stenosis) with right ventricular hypertrophy.

50. This ECG shows:
- P—absent.
- Rhythm—irregular.
- Pathological Q in V_1 to V_3.

Diagnosis: Old anteroseptal myocardial infarction with atrial fibrillation.

51. This ECG shows:
- P—absent.
- Rhythm—irregular.
- ST depression in lead I, aVL, V_5 and V6.
- $S V_1 + R V_6 > 35$ (note the half voltage in V_4 to V_6).

Diagnosis: Atrial fibrillation with left ventricular hypertrophy with strain.

52. This ECG shows:
- Pathological Q with ST elevation in lead II, III and aVF.
- Pathological Q in V_1 to V_4.
- Tall R in aVL (>13 mm).

Diagnosis: Acute inferior and old anteroseptal myocardial infarction with left ventricular hypertrophy.

53. This ECG shows:
- Pathological Q with ST elevation in lead II, III and aVF.
- T inversion in lead II, III and aVF.

Diagnosis: Acute inferior myocardial infarction.

54. This ECG shows:
- P—absent.
- Rhythm—irregular.
- Pathological Q in V_1 to V_3.

Diagnosis: Atrial fibrillation with old anteroseptal myocardial infarction.

55. This ECG shows:
- S V_1 + R V_6 > 35 mm (here it is 48).
- P, QRS, T—normal.
- Heart rate—130/min.
- Rhythm—regular.

Diagnosis: Left ventricular hypertrophy with sinus tachycardia.

56. This ECG shows:
- ST elevation with upward concavity in lead II, III, aVF and V_4 to V_6.

Diagnosis: Acute pericarditis (in acute MI, ST is elevated with upward convexity).

57. This ECG shows:
- Pathological Q in lead II, III and aVF.
- Tall R in V_1 and V_2.
- Poor R wave progression.

Diagnosis: Old inferior myocardial infarction with right ventricular hypertrophy.

58. This ECG shows:
- Heart rate—56/min.
- P, QRS, T—normal.
- wave in lead II, V_4 to V_6.

Diagnosis: Sinus bradycardia.

59. This ECG shows:
- S V_1 + R V_6 > 35 mm (here it is 48).
- U wave in V_2 to V_6.

Diagnosis: Left ventricular hypertrophy with hypokalemia.

60. This ECG shows:
- P inverted in lead I.
- Deep S in V_4 to V_6.

Diagnosis: Dextrocardia.

Differential Diagnosis: Arm leads reversed. See also ECG No. 110.

61. This ECG shows:
- Heart rate—150/min.
- P is absent, but QRS, T—normal.
- Rhythm—regular.

Diagnosis: Supraventricular tachycardia.

62. This ECG shows:
- P—absent.
- QRS, T—normal.
- Heart rate—98/min.
- Rhythm—regular.

Diagnosis: Nodal tachycardia.

63. This ECG shows:
- P-R interval—short (0.08 second).
- Delta wave in V_4 to V_6.
- Deep S in V_1.

Diagnosis: WPW syndrome type B (deep S in V_1).

64. This ECG shows:
- Ectopic beats in all leads.

Diagnosis: Atrial ectopics.

65. This ECG shows:
- In the upper tracing—first half shows ventricular ectopics, second half shows runs of ectopics (ventricular tachycardia).
- In the middle tracing—ventricular tachycardia.
- In the lower tracing—first half shows torsades de pointes, second half shows ventricular fibrillation.

66. This ECG shows:
- S V_1 + R V_6 > 35 mm (here it is 64 mm).
- T inversion in V_4 to V_6.

Diagnosis: Left ventricular hypertrophy with strain.

67. This ECG shows:
- Pathological Q in lead III and aVF.
- Multiple ventricular ectopics.
- Every three normal beat is followed by a ventricular ectopic.

Diagnosis: Old inferior myocardial infarction with ventricular quadrigeminy.

68. This ECG shows:
- Multiple ventricular ectopics.
- Every normal beat is followed by a ventricular ectopic.

Diagnosis: Ventricular bigeminy.

69. This ECG shows:
- Multiple ventricular ectopics.
- Every two normal beat is followed by a ventricular ectopic.

Diagnosis: Ventricular trigeminy.

70. This ECG shows:
- First tracing shows prolonged P-R interval—first degree AV block.
- Second tracing shows progressive lengthening of the P-R interval followed by a drop—Mobitz type I second degree AV block (Wenckebach's phenomenon).
- Third tracing shows every three P, QRS, T is followed by a drop beat—Mobitz type II second degree AV block (3:1).
- Fourth tracing shows complete dissociation between P and QRS—complete heart block.

71. This ECG shows:
- P—absent.
- Rhythm—irregular.
- ST depression with thumb impression appearance.

Diagnosis: Atrial fibrillation with digoxin effect.

72. This ECG shows:
- Tall R in lead I and deep S in lead III (indicates left axis deviation).
- Tall R in V_1 and V_2 (right ventricular hypertrophy).
- Tall R in aVL (here it is 17 mm)—indicates left ventricular hypertrophy.

Diagnosis: Biventricular hypertrophy.

73. This ECG shows:
- Tall R in lead I and deep S in lead III (indicates left axis deviation).
- RSR'/ M pattern with wide QRS in V_1.

Diagnosis: Right bundle branch block with left anterior hemiblock (bifascicular block).

74. This ECG shows:
- Deep S in lead I, tall R in lead III (indicates right axis deviation).
- Tall R in V_1 and V_2 with T inversion (indicates right ventricular hypertrophy).

Diagnosis: Right ventricular hypertrophy with strain with left posterior hemiblock.

75. This ECG shows:
- Tall R in lead I, deep S in lead III (indicates left axis deviation).
- RSR'/ M pattern in V_1 with wide QRS.

Diagnosis: Right bundle branch block with left anterior hemiblock (bifascicular block).

76. This ECG shows:
- Pathological Q in lead II, III, aVF and also in V_1 to V_3.

Diagnosis: Old inferior and anteroseptal myocardial infarction.

77. This ECG shows:
- Deep S in lead I and tall R in lead III (indicates right axis deviation).
- Tall P in lead II (P-pulmonale).
- Bifid P in V_1 with tall upward deflection.
- Tall R in V_1 to V_3 with T inversion in V_1 to V_4.

Diagnosis: Right ventricular hypertrophy with right atrial hypertrophy.

78. This ECG shows:
- Pathological Q in lead II, III and aVF.

Diagnosis: Old inferior myocardial infarction.

79. This ECG shows:
- RSR' in V_1.
- QRS is normal (0.08 second).

Diagnosis: Partial right bundle branch block.

80. This ECG shows:
- Tall P in lead II (P- pulmonale).
- Bifid P in V_1.
- Wide notched P in V_2 to V_4 (P-mitrale).

Diagnosis: Biatrial hypertrophy.

81. This ECG shows:
- Low voltage tracing.
- Occasional ventricular ectopics.
- P-R interval—prolonged (0.24 sec).

Diagnosis: First degree heart block with ventricular ectopics with low voltage tracing.

82. This ECG shows:
- Deep S in lead I.
- Deep Q and T inversion in lead III.

Diagnosis: Pulmonary embolism (typical $S_I Q_{III} T_{III}$ pattern).

83. This ECG shows:
- P—absent.
- Rhythm is irregular.
- Pathological Q in lead II, III, aVF and also in V_1 to V_4.
- QRS—0.12 second.
- RSR′/ M pattern in lead I, aVL, V_5 and V_6.

Diagnosis: Old inferior and anteroseptal myocardial infarction with atrial fibrillation with partial left bundle branch block.

84. This ECG shows:
- P—absent.
- Rhythm is irregular.
- Heart rate—110/min

Diagnosis: Fast atrial fibrillation.

85. This ECG shows:
- Pathological Q in lead II, III and aVF.
- Tall R in V_1 and V_2.

Diagnosis: Old inferior myocardial infarction with right ventricular hypertrophy.

86. This ECG shows:
- P-R interval is prolonged (0.24 second).
- Pathological Q in lead II, III and aVF, also in V_1 to V_3.
- Tall R in V_1.
- QRS—wide (0.16 second).

Diagnosis: Old inferior and anteroseptal myocardial infarction with first degree heart block with right bundle branch block.

87. This ECG shows:
- Tall R in lead I, deep S in lead III (indicates left axis deviation).
- Tall P in lead II (right atrial hypertrophy).
- Bifid P with deeper downward deflection in V_1 (left atrial hypertrophy).
- SV_1 + RV6 > 35 mm (here it is 40 mm), also tall R in aVL (> 11 mm).
- T inversion in lead I, aVL, V_5 and V_6.

Diagnosis: Left ventricular hypertrophy with strain and right atrial hypertrophy with left atrial hypertrophy (biatrial).

88. This ECG shows:
- Complete dissociation between P and QRS.
- Pathological Q with ST elevation in V_1 to V_3.

Diagnosis: Acute anteroseptal myocardial infarction with complete heart block.

89. This ECG shows:
- P-R interval is prolonged (0.24 second).
- Pathological Q in lead III and aVF.
- Symmetrical T inversion in V_1 to V_6.
- Tall R in aVL (17 mm).

Diagnosis: Old inferior myocardial infarction with subendocardial myocardial infarction with first degree heart block with left ventricular hypertrophy.

90. This ECG shows:
- P—absent.
- Rhythm—irregular.
- Pathological Q in lead II, III, aVF and also in V_1 to V_4.

Diagnosis: Old inferior and anteroseptal myocardial infarction with fast atrial fibrillation.

91. This ECG shows:
- Pathological Q and ST elevation in V_1 to V_4.
- RSR′/M pattern in V_5 and V_6.
- QRS is 0.12 sec.
- Heart rate–102/min.

Diagnosis: Acute anteroseptal myocardial infarction with partial left bundle branch block with sinus tachycardia.

92. This ECG shows:
- P—absent and saw tooth appearance in V_1.
- Rhythm is irregular.
- RSR'/M patter in V_6.
- QRS—0.12 second.

Diagnosis: Atrial flutter with fibrillation with partial left bundle branch block.

93. This ECG shows:
- P wave is absent.
- Multiple ventricular ectopics.
- Rhythm is irregular.

Diagnosis: Atrial fibrillation with multiple ventricular ectopics.

94. This ECG shows:
- Every 2 P wave is followed by absent QRS complex.

Diagnosis: Mobitz type II, second degree AV block (2:1).

95. This ECG shows:
- ST elevation with pathological Q in V_1 to V_5.
- Multiple ventricular ectopics.
- QRS wide (0.20 second) in V_1 with RSR'/M pattern.
- Prolonged absence of P, QRS and T in rhythm strip.

Diagnosis: Acute anterior myocardial infarction with right bundle branch block with multiple ventricular ectopics with sinus arrest.

96. This ECG shows:
- Heart rate—150/min.
- Pathological Q with ST elevation in lead II, III and aVF.
- RSR'/M pattern in V_1 with wide QRS (0.16 sec.).

Diagnosis: Acute inferior myocardial infarction with right bundle branch block with sinus tachycardia.

97. This ECG shows:
- P—absent.
- Rhythm—irregular.
- Multiple ventricular ectopics.
- Pathological Q in V_1 to V_4.

Diagnosis: Atrial fibrillation with multiple ventricular ectopics with old anteroseptal myocardial infarction.

98. This ECG shows:
- Pathological Q in lead III and aVF.
- S V_1 + R V_6 > 35 mm.
- Tall R in aVL, T inversion in 1, aVL, V_6.

Diagnosis: Old inferior myocardial infarction with left ventricular hypertrophy with strain.

99. This ECG shows:
- Pathological Q in lead III and aVF.
- ST elevation and pathological Q in V_1 to V_3.
- Tall R in V_1 and V_2.
- QRS is wide (0.26 second).

Diagnosis: Old inferior and acute anteroseptal myocardial infarction with right bundle branch block.

100. This ECG shows:
- Progressive lengthening of PR interval followed by drop beat.
- RSR' in V_1 with QRS 0.12 sec.

Diagnosis: Wenckebach's phenomenon with partial right bundle branch block.

101. This ECG shows:
- P wave—absent.
- Rhythm—irregular (RR interval irregular).
- QRS—wide > 0.12 (here it is 0.16).
- Delta wave in V_4, V_5 and V_6.

Diagnosis: WPW syndrome with atrial fibrillation.

102. This ECG shows:
- ST elevation and pathological Q in lead II, III and aVF.
- Pathological Q in V_4, V_5 and V_6.

Diagnosis: Acute inferior and old lateral myocardial infarction.

103. This ECG shows:
- P—absent.
- Rhythm—irregular (RR interval is irregular).
- RSR'/M pattern in V_5 and V_6.
- QRS—wide > 0.12 second (here—0.16).

Diagnosis: Left bundle branch block with atrial fibrillation.

104. This ECG shows:
- PR interval—0.22 sec.
- Pathologi cal Q in lead I I , I I I and aVF.
- RSR'/M pattern in V_1 and V_2.
- QRS—wide > 0.12 second (here–0.16).

Diagnosis: Old inferior myocardial infarction with 1st degree heart block with right bundle branch block (bifascicular block).

105. This ECG shows:
- P—bifid and wide (0.12).
- Tall R in V_1.
- Tal l R in V_5 (32).

Diagnosis: Biventricular hypertrophy with left atrial hypertrophy or enlargement.

106. This ECG shows:
- Multiple unifocal ventricular ectopic.
- Pathological Q in C_1, C_2 and C_3.

Diagnosis: Old anteroseptal myocardial infarction with ventricular ectopics.

107. This ECG shows:
- Pacemaker spike.
- One spike before P wave and another spike before QRS.

Diagnosis: Dual chamber pacing.

108. This ECG shows:
- P—absent.
- Rhythm—irregular (RR interval is irregular).
- ST—depression in lead II, III, aVF, V_1 to V_6.
- RSR′/M pattern in V_1 and V_2 with QRS 0.12 sec.

Diagnosis: Atrial fibrillation with digoxin effect with partial right bundle branch block.

109. This ECG shows:
- Left axis deviation (tall R in lead I and deep S in III).
- Tall R in aVL (18 mm).
- RSR′/M pattern in V_5 and V_6 with QRS 0.10 sec.
- T-inversion in lead I, aVL, V_3 to V_6.

Diagnosis: Left ventricular hypertrophy with strain with partial left bundle branch block.

110. This ECG shows:
- P-inverted in lead I.
- QRS in chest leads—normal.

Diagnosis: Arms leads reversed or incorrectly placed arms lead (see also ECG No. 60).

111. This ECG shows:
- Left axis deviation (tall R in lead I and deep S in III).
- Tall R in aVL (19 mm).
- RSR′/M pattern in V_1 and V_2 with QRS 0.16 sec.
- Tall R in V_5 (30 mm) with T inversion in V_5 and V_6.

Diagnosis: Left ventricular hypertrophy with strain with right bundle branch block with left anterior hemiblock.

112. This ECG shows:
- P wave—absent.
- Rhythm—irregular (RR interval is irregular).
- ST—depression in lead II, III, aVF, V_1 to V_6.
- RSR′/M pattern in V_1 and V_2 with QRS 0.16 sec.

Diagnosis: Atrial fibrillation with with right bundle branch block.

113. This ECG shows:
- ST elevation and pathological Q in lead II, III and aVF.
- ST elevation in V_1 to V_6 (right side).

Diagnosis: Acute inferior and right ventricular infarction (right ventricular infarction is associated with inferior myocardial infarction, seen in V_1, also RV_3 and RV_4).

114. This ECG shows:
- P—absent.
- Rhythm—irregular (RR inverval is irregular).
- Unifocal ventricular ectopics in V_1 to V_5.
- Occasional supraventricular ectopics in lead I, II, III, aVR, aVL, aVF and V_6.

Diagnosis: Atrial fibrillation with ventricular ectopics with supraventricular ectopics.

115. This ECG shows:
- Left axis deviation (tall R in lead I and deep S in III).
- Unifocal ventricular ectopics in V_1 to V_6.
- Occasional supraventricular ectopics.
- Tall R in V_1 to V_2 with QRS 0.16.

Diagnosis: Right ventricular hypertrophy with right bundle branch block with ventricular ectopics with supraventricular ectopics.

116. This ECG shows:
- Heart rate—28/min.
- Left axis deviation (tall R in lead I and deep S in III).
- Tall R in aVL (15 mm).
- RSR′/M pattern in V_1 and V_2 with QRS 0.16.

Diagnosis: Severe sinus bradycardia with left ventricular hypertrophy with right bundle branch block.

117. This ECG shows:
- Left axis deviation (tall R in lead I and deep S in III).
- Tall R in aVL (16 mm).
- Absent QRS in some lead.
- RSR'/M pattern in V_1 and V_2 with QRS 0.16.

Diagnosis: Left ventricular hypertrophy with right bundle branch block with SA block.

118. This ECG shows:
- ST elevation in lead III and aVF, also V_3 to V_6.
- Pathological Q in lead I, aVL, V_5 and V_6.
- Few supraventricular ectopic in L_{II}.

Diagnosis: Acute inferior and anterolateral myocardial infarction with supraventricular ectopic.

119. This ECG shows:
- Absent of PQRS in some leads.
- T inversion in lead I and V_3 to V_6.

Diagnosis: Sinus arrest with lateral ischemia.

120. This ECG shows:
- Heart rate—130/min.
- Low voltage tracing (R < 5 mm in limb leads and < 10 mm in chest leads).

Diagnosis: Low voltage tracing with sinus tachycardia.

121. This ECG shows:
- Multiple unifocal ventricular ectopics.
- Every one normal beat is followed by an ectopic beat.

Diagnosis: Ventricular ectopics with bigeminy pattern.

122. This ECG shows:
- P inverted in L_1.
- Deep S in V_2 to V_6.

Diagnosis: Dextrocardia.

Differential Diagnosis: Arms leads reversed, see page 263 and 267.

123. This ECG shows:
- Every two P, QRS, T is followed by a drop beat—Mobitz type II second degree AV block (2:1).

124. This ECG shows:
- Two consecutive pacemaker spikes followed by QRS.

Diagnosis: Dual chamber pacemaker.

125. This ECG shows:
- Atrial rate—100/min.
- Ventricular rate —50/m.
- Complete dissociation between P and QRS.

Diagnosis: Complete heart block.

126. This ECG shows:
- P—absent.
- Rhythm—irregular.
- Pathological Q in V_1 to V_3.
- One ventricular ectopic beat.

Diagnosis: Old anteroseptal myocardial infarction with atrial fibrillation with ventricular ectopic beat.

127. This ECG shows:
- P—absent.
- Rhythm—irregular.
- Pathological Q in III and aVF, also in V_1 to V_3.

Diagnosis: Old inferior and anteroseptal myocardial infarction with atrial fibrillation.

128. This ECG shows:
- Pacemaker spike followed by QRS.
- One ventricular ectopic beat.

Diagnosis: Ventricular pacemaker with ventricular ectopic.

129. This ECG shows:
- Low voltage tracing (R < 5 mm in limb leads and < 10 mm in chest leads).
- Pathological Q in V_1 to V_3.

Diagnosis: Old anteroseptal myocardial infarction with low voltage tracing.

130. This ECG shows:
- Pathological Q in V_1 to V_3.
- S V_1+ R V_6 > 35.

Diagnosis: Old anteroseptal myocardial infarction with left ventricular hypertrophy.

131. This ECG shows:
- S V_1 + R V_6 > 35 mm.
- U wave in V_3 to V_6.

Diagnosis: Left ventricular hypertrophy with hypokalemia.

132. This ECG shows:
- P—absent.
- Rhythm—irregular.
- Ventricular ectopics in V_1 to V_6.

Diagnosis: Atrial flutter with fibrillation with ventricular ectopics (confuses with Ashman phenomenon).

133. This ECG shows:
   - Pathological Q in lead III and aVF.
   - Heart rate—50/min.
   - P, QRS, T—normal.

Diagnosis: Sinus bradycardia with old inferior myocardial infarction.

134. This ECG shows:
   - Heart rate—58/min
   - Pathological Q in lead III and aVF.
   - Pathological Q in V_1 to V_6.

Diagnosis: Old inferior and anterior myocardial infarction with sinus bradycardia.

135. This ECG shows:
   - Pathological Q with ST elevation in V_1 to V_3.
   - Tall R in V_6 (> 25).
   - T inversion in V_2 to V_6.

Diagnosis: Acute anteroseptal myocardial infarction with left ventricular hypertrophy with strain.

136. This ECG shows:
   - Tall R in lead I and deep S in lead III (indicates left axis deviation).
   - RSR′/ M pattern with wide QRS in V_1.
   - Tall R in V_1 and V_2 (indicates right ventricular hypertrophy).
   - Tall R in aVL (> 11).

Diagnosis: Right bundle branch block with left anterior hemiblock (bifascicular block) with left ventricular hypertrophy.

137. This ECG shows:
   - Short PR interval.
   - Tall R in lead I and deep S in lead III (indicates left axis deviation).
   - RSR′/ M pattern with wide QRS in V_1.
   - Tall R in V_1.
   - Tall R in aVL (> 11).

Diagnosis: Right bundle branch block with left anterior hemiblock (bifascicular block) with left ventricular hypertrophy with short PR interval.

138. This ECG shows:
   - Pathological Q with ST elevation in lead III and aVF.
   - ST depresion in lead I, aVL, V_2 to V_6.

Diagnosis: Acute inferior myocardial infarction with anterolateral ischemia.

139. This ECG shows:
   - P—absent.
   - Rhythm is irregular (R-R interval is irregular).
   - RSR′/ M pattern with wide QRS in V_1 to V_4.
   - ST depression in V_2 to V_6 (thumb impression or reversed tick appearance).

Diagnosis: Atrial fibrillation with digoxin effect with right bundle branch block.

140. This ECG shows:
   - Atrial ectopics in lead II, III.
   - Ventricular ectopics in lead I, aVL, aVF, V_1 to V_6.
   - RSR′ in V_1 and V_2.

Diagnosis: Atrial ectopics with ventricular ectopics with right bundle branch block.

141. This ECG shows:
   - P—absent.
   - Rhythm is irregular.
   - Pathological Q in lead III and aVF.
   - RSR′/ M pattern in V_1 to V_3.

Diagnosis: Old inferior myocardial infarction with atrial fibrillation with right bundle branch block.

142. This ECG shows:
   - Heart rate—50/min.
   - P, QRS, T—normal.
   - Supraventricular ectopics in V_1 to V_6.

Diagnosis: Sinus bradycardia with supraventricular ectopics.

143. This ECG shows:
   - P wave is absent, some fibrillary f wave in lead III.
   - Rhythm is irregular.
   - Few flutter waves in II, III aVF.
   - $SV_1 + RV_6$ > 35.
   - Heart rate > 100/min.

Diagnosis: Fast atrial flutter fibrillation with left ventricular hypertrophy.

144. This ECG shows:
- Tall R in lead I and deep S in lead III (indicates left axis deviation).
- Tall R in V_1 and V_2 (right ventricular hypertrophy).
- Tall R in aVL (indicates left ventricular hypertrophy).
- Pathological Q in V_1 to V_6.

Diagnosis: Biventricular hypertrophy with old extensive anterior myocardial infarction.

145. This ECG shows:
- P—absent.
- Rhythm is irregular.
- Pathological Q in V_1 to V_3.
- Tall R in V_6.

Diagnosis: Fast atrial flutter fibrillation with left ventricular hypertrophy with old anteroseptal myocardial infarction.

146. This ECG shows:
- ST elevation with pathological Q in lead II, III and aVF.
- One ventricular ectopic in II.
- Heart rate—130/min.

Diagnosis: Acute inferior myocardial infarction with ventricular ectopic with sinus tachycardia.

147. This ECG shows:
- Pathological Q in V_1 to V_4.
- Absent of P, QRST.

Diagnosis: Old anteroseptal myocardial infarction with SA block.

148. This ECG shows:
- Tall R in L_{III}, deep S in L_I.
- RSR'/ M pattern in V_1 to V_3.
- Tall R in V_6.

Diagnosis: Right bundle branch block with left posterior hemiblock with left ventricular hypertrophy.

149. This ECG shows:
- P-R interval—short (0.08 second).
- Delta wave in V_1.
- Pathological Q in II, III and aVF.

Diagnosis: WPW syndrome type A.

150. This ECG shows:
- Tall R in aVL.
- Absent of P, QRST.

Diagnosis: Left ventricular hypertrophy with SA block.

Suggested Reading

1. Chung Edward K. Pocket Guide to ECG Diagnosis, 1st edition: 1996; Oxford University Press.
2. Dennis L, Kasper, Anthonys, Fauci et al. Harrison's Principles of Internal Medicine, 16th edition: 2005; McGraw Hill.
3. Dunn Marvin I, Lipman Bernard S. Lipman-Massie Clinical Electrocardiography, 8th edition: 1989; Yearbook Medical Publishers Inc.
4. Goldberger Ary L, Goldberger Emanuel. Clinical Electrocardiography, A Simplified Approach, 3rd edition: 1990; Jaypee Brothers Medical Publishers (P) Ltd.
5. Goldman MJ. Principles of Clinical Electrocardiography, 10th edition: 1979; Lange Medical Publications.
6. Hampton John R. The ECG Made Easy, 5th edition: 1997; Churchill Livingstone.
7. Houghton, Andrew R, Gray, David. Making Sense of the ECG, 2nd edition: 1998; Oxford University Press.
8. Julian DG, Cowan JC, McLenachan JM. Cardiology, 8th edition: 2005; Elservier Ltd.
9. Kumar and Clark. Clinical Medicine, 6th edition: 2005; Elsevier Saunders.
10. Lipman Bradford C. Lipman Bernard S. ECG Pocket Guide, 1st edition: 1990; Jaypee Brothers Medical Publishers (P) Ltd.
11. Nicholas A Boon et al. Davidson's Principles and Practice of Medicine, 20th edition: 2006; Elsevier Science Ltd. Churchill Livingstone.
12. Schamroth Leo. An Introduction to Electrocardiography, 7th edition: Blackwell Science Ltd. 1990.

Index